Treatment Protocols
for
Articulation and Phonologic Disorders

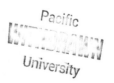

Treatment Protocols
for
Articulation and Phonologic Disorders

M. N. Hegde
Adriana Peña-Brooks

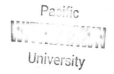
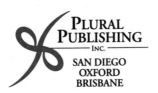
PLURAL
PUBLISHING
INC.
SAN DIEGO
OXFORD
BRISBANE

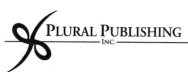

5521 Ruffin Road
San Diego, CA 92123

e-mail: info@pluralpublishing.com
Web site: http://www.pluralpublishing.com

49 Bath Street
Abingdon, Oxfordshire OX14 1EA
United Kingdom

Typeset in 10/12 Bookman by Flanagan's Publishing Services, Inc.
Printed in the United States of America by Bang Printing

ISBN-13: 978-1-59756-084-9
ISBN-10: 1-59756-084-7

Library of Congress Cataloging-in-Publication Data

Hegde, M. N. (Mahabalagiri N.), 1941-
   Treatment protocols for articulation and phonological disorders /
M.N Hegde, Adriana Peña-Brooks.
      p. ; cm.
   Includes bibliographical references and index.
   ISBN-13: 978-1-59756-084-9 (softcover)
   ISBN-10: 1-59756-084-7 (softcover)
   1. Articulation disorders. 2. Voice disorders. 3. Speech therapy.
I. Peña-Brooks, Adriana. II. Title.
   [DNLM: 1. Articulation Disorders--therapy. 2. Clinical Protocols.
WL 340.2 H462t 2006]
RC424.7.H44 2006
   616.85'506--dc22   2006019411

Contents

Part II. Phoneme Clusters

Initial Clusters

L-clusters

R-clusters

S-clusters

Final Clusters

L-clusters

Preface

The *Webster's II New College Dictionary* defines a protocol as "a plan for a scientific experiment or treatment." An effective plan for treatment needs to be as clear and precise as a scientific experiment. The concept of protocols, therefore, is eminently suitable for treatment plans in speech-language pathology.

Treatment in communication disorders is primarily a matter of planned social interaction. These interactions can be envisioned as dynamic relationships in which the clinician and the client affect each other. A single observation of a treatment session will convince us that, in any treatment session, the clinician and the client play out their respective roles and come out of successful treatment as changed people. It is this view of treatment that has inspired these protocols.

If treatment is a set of scenarios in which the clinician and the client play out their roles, protocols are scripts they follow to achieve improved patterns of communication. Therefore, these protocols are written as scripts that help the clinician and the client play their roles effectively, efficiently, and with a reasonable expectation of positive outcomes for the child and his or her family.

Another in a series of protocols for treating various communication disorders, this book offers treatment protocols for articulation and phonologic disorders in children. The book follows the general pattern established in the earlier *Treatment Protocols for Language Disorders in Children, Volume I (Essential Morphologic Skills)* and *Volume II (Social Communication)*.

These protocols for teaching articulation and phonologic skills in children include all English consonants that may be treatment targets. Articulation and phonologic disorders are among the most common speech disorders that clinicians treat in various professional settings—especially in public schools. Treatment of these disorders requires extensive preparation of stimulus materials. Multiple target words need to be carefully selected for teaching correct production of various singleton consonants and consonant clusters. These protocols list words that contain target singleton consonants in the initial, and when appropriate, final positions. Word lists for syllabic /ɚ/ contain the target sound in the medial and final positions. The syllabic /ɝ/ words are only in the medial word-positions. Target words for clusters are organized according to initial and final clusters. Unfolding scripts that illustrate baserate, treatment, and probe sessions provide detailed protocols to treat most articulatory targets.

Introduction to Treatment Protocols and the CD Resource

These protocols for treating articulation and phonologic disorders in children are written as scenarios that unfold in teaching speech sound production skills to children. Clinicians treating children with articulation and phonologic disorders spend significant amounts of time and effort in establishing speech sound production skills in them.

In selecting articulation and phonologic treatment procedures for the protocols, the overriding concern has been efficacy. The protocols, therefore, include a core set of treatment procedures for which there is plenty of replicated positive evidence.

Evidential Basis of the Treatment Protocols

Treatment in speech-language pathology ought to be based on evidence generated by controlled scientific experiments that evaluate the effects of individual procedures. Such evidence should be replicated in varied settings. Treatment procedures that receive controlled and replicated experimental support may be recommended for general practice. If the evidence is widely replicated, the procedures may be somewhat standard and consistent across varied target behaviors. In preparing these protocols, evidence has been the most overriding concern. The *Individuals with Disabilities Education Improvement Act—2004* requires a statement that the services provided to the child within an *Individualized Education Program* are based on peer-reviewed research (Wright, 2004). School-based clinicians can be confident that these treatment protocols go over and beyond that requirement because the protocols contain evidence-based treatment procedures that have stood the test of time.

Over the past several decades, the treatment of articulation and phonologic disorders has undergone many theoretical changes. Changing perspectives have suggested individual phonemes, distinctive features, and phonologic processes as targets of intervention.

Currently popular approaches seek to eliminate inappropriately persisting phonologic processes. Fortunately for the clinicians, a constant feature of these changing perspectives is the treatment techniques themselves. Each new perspective on articulation and phonologic disorders has not resulted in newer treatment techniques. For the most part, each new perspective has suggested new ways of conceptualizing or analyzing articulatory skills in children. How those skills are taught has not changed much over the years.

Currently popular phonologic treatment approaches still require the clinician to teach the production of individual speech sounds. It is only by teaching the production of individual sounds that a clinician can remediate an inappropriate phonologic process in a child. The initial or the final consonant deletion processes, for example, cannot be eliminated without teaching at least a few of the missing initial or final consonants. Similarly, remediation of the cluster reduction process, the unstressed syllable deletion process, or any of the several substitution processes requires the clinician to teach the production of individual sounds classified within those processes. Whether the clinician conceptualizes treatment in terms of individual speech sound productions or elimination of phonologic processes, immediate treatment targets are always the correct production of specific sounds that exemplify either individual errors or patterns of errors. Therefore, protocols to teach individual sounds are essential in remediating articulation and phonologic errors in children.

Teaching individual sound productions either as the final targets by themselves or as a means to eliminate phonologic processes is accomplished by such behavioral techniques as modeling, prompting, manual guidance, fading, shaping, positive reinforcement, and corrective feedback. Furthermore, such varied programs as the traditional approach, the multiple-phoneme approach, the sensory-motor approach, and the so-called linguistic approaches (including the distinctive feature and phonologic approaches), have, at their core, only behavioral treatment techniques (Peña-Brooks & Hegde, 2007). Effects of the behavioral techniques have been historically well documented. Initial experimental studies on the effectiveness of behavioral procedures in treating articulation disorders in children were published in the 1970s and 1980s (Bailey, Timbers, Phillips, & Wolf, 1971; Baker & Ryan, 1971; Bennett, 1974; Costello & Onstine, 1976; Elbert, Dinnsen, Swartzlander, & Chin, 1990; Elbert & McReynolds, 1975; Fitch, 1973; Gierut, 1989, 1990, 1998; Koegel, Koegel, & Ingham, 1986; Koegel, Koegel, Voy, & Ingham, 1988; McReynolds & Elbert, 1981; Mowrer, 1989. Williams & McReynolds, 1975). In subsequent years, evidence supporting the behavioral techniques has continued to be published (see Gierut, 1998; Peña-Brooks & Hegde, 2007; Sommers, Logsdon, & Wright, 1992 for reviews). Consequently, the behavioral treatment procedures with discrete trials are now firmly established with sufficient controlled and replicated evidence (Bernthal & Bankson, 2004; Creaghead, Newman, & Secord, 1989; Peña-Brooks & Hegde, 2007). Therefore, the protocols suggest the use of the discrete trial method, which incorporates modeling, positive reinforcement, corrective feedback, fading of modeling, and evoked (spontaneous) productions in treating articulation and phonologic disorders in children.

What the Protocols Offer

Treatment protocols are common in medicine, where such protocols are more prescriptive. Treatment plans in speech-language pathology need to be flexible and adaptable to individual clients. Nonetheless, a general pattern of baserate, treatment, and probe sequence is basic to treating all communication disorders, including articulation and phonologic disorders. Such protocols may easily be modified to suit individual children. The protocols described in this book leave much room for the clinician's innovation, adaptation, and modification. The protocols for each target phoneme and phoneme clusters (blends) are described as a separate and complete entity. All phonemes and phoneme clusters may be taught in a simple and predictable manner. For instance, protocols show that treating each target articulatory skill requires the following five elements:

- **A protocol to establish baserates** of articulation treatment target. The baserates help establish the need for treatment and provide an objective and quantitative basis to evaluate the child's progress in treatment.

- **A baserate recording sheet** that lists up to 20 exemplars for a phoneme or cluster with columns for two types of baserate trials: a set of evoked trails and a set of modeled trials; the clinician may copy the page and use it in the clinic to obtain reliable baserates.

- **A protocol to teach sound production** that provides unfolding scenarios for treatment; the protocols are detailed enough for the clinician to implement treatment with little or no modifications; the protocols are written in the form of scripts for both the clinician and the child; in essence, these treatment protocols allow the clinician and the client to play their respective roles.

- **A treatment recording sheet** that lists up to 10 target articulatory exemplars that may be taught in discrete trials or more naturalistic interactions; the recording sheet provides for objective measurement of each attempt the child makes on modeled and evoked treatment trials.

- **A protocol to probe for and record generalized production** of new and untrained articulatory targets in the absence of treatment; these probe protocols, too, are written in the form of scripts that assign roles the clinician and the child play; the protocol sheet also contains a recording form to document the percent correct generalized response of the sound production just taught; these probe protocols help determine whether the child needs to be taught additional individual sound or cluster exemplars; if the child meets the probe criterion, the clinician then can move on to other sounds, other clusters, or to a higher level of training on target skills already trained at the word level.

Protocols for individual speech sounds are provided first, followed by those for sound clusters. The order in which the sound- and cluster-protocols are given is not meant to suggest a treatment sequence. Clinicians may sequence the target articulatory skills in any number of ways to suit the individual child. The entry point for a child may be anywhere within the sequence; the child's errors or error patterns will suggest a useful or necessary entry point and a sequence with which all target sounds or clusters are taught.

Clinicians may use the recording sheets to document the child's progress in treatment. By recording correct and incorrect responses the child gives in each session, the clinician can document systematic changes that may take place in the child's articulatory and phonologic skills across treatment sessions. Because they are objective and show positive changes from the baserate level of the skill, the data recorded will help document the improvement under treatment and support any claims for third-party reimbursement for services.

The various recording sheets may be photocopied for clinical use. For instance, the clinician can photocopy a baserate or treatment recording sheet that contains 20 word exemplars for a target speech sound or cluster. The treatment and probe recording sheets also have the articulatory targets at the word level. This will save the treatment planning and preparation time as well as considerable effort involved in generating extensive exemplars (words that contain various target sounds in initial and final positions and clusters in initial and final positions). The baserate, treatment, and probe recording sheets are also provided in Appendixes that the clinician can photocopy for personal use. Furthermore, the clinician can use the accompanying CD as described next in getting prepared for treatment sessions.

The book includes a Glossary that is more detailed than the usual. All treatment terms are defined and described. Clinicians who are unfamiliar with some of the terms used in the protocols are encouraged to review the detailed Glossary.

How to Use the Accompanying CD

The CD that accompanies the book contains all the baserate, treatment, and probe recording sheets. All the files on the CD are modifiable. The clinician can type in new information or delete what is on them. This will make it possible for the clinician to individualize articulatory targets and the recording forms for particular children. For instance, the clinician can easily delete a consonant or cluster exemplar and type in one that is more specific to the child. On the baserate, treatment, and probe recording sheets, the clinician can type in the names of family members, teachers, pets, friends, favorite food items, favorite activities, and so forth that contain the target sounds. Such modifications will result in client-specific and functional target articulatory skills to be used in baserate, treatment, and probe segments. While individualizing the recording sheets in this manner, the clinician can retain the standard recording sheet given in the CD.

To further individualize the recording sheets, the clinician can type in the name of the clinic or the school, the child's name, the clinician's name, date of treatment session, and such other clinician- and child-specific information that are typically included in recording sheets. Unlike the typical forms given in resource books, the modifiable and printable forms do not have page numbers, book chapter titles, and such other information that will make it inappropriate to place in a client's folder. Forms so modified and printed from the CD provided in the book will look like the clinician's clinic stationery.

For the clinician's convenience, the CDs are prepared in simple MS-Word format that most clinicians are familiar with; the CD is not encrypted in any way to facilitate quick access and easy use of the documents on it. Once again, the use of the CD will help the clinician save planning time and effort involved in getting prepared for treatment sessions.

How to Use the Companion Books of Stimulus Pictures

These articulation and phonologic treatment protocols specify various kinds of stimuli to evoke the target phoneme productions. Finding pictures to evoke target phoneme productions can be an extremely time-consuming task for the busy clinician. The protocols themselves might be more efficiently used with little preparation if the stimulus items also were provided. However, it was impractical to include the pictures in the protocols. The size of the protocols would have been unmanageable to the clinician. Therefore, stimuli needed to teach all the sounds and sound clusters described in these protocols have been drawn and published as separate *stimulus* books. The companion books, each entitled Sound Stimuli Books (volumes 1 through 8) for *Treatment Protocols for Articulation and Phonologic Disorders* contain all the words listed in the baserate, treatment, and probe protocols of this book. Large pictures included in the book facilitate easy evocation of target words. For a few nonpicturable words that had to be included in the protocols, printed words themselves serve as stimuli. With no additional training, the clinician can evoke the word with the help of the printed stimulus if the child is a reader. If not, the clinician may give a few trials on which the child is taught to say the word in relation to the printed word stimulus.

Because each card contains a printed word, the clinician may also use these cards in literacy training. Such training may be integrated into articulation treatment or may be independent of it. Depending on the treatment plan written for a child, words the child does not know may be taught on a few trials and then one may move on to either articulation training or other cards for literacy training.

It is hoped that when used in combination, the treatment protocols and the stimulus picture books will make it much easier to plan for and treat articulation and phonologic disorders in children. The clinician may personalize the baserate, treatment, and probe recording sheets and will be ready to treat and document the child's response rates with no additional time spent on searching for stimulus items.

An Overview of Treatment of Articulation and Phonologic Disorders

The protocols describe procedures for treating articulation and phonologic disorders in children. They include target phonemes and their exemplars in word-initial and word-final positions. The protocols give the clinician a core set of articulatory targets that may be adapted in various ways to teach either only a few sounds or several sounds. These protocols may be used to remediate phonologic processes as well. As noted in the *Introduction*, the procedures are supported by treatment efficacy research. The protocols assume that an assessment of articulation or phonologic disorders has been completed.

Selecting Treatment Targets

Treatment targets for articulatory and phonologic treatment are those skills, that when taught, significantly enhance the child's overall communicative effectiveness by improving the speech sound production skills. To begin with, the clinician may set some *short-term objectives* that are targeted in the initial period of intervention. The *long-term goal* of treatment is the final outcome of treatment: normal or improved speech intelligibility and communicative effectiveness (Peña-Brooks & Hegde, 2007).

Careful Selection of Treatment Targets Is Important

To meet the short-term and long-term goals, the clinician should carefully select articulatory or phonologic treatment targets. Some general guidelines, when followed, will help one efficiently achieve both the short-term and long-term goals. First, the targets selected should make an immediate difference in the child's speech intelligibility. Sounds the child most frequently misarticulates, when effectively treated, will improve communication better than those that are infrequently misarticulated. Second, the clinician may select targets that are most useful to communicate effectively in natural settings. Various speech sounds may be taught in arcane words or nonsense syllables. But teaching the same sounds in functional, everyday words will be more effective because these words are likely to be produced and reinforced in home, school, and other natural settings. Third, the targets selected for children should be culturally and linguistically appropriate for them. For all children, selected articulatory and phonologic targets should reflect the child's language and culture. In case of culturally and linguistically diverse children, the selected targets should reflect the unique phonologic patterns of language or dialect spoken at home (Peña-Brooks & Hegde, 2007).

Generally, a child-specific strategy of selecting treatment targets is superior to a canned approach. The former strategy considers the child and the family's ethnocultural background, family communication patterns, usefulness of specific treatment targets, and potential for rapid improvement in communicative effectiveness.

Various Criteria Help Select Treatment Targets

At least for initial treatment target selection clinicians have used several guidelines. A historically well-established guideline is based on **normative data**. Those who rely on this approach believe that age-based norms are the best guidelines for selecting treatment targets. Although popular, this approach has certain limitations. Available normative data sometimes may be inappropriate for children of ethnoculturally diverse backgrounds. Even for the mainstream children, age-based norms may not always suggest the best possible treatment targets because they do not consider a child's unique pattern of disorder and specific academic and family communicative needs. Furthermore, there is experimental evidence that suggests that teaching children advanced and later-acquired speech sounds in relation to their chronologic age may result in positive changes in untreated sound classes (Gierut et al., 1996).

Another guideline clinicians have followed is the ease of teaching certain phonemes. At least in the initial stages of treatment, the clinician may select phonemes that are easier to teach. For instance, sounds that are visible on the articulators, error sounds that are occasionally produced correctly, or those that are imitated (stimulable) may be selected on the assumption that they are easier to teach. This guideline prompts the clinician to select phonologic processes whose frequency is less than 100%; in essence, the processes are less severe, perhaps easier to eliminate. Early success may better prepare the child to tackle more difficult sounds later in treatment. Although this is a common assumption, some recent research suggests that easier-to-teach sounds may not always be the best targets because more difficult sounds, when taught, may lead to more extensive generalization of correct production.

Potential for extensive generalization has been a more recently advocated guideline. Possibly, treatment of sounds that are maximally opposed produces more extensive generalization than treating sounds that are minimally opposed (Gierut, 1990). Unfortunately, studies on generalization of treated sounds have produced somewhat inconsistent results (see Peña-Brooks & Hegde, 2007, for a review of studies). Additional research is needed to suggest the kinds of sounds that when treated will produce extensive generalization.

Improved intelligibility is an important treatment goal. This has led to yet another guideline which suggests that the clinicians should select speech sounds or phonologic processes that affect intelligibility the most. Correct production of such sounds or elimination of such processes will have a significant positive effect on intelligibility. This guideline generates targets for a child that are opposite of the *easier-to-teach* guideline. According to the guideline of improved intelligibility, sounds that are consistently omitted or incorrectly produced are the first targets; those that are produced correctly in some contexts would only be later targets. Phonologic processes that are evident 100% in a child's speech would be priority targets, not those that are evident at significantly below that level (Peña-Brooks & Hegde, 2007). Processes that result in homonymy (replacement of a single word for multiple words; see *Glossary*) would also be priority targets. This guideline does make intuitive sense and is consistent with the common sense approach that if the most severe types of errors are eliminated, speech intelligibility would improve most significantly.

Practicing clinicians may favor one guideline over others. For instance:

- If initial treatment success is important, the clinician is likely to select easier-to-teach phonemes. The clinician then is likely to select for immediate intervention stimulable (imitated) sounds, sounds that are correctly produced on some baseline trials, sounds that are inconsistently produced in a speech sample, sounds that are visible on the face, and phonologic processes that are well below 100% in their occurrence.

- If delayed success is acceptable to both the clinician and the child then the goal would be to achieve more extensive generalization or marked positive effect on intelligibility. To achieve this goal, the clinician may select as initial treatment targets sounds that are complex, sounds that are consistently misarticulated, sounds that are totally absent in the child's repertoire, phonologic processes that affect the greatest number of sounds, processes that are evident at 100%, and processes that result in homonymy.

- Regardless of any of the other strategies used, the clinician should select sounds that are ethnoculturally appropriate for the child. Sounds that are in the child's dialect will be important for children who speak a varied dialect of English. For all children, words selected to teach sounds should be screened for academic relevance and success.

- When priority targets selected for initial treatment are taught, the clinician should teach sounds that are still in error. No previous guideline should leave a child without treatment for an articulation problem, whether it is of high or low frequency.

Clinicians who carefully read and critically evaluate treatment research will be able to select treatment targets that will produce the most beneficial effects for the children they serve. In some cases, treatment research results may suggest strategies that are counterintuitive. Results may contradict traditional practice or common sense. Ultimately, only controlled and replicated clinical treatment research will suggest effective treatment targets as well as treatment procedures.

Establishing the Baserates

Following the assessment and selection of treatment targets, the clinician's first job is to baserate the articulatory skills that will be taught in the initial treatment sessions. **Baserates** are in-depth assessments of selected target skills conducted just prior to treatment initiation. Going beyond the traditional assessment, baserates help ensure that the child indeed needs treatment to improve articulatory skills. Because each articulatory target (a single phoneme or a phonemic cluster) is baserated with some 20 or so exemplars (opportunities to produce the skill), the results of baserate procedures are more extensive and reliable than the traditional assessment results. In addition, baserates, being measures of target skills just before treatment initiation, help assess the child's improvement during the treatment process. Even more importantly, baserates help justify positive outcomes for the child and thus support claims for reimbursement.

When treatment fails to produce significant improvement over the baserate levels, the clinician can modify the treatment procedure. For example, the clinician may select more effective reinforcers for the child, simplify the target skills, select another target skill, model more frequently, use the shaping procedure, and so forth. Without a reliable base rate, prompt treatment modifications are difficult to make because the clinician would not know whether the skills being treated are improving or not.

There are two kinds of baserate trials: **modeled** and **evoked**. In the modeled trials, the clinician asks a question and immediately produces the correct response for the child to imitate. On evoked trials, the clinician does not model. Both kinds of trials are administered for each exemplar.

Each kind of baserate trial has a standard structure. On the modeled baserate trial, the clinician:

- Presents a stimulus picture or object; for example, in teaching /p/ in word-initial positions, the clinician presents the picture of a pan to the child;

- Points to the stimulus and asks a question; for example, "Sam, what is this?"

- Immediately after asking the question, the clinician models the correct response; for example, the clinician says, "Sam, say, *pan*" and waits for a few seconds for the child to respond;

- The clinician scores the child's response as correct, incorrect, or absent (no response); then waits for a few seconds to initiate the next trial

- The clinician then introduces the next trial; presents a different picture (e.g., the picture of a pail), asks the question, models the response, scores the child's response, and moves on to the next exemplar.

On evoked baserate trials, the clinician simply skips modeling. After presenting the stimulus, the clinician asks a question, waits for the child to respond, and scores the response.

An important aspect of baserates is that the child receives no differential feedback (reinforcement or corrective feedback) for correct or incorrect responses. Absence of such feedback distinguishes a baserate trial from a treatment trial.

The baserate recording sheets provide 20 exemplars to most articulatory targets. A few articulatory targets have fewer than 20 exemplars because of the paucity of words beginning or ending with certain English sounds. The clinician baserates the production of the articulatory targets in each of the exemplars provided. It is recommended that the clinician first administer the evoked trials on all the exemplars, followed by modeled baserate trials. This sequence helps assess whether the child can produce the phoneme without modeling, and failing that, whether the child can benefit from modeling.

Implementing Treatment

After establishing the baserates, the clinician initiates treatment. In the protocols, the baserate and treatment trials have a similar structure. The treatment trials include all steps of baserate trials; in addition, they include verbal praise or corrective feedback.

Treatment Begins with Modeling

Most children benefit from modeling. Therefore, it is essential to begin treatment trials with modeling. Eventually, modeling is faded to introduce the evoked trials. On a modeled treatment trial, the clinician:

- Presents a stimulus picture or object; for example, in teaching /p/ in word-initial positions, the clinician presents the picture of a pan to the child.

- Points to the stimulus and asks a question; for example, "Sam, what is this?"

- Immediately after asking the question, the clinician models the correct response; for example, the clinician says, "Sam, say, *pan*," vocally emphasizes the target phoneme, and waits for a few seconds for the child to respond.

- Reinforces the child's correct responses (e.g., "Excellent!" or "That was correct!") or offers corrective feedback (e.g., "No, that was not correct! You forgot to include the *p* sound at the beginning of the word . . . ").

- The clinician scores the child's response as correct, incorrect, or absent (no response); then waits for a few seconds to initiate the next modeled trial.

- The clinician then introduces the next modeled trial; presents a different picture (e.g., the picture of a pail), asks the question, models the response, scores the child's response, and moves on to the next exemplar.

Modeled Trials Are Faded into Evoked

When the child gives five correctly imitated responses in a sequence, the clinician fades modeling to introduce the evoked trials. Responses are *evoked* when there is no modeling and *imitated* when there is modeling. Two methods of fading a modeled trial into an evoked trial are provided in the protocols.

One method of fading modeling into an evoked trial is a verbal prompt to remind the child of the target phoneme soon after asking the child to name the stimulus picture. For example, the clinician might ask, "What is this?" and immediately say, "Don't forget the *p* at the beginning." In this instance, the modeling of the word *pan* is omitted, but the child is prompted of the target sound. The child's success on a few trials with a verbal prompt leads the clinician to drop it to move on to the evoked trials in which the clinician simply asks the typical question: "What is this?"

Another method of fading modeling into an evoked trial includes nonverbal prompts. A nonverbal prompt in articulation treatment is a partial model—model of an articulatory posture in the absence of sound. For example, after asking the question, "What is this?" the clinician may say, "It starts with . . . " and then show the child the silent articulatory posture of lip closure needed to produce the /p/. When the silent modeling of an articulatory posture is successful in evoking the target phoneme on a few trials, the clinician omits the silent model to transition the child to evoked trials.

If the child fails to respond correctly within a fading sequence, the clinician reinstates either the verbal or nonverbal prompts, and if necessary, the full model of the target phoneme. After a few successful trials, the clinician once again tries to fade the modeling or the prompts into evoked trials.

Providing Effective Feedback

The most critical treatment variable is effective and functional feedback. Children in treatment sessions need precise and prompt information on how they are doing. The protocols suggest verbal praise—a form of social reinforcement—as the most easily administered positive reinforcer for correct responses. Verbal praise is natural, inherent to most communicative situations, and can be delivered as soon as the child gives a correct response. It is known to be effective, and it does not cost anything. Children rarely get tired of honest verbal praise offered when their performance meets specified standards.

Delivery of Reinforcers Should Be Prompt and Functional

A reinforcer is effective and functional only when it results in an increased rate of responses for which it is being offered. Therefore, clinicians need to have options in case verbal praise proves ineffective with a child. With most children, a good option is the token system of reinforcement. Tokens are known as *conditioned generalized reinforcers* because they may be exchanged for a variety of reinforcers. The clinician may give a token for every correct response and let the child exchange the tokens for a small gift (the backup reinforcer) at the end of the session. Stickers and points given for correct responses also may be effective, especially if they are exchanged for a gift of the child's choice.

In treating children with severe developmental disabilities, very young children, and children with brain injury, the clinicians may use such primary reinforcers as food items. Before deciding to use food items, the clinician should consult with the parent to obtain their clearance and to get suggestions for selecting healthful edibles that may be the child's favorite, hence more likely to be effective.

Activities children enjoy also may be used to reinforce correct production of speech sounds. Children like to listen to stories or nursery rhymes, draw on the blackboard, color printed drawings, work on puzzles, paint, play with a favorite toy, work on a craft or art project, and so forth. Such activities are high probability behaviors in that the child is very likely to engage in them. Working on speech sound production is often a low-probability behavior in that the child needs strong reinforcement to engage in it. If access to a desired (high-probability) activity is given only when the child completes a block of speech training trials, the speech sound production under training is likely to increase significantly.

Initially, the clinician offers reinforcement for every correct response. However, the amount of reinforcement offered to a child should eventually approach what is typically offered in social situations. Therefore, the continuous reinforcement the clinician initially uses should be faded to an intermittent reinforcement schedule in which every second, third, or fourth response is correctly reinforced. This is easily accomplished when training moves to conversational speech in which the clinician only occasionally reinforces correct responses.

Corrective Feedback Should Be Prompt and Functional

Prompt and effective corrective feedback for incorrect responses is equally important. Children may be simply told that the response was incorrect or that something specified was missing. In the initial treatment sessions, the corrective feedback should be explicit and verbal. The clinician might say, "No, that was not correct," "You missed the *s* sound at the beginning of the word," "Did you forget the *s* sound?," or "You said *top* instead of *stop*," or "You should say *bread*, not *bed*" to decrease the production of incorrect responses.

In later treatment sessions, corrective feedback may be less explicit, and in most cases, may be just gestural. A raised eyebrow, a raised finger, a facial gesture that suggests an error might be just as effective as a verbal corrective feedback.

Children readily accept corrective feedback when it is fair, delivered objectively, and immediately followed by helpful modeling or repetition of a trial in which the child succeeds. Although verbal corrective feedback is most commonly used—and hence is a part of the protocols, there are other forms in case the need arises.

Withdrawal of a token is an effective strategy that may be combined with verbal corrective feedback. The clinician who awards a token for a correct response may withdraw one for an incorrect response. This strategy is known as *response cost.*

Excessive need to offer corrective feedback implies some problem with the treatment procedure. Perhaps the target skill needs to be simplified; maybe another target is suitable. The clinician may have to shape the child's behavior in small steps, so that the child experiences success at each step. This strategy helps avoid excessive or perhaps detrimental use of corrective feedback. As the correct responses increase during treatment, the need for corrective feedback will automatically diminish.

Sequencing Treatment

Several clinical criteria help move the child in a smooth and efficient manner through the various stages of treatment. Essentially, the clinician should judge when to discontinue modeling on a given exemplar, when to stop teaching a given exemplar, when to probe for generalized productions, and when to move on to the next level of training involving the same target skill or when to move on to the next (different) target skill.

Some Criteria Are Independent of Different Sequences

We will soon address some traditional and novel methods of sequencing treatment targets. Regardless of options for sequencing treatment stages, the clinician needs to make certain decisions to move the child through whatever the sequence selected. The following clinical criteria help move the child through treatment stages that may be inherent to different sequences:

- **When to discontinue modeling.** When the child gives five consecutively correct, imitated responses on a given exemplar, the clinician should fade modeling with partial modeling or hints. Exemplars may be words, phrases, or sentences. Protocols show this strategy of discontinuing modeling.

- **When to reintroduce modeling.** When the child makes errors on the first few evoked trials, the clinician should reintroduce modeling and fade it again after about five correct, imitated responses.

- **When to stop teaching an exemplar.** When the child gives 10 consecutively correct, evoked responses on a given exemplar (e.g., correct production of /s/ in the word *sack* or in a sentence *this is a sack*), the clinician may stop teaching that exemplar. This guideline is the *tentative training criterion*. It is tentative because the /s/ production has been mastered only at the word level, that too, in a single word.

- **When to teach the next exemplar.** When an exemplar for a single phoneme (e.g., /s/ in the word *sand* or the same phoneme in a word produced in a sentence) or a phoneme cluster (e.g., *br* in the word *bread* or the same target produced in a sentence) meets the tentative training criterion (10 consecutively correct evoked responses), the clinician should move on to teaching the next exemplar containing the same phoneme or phoneme cluster.

- **When to probe for generalized productions.** The clinician should probe for generalized productions as soon as the child has met the tentative training criterion for each of some six to eight exemplars for a given phoneme or phoneme cluster (each exemplar is produced without the help of modeling on 10 consecutive trials).

- **When to go back to training more exemplars.** When the child's correct production of the target phoneme on probe exemplars falls short of the probe criterion (90% correct or 9 out of 10 correct probe responses), the clinician should teach additional exemplars taken from the list of baserated exemplars.

- **When to initiate training on a new skill.** When the child meets the probe criterion (90% correct in untrained contexts) for a given phoneme (e.g., production of /s/) or phoneme cluster (e.g., production of /br/), the clinician should initiate training on a new phoneme (e.g., /g/) or a new phoneme cluster (e.g., /st/).

- **When to shift training to a higher level of response complexity.** When the child meets the probe criterion for a given level (e.g., /s/ or *st* blend in words, phrases, or sentences), the clinician should shift training to the phrase or sentence level; however, as noted in the previous bulleted list, the clinician at this stage has the option of introducing a new phoneme or phoneme cluster.

- **When to consider a particular skill mastered.** When the child produces all the target phonemes and phoneme clusters in new and varied verbal contexts and in conversational speech produced in naturalistic social situations (e.g., home, school), the clinician may consider clinically targeted articulatory skills as mastered. It is assumed that the clinician will have trained at all levels of response topography either sequentially or concurrently (words, phrases, sentences, and conversational speech).

In essence, the clinician initially baserates the target skill with multiple exemplars, teaches several exemplars, probes to see if the skill is generalized, offers treatment on additional exemplars if the probe criterion is not met, and probes again. Training and probing are alternated until the child meets the probe criterion (90% correct responses when untrained stimuli are presented). The child is dismissed from treatment when all the articulatory and phonologic targets needed for that child are taught with multiple exemplars and the child has met the probe criterion for each target.

There Are Options to Sequence Levels of Treatment

The **levels of treatment** refer to response topography: words, phrases, sentences, or conversational speech. Traditionally, clinicians have taught the sound at the level of words, phrases, and sentences—in that sequenced order. Some clinicians and in some articulation treatment approaches, nonsense syllables or *phoneme-in-isolation* may be the initial target. Within this approach, most speech sounds or blends may be taught at the basic level—perhaps the word or phrase level. It is only when the client has met the probe criterion for the initial level of training that a clinician would move the child to the next level. In essence, in this common and standard procedure, the child is moved through the levels of words, phrases, and sentences, and conversational speech.

The clinician need not necessarily adopt the standard topographic sequence of words-before-phrases, phrases-before-sentences, and (isolated) sentences-before-conversational speech. There is some emerging evidence that the child may be **concurrently** taught at different topographic levels. Skelton (2004) has demonstrated that it is possible to get good outcome when the children are simultaneously taught target phonemes at all levels of response topography—including words, phrases, sentences, and evoked (nonimitative) sentences. In the concurrent treatment approach, all levels of response complexity are randomly intermixed.

These protocols illustrate the word level as the starting point of training, which is most appropriate for children who imitate the target consonant or cluster with at least 20% accuracy during baserate trials. Children whose imitation accuracy is limited to 0 to 10% likely will need initial training at a lower response topography. The clinician may need to first establish the motor production of the treatment target through the use of one or more special techniques, including phonetic placement, successive sound approximation, verbal instructions, physical manipulation of the articulators, mirror work, and so forth (see Peña-Brooks & Hegde, 2007 for details on these procedures). Production training may begin by teaching the child how to make the sound in isolation and then progressing to more complex levels as the child's productions are stabilized at this most basic level.

There Are Options to Treat One or More Phonemes or Processes

Initially, some clinicians select only one or just a few speech targets to teach in a given session. For instance, the clinician may select the correct production of /s/ as the initial treatment target. It is only when the child meets the probe criterion for sentences for the initially selected phoneme that a clinician would target another phoneme for intervention.

Even when a clinician begins treatment for a single phoneme, treatment eventually may involve multiple phonemes in a single session. For instance, when the child meets the probe criterion for /s/ at the word level (a single phoneme), the clinician may shift training for that phoneme at the phrase level. While spending some treatment time on teaching the /s/ at the phrase level, the clinician may initiate treatment for a different phoneme at the word level (e.g., /t/). In this case, the child will be receiving treatment in the same session for two sounds at two levels of response complexity: /s/ at the phrase level and /t/ at the word level. Eventually, the clinician may be teaching different skills at vastly different levels (some at the phrase, others at the simple sentence, and still others at the extended sentence levels or conversational speech).

An alternative is to introduce multiple phonemes or phoneme blends from the beginning of treatment. The multiple phoneme approach has always advocated this strategy (McCabe

& Bradley, 1975). Similarly, in the more recent multiple oppositions approach the clinician targets multiple phonemes in each treatment session (Williams, 2000, 2003).

Individual children may well differ in their response to either single or multiple targets addressed in the same session. There is not much experimental data to suggest who would be the best candidate for a multiple phoneme approach.

Measuring the Child's Progress

Clinicians appreciate the necessity of documenting the progress children (or adult clients) make in treatment sessions. This is especially critical for third-party payers. Regardless of payment issues, measurement of skills being taught is a necessary scientific task. The protocols make it easier to track children's responses during treatment so that clinicians have precise quantitative information that they can analyze in relation to the baserates. Virtually everything clinicians teach is quantifiable; if the client's responses are not quantified, no one can be sure what is going on in treatment.

The recording sheets available on the accompanying CD include recording sheets that the clinicians can use to document the child's production of phonemes in baserates, during treatment, and during probes. Diligently used, these recording sheets will give precise numbers of correct and incorrect responses a child gives in baserate, treatment, and probe sessions. The clinician can contrast the child's response rates before, during, and after treatment. The clinician thus will have precise and objective data to document a child's progress. For example, a child's baserate production of a particular phoneme may be at 10%; but it may increase to 90% or better during treatment; and may meet the 90% probe criterion at the end of treatment. Such quantitative data help quell any doubts about the need for treatment and the improvement that did take place as a result of treatment. The *Individuals with Disabilities Education Improvement Act—2004* requires a description of how the child's progress toward meeting the annual goals will be measured (Wright, 2004). The recording sheets given for baserates, treatment, and probes can be an effective means for the school-based clinician to objectively measure and convincingly document the child's progress.

The recording sheets on the CD may be individualized for the clinic, the clinician, and the child. Because all recording sheets are simple *MS-Word* documents, they can be personalized to any professional setting. The CD helps generate clinic-specific stationery on which the child's responses are recorded.

How to Use These Protocols in Remediating Phonologic Processes

By looking at the protocols, one may gain an initial impression that they are designed to treat only articulation disorders, not phonologic disorders. However, as pointed out in the *introduction*, it is only by teaching individual phonemes that a clinician can remediate inappropriate phonologic processes. The protocols may be efficiently used to teach individual phonemes as well as to remediate phonologic processes.

Phonologic process remediation does not require unique treatment procedures. It does require a slightly different organization of teaching tasks and probing for untreated tasks. Phonologic process remediation is more a matter of treatment data analysis than treatment itself (Peña-Brooks & Hegde, 2007).

Individual Phoneme Teaching Versus Phonologic Process Remediation

A significant difference between teaching individual phonemes with no phonologic pattern and eliminating an inappropriate pattern (process) is the **sequence** in which the treatment and probes are administered. In teaching individual sounds with no pattern, the clinician will first teach a sound to the adopted mastery criterion, and then probe for its generalized production. When the probe criterion is met for that sound, the clinician will train another sound and then probe for its generalized production. In this manner, the clinician will teach and probe the unpatterned sound productions that are clinical targets for a given child. In essence, in remediating individual phonemes, **all sounds are treated and probed**. The protocols provided in this book show this sequence for each phoneme: the probe protocol/recording sheet is provided following a treatment protocols sheet and a recording sheet.

In eliminating a pattern of errors, the clinician **does not teach all the sounds within the pattern**. The clinician will teach a few of the sounds within the pattern. However, teaching each sound and probing for generalized production of just-taught sound will follow the same sequence as that needed to teach sounds with no phonologic pattern. Therefore, the protocols are essential for this purpose. The main and perhaps the only distinguishing feature of pattern-based treatment is this: **It requires the clinician to probe for generalized productions of baserated but untreated sounds within a pattern**. For instance, in eliminating the final consonant deletion process in a child who omits some eight phonemes in word-final positions, the clinician will teach three or four phonemes, probe for generalized production of each phoneme following its teaching, and then **probe for generalized productions of four or five untreated phonemes** that the child did not produce in word-final positions before treatment. In remediating individual phonemes, the clinician almost never probes for generalized production of untreated phonemes as such generalization is not expected, although this position is by no means fully confirmed by experimental treatment research. Similarly, the expectation that untreated phonemes within various processes always are produced on the basis of generalization is also not universally and strongly supported by experimental research. Nonetheless, these are the expected practices within the individual-phoneme or pattern-based approaches to treatment.

Conclusion

In summary, the protocols may be used in the following manner to remediate phonologic processes:

- Following a thorough assessment, the clinician selects the phonologic processes for remediation. For a given child, for instance, processes targeted for elimination may be initial and final consonant deletions. The assessment will have identified the individual word-initial and word-final consonants that are missing from the child's phonemic inventory.

- Following the selection of initial and final consonant deletion for remediation, the clinician then baserates the production of missing sounds in word-initial and word-final positions as provided for in the protocols.

- The clinician then may begin teaching some of the missing consonants in the word-initial positions. For instance, if the child omitted some eight phonemes in the word-initial positions, the clinician may teach three of them. Each phoneme taught will immediately be probed for its generalized production as provided for and sequenced in the protocols. After teaching and probing three phonemes, the clinician will then go directly to the baserate sheets for the five untrained (and initially baserated) phonemes to probe their generalized production because of the effects of training the three phonemes within the process. Because at this point, the clinician will use the *Baserate Exemplars and Recording Sheets* to assess generalized productions, the clinician may use the CD to modify the sheet. The clinician may rename the form as *Probe Recording Sheet.*

- If the child correctly produced the untreated five phonemes because of the effect of the three treated phonemes in the word-final position, the clinician may consider the final consonant deletion process eliminated at this stage of treatment (in words). The clinician then may probe for the correct production of all the missing phonemes in sentences or conversational speech. Additional treatment will be offered as needed.

- If the child did not correctly produce any or all of the untreated sounds within the process, the clinician will offer additional treatment for selected phonemes. The treatment will stop when all the phonemes within the process are produced to an acceptable criterion of performance.

The protocols, therefore, offer a structure within which various phonologic processes may be remediated. To facilitate this process, the clinician may use the CD in the following manner:

- The clinician may first print all the baserate, probe, and treatment recording sheets for the sounds specified within a phonologic process.

- The clinician will then baserate the production of each sound with the help of 20 exemplars provided. The clinician may individualize the target words by typing in new exemplars on the *Baserate Exemplars and Recording Sheet.*

- The clinician will teach a few of the phonemes within a phonologic pattern. As noted before, each treated phoneme will be probed on the *Probe Protocols and Recording Sheet* individualized and printed from the CD.

- When each of the selected phonemes meets the training and the probe criterion, the clinician is ready to probe for generalized production of untreated phonemes within the process. To accomplish this task, the clinician will return to the CD and rename the *Baserate Exemplars and Recording Sheet* as *Probe Exemplars and Recording Sheet.* Printing out the renamed sheets, the clinician will probe the untreated phonemes within the process to see if the process is now eliminated. Depending on the probe results, additional treatment may be offered for a few more phonemes within the process or it may be concluded that the process is no longer evident.

- The provided *Probe Protocols and Recording Sheet* are intended to assess generalized production of treated phonemes. This sheet contains fewer exemplars than the *Baserate Exemplars and Recording Sheet.* To be sure that untreated phonemes within a pattern are correctly produced as a function of generalization, the clinician may need to probe them with all the words initially baserated. Therefore, we recommend that the clinician rename and reuse the *Baserate Exemplars and Recording Sheet* to assess generalized production of untreated phonemes to judge whether a pattern still exists or not.

In essence, protocols help teach selected phonemes within a process, asses the generalized correct production of untreated phonemes within the process, teach additional phonemes within the process if there is a failure to generalize, and probe again for generalized productions of untreated phonemes. The basic treatment procedure inherent to protocols is an *alternation of treatment and probe assessment.* When phonemes are grouped according to a pattern within the speech of a child, such an alternation is all that is needed to remediate phonologic processes.

Part I

Teaching Individual Sounds

/p/ in Word-Initial Positions

Baserate Protocols

*Use stimuli from the **Stimulus Book, Volume 1**.*

At the beginning of each trial, place a relevant stimulus (an object, a picture, or a printed word) in front of the child. Point to the stimulus as you ask an evoking question. Do not respond in any way to the child's correct, incorrect, or lack of responses.

Scripts for Evoked Baserate Trial		Note
Clinician	[*stimulus: pan*] "What is this?"	Evoked trial
Child	"an."	Omission of initial /p/
Clinician	Pulls the stimulus toward her; records the response.	No corrective feedback
Clinician	[*stimulus: pail*] "What is this?"	The next evoked trial
Child	"ail."	Omission of initial /p/
Clinician	Pulls the stimulus toward her; records the response.	No corrective feedback

Administer the modeled baserate trials only after completing the evoked trials on all 20 (or more) exemplars.

Scripts for Modeled Baserate Trial		Note
Clinician	[*stimulus: pan*] "What is this? Say, pan."	Modeled trial
Child	"Pan."	Correct response
Clinician	Pulls the stimulus toward her; records the response.	No reinforcement
Clinician	[*stimulus: pail*] "What is this? Say, pail."	The next modeled trial
Child	"ail."	Omission of initial /p/
Clinician	Pulls the stimulus toward her; records the response.	No corrective feedback

Use the recording sheet with exemplars shown on the next page to establish the baserates; print it from the CD.

/p/ in Word-Initial Positions

Baserate Exemplars and Recording Sheet

Use stimuli from the **Stimulus Book,** *Volume 1.*

Print this page from the CD or photocopy this page for your clinical use.

Name/Age:	Date:
Goal: To establish the baserate production of /p/ in word-initial positions.	Clinician:

Scoring: Correct: ✓   Incorrect or no response: X

/p/ in word-initial positions	Evoked	Modeled
1. pan		
2. pail		
3. pea		
4. peach		
5. paw		
6. pajamas		
7. pelican		
8. penny		
9. piano		
10. ponytail		
11. pear		
12. pill		
13. pony		
14. pot		
15. pie		
16. pedal		
17. policeman		
18. potato		
19. pyramid		
20. pillow		
Percent correct baserate		

Replace or add new exemplars as you see fit for a given child. After establishing the baserates, begin production teaching. Follow the protocols given on the next page.

/p/ in Word-Initial Positions

Treatment Protocols

Use stimuli from the **Stimulus Book, Volume 1.**

Teach 6 to 8 exemplars using the following script.

Place a relevant stimulus in front of the child (an object, a picture, or a printed word) and ask a question as you point to the stimulus.

Scripts for Modeled Discrete Trial Training		Note
Clinician	[*stimulus: pan*] "What is this? Say, **pan.**"	Modeling; the target vocally emphasized
Child	"an."	A wrong response
Clinician	"No. That's not correct. You said *an*, but it's a **pan**."	Corrective feedback
Clinician	[*the same stimulus*] "What is this? Say, **pan.** Don't forget the *p* at the beginning."	The next trial
Child	"Pan."	A correct response
Clinician	"Excellent! You didn't miss the *p* this time!"	Verbal praise

Repeat the trials until the child gives 5 consecutively correct, imitated responses.

When the child imitates 5 correct responses in sequence, fade the modeling.

Scripts for Fading the Modeling		Note
Clinician	[*stimulus: pan*] "What is this? Don't forget the *p* at the beginning."	Only a prompt
Child	"an."	A wrong response
Clinician	"Gee, you forgot the *p* this time! It's a *pan*, not *an*. Put the *p* at the beginning."	Corrective feedback
Clinician	[*the same stimulus*] "What is this? It starts with . . . [*silently models the lip posture for the target sound.*]	The next trial; a partial modeling
Child	"Pan."	A correct response
Clinician	"That's great! You said *pan*, not *an*."	Verbal praise
Clinician	[*the same stimulus*] "What is this?"	Typical question; evoked trial
Child	"Pan."	A correct response
Clinician	"Great job! You said it correctly!"	Verbal praise

If the wrong responses persist on 4 to 5 evoked trials, reinstate partial or full modeling for a few trials, again fade the modeling, and re-present the evoked trials.

When the child meets the tentative learning criterion of 10 consecutively correct, nonimitated responses for a given stimulus item, move on to the next stimulus item. With this procedure, teach 6 to 8 exemplars shown on the following recording sheet. Use different exemplars as you see fit for a given child.

/p/ in Word-Initial Positions

Treatment Exemplars and Recording Sheet

Use stimuli from the **Stimulus Book, Volume 1**.

Print this page from CD or photocopy this page for your clinical use.

Name/Age:	Date:
Goal: Production of /p/ in word-initial positions with 90% accuracy when asked an evoking question while showing a stimulus.	Clinician:

Scoring: Correct: ✓   Incorrect or no response: X

Target skills	Discrete Trials														
	1	2	3	4	5	6	7	8	9	10	11	12	13	14	15
1. pan															
2. pail															
3. pea															
4. peach															
5. paw															
6. pajamas															
7. pelican															
8. penny															

When the child has met the learning criterion of 10 consecutively correct evoked (nonimitated) responses for each of the 6 to 8 target exemplars, conduct a probe to see if the production has generalized to previously baserated but untrained exemplars.

If the probes do not meet the 90% correct criterion for untrained exemplars, teach additional exemplars and then probe again.

/p/ in Word-Initial Positions

Probe Protocols and Recording Sheet

Use stimuli from the **Stimulus Book,** *Volume 1.*

Print this page from the CD or photocopy this page for your clinical use.

On the probes, present only the untrained exemplars (UT). When the child fails to meet the 90% correct probe criterion, either teach 2 to 4 new exemplars or give additional training trials on already trained stimuli. If needed, select new exemplars for probes. Probe at least 10 untrained exemplars. Alternate probes and treatment until the probe criterion is met.

Scripts for Probe Trials		Note
Clinician	[*untrained stimulus: a piano*] "What is this?"	No modeling or prompts
Child	"Piano."	A correct, generalized response
Clinician	Scores the response as correct.	No reinforcement
Clinician	[*untrained stimulus: a ponytail*] "What is this?"	The second probe trial
Child	"onytail."	A wrong probe response
Clinician	Scores the response as incorrect.	No corrective feedback

Name:	Date:	Session #:
Age:	**Clinician:**	
Diagnosis: Articulation/Phonologic Disorder	**Word-initial /p/ probe**	
Untrained Stimuli	**Score: + correct; – incorrect or no responses**	
1. piano		
2. pear		
3. ponytail		
4. pill		
5. pony		
6. pot		
7. pie		
8. pedal		
9. policeman		
10. potato		
11. pyramid		
12. pillow		
Percent correct: (Criterion: 90%)		

If the child does not meet the probe criterion, give additional training on already trained exemplars or teach a few new exemplars. Subsequently, readminister the probe trials. When the child meets the 90% correct probe criterion for the exemplars, shift training to the sentence or conversational level or to another phoneme.

/p/ in Word-Final Positions

Baserate Protocols

Use stimuli from the **Stimulus Book, Volume 1**.

At the beginning of each trial, place a relevant stimulus (an object, a picture, or a printed word) in front of the child. Point to the stimulus as you ask an evoking question. Do not respond in any way to the child's correct, incorrect, or lack of responses.

Scripts for Evoked Baserate Trial		Note
Clinician	[*stimulus: a cap*] "What is this?"	Evoked trial
Child	"cæ."	Omission of final /p/
Clinician	Pulls the stimulus toward her; records the response.	No corrective feedback
Clinician	[*stimulus: a cup*] "What is this?"	The next evoked trial
Child	"cə."	Omission of /p/
Clinician	Pulls the stimulus toward her; records the response.	No corrective feedback

Administer the modeled baserate trials only after completing the evoked trials on all 20 (or more) exemplars.

Scripts for Modeled Baserate Trial		Note
Clinician	[*stimulus: a cap*] "What is this? Say, *cap*."	Modeled trial
Child	"Cap."	Correct response
Clinician	Pulls the stimulus toward her; records the response.	No reinforcement
Clinician	[*stimulus: a cup*] "What is this? Say, *cup*."	The next modeled trial
Child	"cə."	Omission of /p/
Clinician	Pulls the stimulus toward her; records the response.	No corrective feedback

Use the recording sheet with exemplars shown on the next page to establish the baserates; print it from the CD.

/p/ in Word-Final Positions

Baserate Exemplars and Recording Sheet

Use stimuli from the **Stimulus Book**, *Volume 1*.

Print this page from the CD or photocopy this page for your clinical use.

Name/Age:	Date:
Goal: To establish the baserate production of /p/ in word-final positions.	Clinician:

Scoring: Correct: ✓   Incorrect or no response: X

/p/ in word-final positions	Evoked	Modeled
1. cap		
2. cup		
3. cop		
4. jeep		
5. map		
6. teacup		
7. tulip		
8. whitecap		
9. warship		
10. lollipop		
11. mop		
12. rope		
13. soup		
14. tap		
15. soap		
16. cantaloupe		
17. mountaintop		
18. envelope		
19. buttercup		
20. videotape		
Percent correct baserate		

Replace or add new exemplars as you see fit for a given child. After establishing the baserates, begin production teaching. Follow the protocols given on the next page.

/p/ in Word-Final Positions
Treatment Protocols

*Use stimuli from the **Stimulus Book, Volume 1**.*

Teach 6 to 8 exemplars using the following script.

Place a relevant stimulus (an object, a picture, or a printed word) in front of the child and point to the stimulus as you ask an evoking question.

Scripts for Modeled Discrete Trial Training		Note
Clinician	[*stimulus: a cap*] "What is this? Say, cap."	Modeling; the target vocally emphasized.
Child	"cæ."	A wrong response
Clinician	"No. That's not correct. You said *cæ*, but it's a *ca**p**.*"	Corrective feedback
Clinician	[*the same stimulus*] "What is this? Say, *ca**p**.* Don't forget the *p* at the end."	The next trial
Child	"Cap."	A correct response
Clinician	"Excellent! You didn't miss the *p* at the end of the word!"	Verbal praise

Repeat the trials until the child gives 5 consecutively correct, imitated responses.

When the child imitates 5 correct responses in sequence, fade the modeling.

Scripts for Fading the Modeling		Note
Clinician	[*stimulus: a cap*] "What is this? Don't forget the *p* at the end."	Only a prompt
Child	"cæ."	A wrong response
Clinician	"Gee, you forgot the *p*! It's a *cap*, not *cæ*. Put the *p* at the end."	Corrective feedback
Clinician	[*the same stimulus*] "What is this? It ends with . . ." [*silently models the lip posture for the target sound.*]	The next trial; a partial modeling
Child	"Cap."	A correct response
Clinician	"That's great! You said *cap*, not *cæ*."	Verbal praise
Clinician	[*the same stimulus*] "What is this?"	Typical question; evoked trial
Child	"Cap."	A correct response
Clinician	"I like it! You said it correctly!"	Verbal praise

If the wrong responses persist on 4 to 5 evoked trials, reinstate partial or full modeling for a few trials, again fade the modeling, and re-present the evoked trials.

When the child meets the tentative learning criterion of 10 consecutively correct, nonimitated responses for a given stimulus item, move on to the next stimulus item. With this procedure, teach 6 to 8 exemplars shown on the following recording sheet. Use different exemplars as you see fit for a given child.

/p/ in Word-Final Positions

Treatment Exemplars and Recording Sheet

Use stimuli from the **Stimulus Book,** *Volume 1.*

Print this page from CD or photocopy this page for your clinical use.

Name/Age:	Date:
Goal: Production of /p/ in word-final positions with 90% accuracy when asked an evoking question while showing a stimulus.	Clinician:

Scoring: Correct: ✓   Incorrect or no response: X

Target skills	Discrete Trials														
	1	2	3	4	5	6	7	8	9	10	11	12	13	14	15
1. cap															
2. cup															
3. cop															
4. jeep															
5. map															
6. teacup															
7. tulip															
8. whitecap															

When the child has met the learning criterion of 10 consecutively correct evoked (nonimitated) responses for each of the 6 to 8 target exemplars, conduct a probe to see if the production has generalized to previously baserated but untrained exemplars.

If the probes do not meet the 90% correct criterion for untrained exemplars, teach additional exemplars and then probe again.

/p/ in Word-Final Positions
Probe Protocols and Recording Sheet

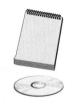

Use stimuli from the **Stimulus Book,** *Volume 1.*

Print this page from the CD or photocopy this page for your clinical use.

On the probes, present only the untrained exemplars (UT). When the child fails to meet the 90% correct probe criterion, either teach 2 to 4 new exemplars or give additional training trials on already trained stimuli. If needed, select new exemplars for probes. Probe at least 10 untrained exemplars. Alternate probes and treatment until the probe criterion is met.

Scripts for Probe Trials		Note
Clinician	[*untrained stimulus: a warship*] "What is this?"	No modeling or prompts
Child	"Warship" ["Ship"]	A correct, generalized response
Clinician	Scores the response as correct.	No reinforcement
Clinician	[*untrained stimulus: a lollipop*] "What is this?"	The second probe trial
Child	"lollipa."	A wrong probe response
Clinician	Scores the response as incorrect.	No corrective feedback

Name:	Date:	Session #:
Age:	**Clinician:**	
Diagnosis: Articulation/Phonologic Disorder	**Word-final /p/ probe**	
Untrained Stimuli	**Score: + correct; – incorrect or no responses**	
1. warship		
2. lollipop		
3. mop		
4. rope		
5. soup		
6. tap		
7. soap		
8. cantaloupe		
9. mountaintop		
10. envelope		
11. buttercup		
12. videotape		
Percent correct: (Criterion: 90%)		

If the child does not meet the probe criterion, give additional training on already trained exemplars or teach a few new exemplars. Subsequently, readminister the probe trials. When the child meets the 90% correct probe criterion for the exemplars, shift training to the sentence or conversational level or to another phoneme.

/b/ in Word-Initial Positions

Baserate Protocols

Use stimuli from the **Stimulus Book,** *Volume 1.*

At the beginning of each trial, place a relevant stimulus (an object, a picture, or a printed word) in front of the child. Point to the stimulus as you ask an evoking question. Do not respond in any way to the child's correct, incorrect, or lack of responses.

Scripts for Evoked Baserate Trial		Note
Clinician	[*stimulus: baby*] "What is this?"	Evoked trial
Child	"eby."	Omission of initial /b/
Clinician	Pulls the stimulus toward her; records the response.	No corrective feedback
Clinician	[*stimulus: balloon*] "What is this?"	The next evoked trial
Child	"əlloon."	Omission of initial /b/
Clinician	Pulls the stimulus toward her; records the response.	No corrective feedback

Administer the modeled baserate trials only after completing the evoked trials on all 20 (or more) exemplars.

Scripts for Modeled Baserate Trial		Note
Clinician	[*stimulus: baby*] "What is this? Say, *baby.*"	Modeled trial
Child	"Baby."	Correct response
Clinician	Pulls the stimulus toward her; records the response.	No reinforcement
Clinician	[*stimulus: balloon*] "What is this? Say, *balloon.*"	The next modeled trial
Child	"əlloon."	Omission of initial /b/
Clinician	Pulls the stimulus toward her; records the response.	No corrective feedback

Use the recording sheet with exemplars shown on the next page to establish the baserates; print it from the CD.

/b/ in Word-Initial Positions

Baserate Exemplars and Recording Sheet

Use stimuli from the **Stimulus Book,** *Volume 1.*

Print this page from the CD or photocopy this page for your clinical use.

Name/Age:	Date:
Goal: To establish the baserate production of /b/ in word-initial positions.	Clinician:

Scoring: Correct: ✓   Incorrect or no response: X

/b/ in word-initial positions	Evoked	Modeled
1. baby		
2. balloon		
3. bear		
4. beach		
5. bun		
6. backpack		
7. backyard		
8. bandana		
9. banana		
10. buffalo		
11. ball		
12. bell		
13. boat		
14. book		
15. bus		
16. battery		
17. birdbath		
18. bicycle		
19. bookshelf		
20. butterfly		
Percent correct baserate		

Replace or add new exemplars as you see fit for a given child. After establishing the baserates, begin production teaching. Follow the protocols given on the next page.

/b/ in Word-Initial Positions
Treatment Protocols

Use stimuli from the **Stimulus Book,** *Volume 1.*

Teach 6 to 8 exemplars using the following script.

Place a relevant stimulus in front of the child (an object, a picture, or a printed word) and ask a question as you point to the stimulus.

Scripts for Modeled Discrete Trial Training		Note
Clinician	[*stimulus: baby*] "What is this? Say, **baby**."	Modeling; the target vocally emphasized
Child	"eby."	A wrong response
Clinician	"No. That's not correct. You said *eby*, but it's a **baby**."	Corrective feedback
Clinician	[*the same stimulus*] "What is this? Say, **baby**. Don't forget the *b* at the beginning."	The next trial
Child	"Baby."	A correct response
Clinician	"Excellent! You didn't miss the *b* this time!"	Verbal praise

Repeat the trials until the child gives 5 consecutively correct, imitated responses.

When the child imitates 5 correct responses in sequence, fade the modeling.

Scripts for Fading the Modeling		Note
Clinician	[*stimulus: baby*] "What is this? Don't forget the *b* at the beginning."	Only a prompt
Child	"eby."	A wrong response
Clinician	"Gee, you forgot the *b*! It's a *baby*, not *eby*. Put the *b* at the beginning."	Corrective feedback
Clinician	[*the same stimulus*] "What is this? It starts with . . . " [*silently models the lip posture for the target sound.*]	The next trial; a partial modeling
Child	"Baby."	A correct response
Clinician	"That's great! You said *baby*, not *eby*."	Verbal praise
Clinician	[*the same stimulus*] "What is this?"	Typical question; evoked trial
Child	"Baby."	A correct response
Clinician	"Wonderful! You said it correctly!"	Verbal praise

If the wrong responses persist on 4 to 5 evoked trials, reinstate partial or full modeling for a few trials, again fade the modeling, and re-present the evoked trials.

When the child meets the tentative learning criterion of 10 consecutively correct, nonimitated responses for a given stimulus item, move on to the next stimulus item. With this procedure, teach 6 to 8 exemplars shown on the following recording sheet. Use different exemplars as you see fit for a given child.

/b/ in Word-Initial Positions

Treatment Exemplars and Recording Sheet

Use stimuli from the **Stimulus Book, Volume 1**.

Print this page from CD or photocopy this page for your clinical use.

Name/Age:	Date:
Goal: Production of /b/ in word-initial positions with 90% accuracy when asked an evoking question while showing a stimulus.	Clinician:

Scoring: Correct: ✓   Incorrect or no response: X

Target skills	Discrete Trials														
	1	2	3	4	5	6	7	8	9	10	11	12	13	14	15
1. baby															
2. balloon															
3. bear															
4. beach															
5. bun															
6. backpack															
7. backyard															
8. bandana															

When the child has met the learning criterion of 10 consecutively correct evoked (nonimitated) responses for each of the 6 to 8 target exemplars, conduct a probe to see if the production has generalized to previously baserated but untrained exemplars.

If the probes do not meet the 90% correct criterion for untrained exemplars, teach additional exemplars and then probe again.

/b/ in Word-Initial Positions

Probe Protocols and Recording Sheet

*Use stimuli from the **Stimulus Book, Volume 1**.*

Print this page from the CD or photocopy this page for your clinical use.

On the probes, present only the untrained exemplars (UT). When the child fails to meet the 90% correct probe criterion, either teach 2 to 4 new exemplars or give additional training trials on already trained stimuli. If needed, select new exemplars for probes. Probe at least 10 untrained exemplars. Alternate probes and treatment until the probe criterion is met.

Scripts for Probe Trials		Note
Clinician	[*untrained stimulus: banana*] "What is this?"	No modeling or prompts
Child	"Banana."	A correct, generalized response
Clinician	Scores the response as correct.	No reinforcement
Clinician	[*untrained stimulus: buffalo*] "What is this?"	The second probe trial
Child	"əffalo."	A wrong probe response
Clinician	Scores the response as incorrect.	No corrective feedback

Name:	Date:	Session #:
Age:	**Clinician:**	
Diagnosis: Articulation/Phonologic Disorder	**Word-initial /b/ probe**	
Untrained Stimuli	**Score: + correct; – incorrect or no responses**	
1. banana		
2. buffalo		
3. ball		
4. bell		
5. boat		
6. book		
7. bus		
8. battery		
9. birdbath		
10. bicycle		
11. bookshelf		
12. butterfly		
Percent correct: (Criterion: 90%)		

If the child does not meet the probe criterion, give additional training on already trained exemplars or teach a few new exemplars. Subsequently, readminister the probe trials. When the child meets the 90% correct probe criterion for the exemplars, shift training to the sentence or conversational level or to another phoneme.

/b/ in Word-Final Positions

Baserate Protocols

Use stimuli from the **Stimulus Book, Volume 1**.

At the beginning of each trial, place a relevant stimulus (an object, a picture, or a printed word) in front of the child. Point to the stimulus as you ask an evoking question. Do not respond in any way to the child's correct, incorrect, or lack of responses.

Scripts for Evoked Baserate Trial		Note
Clinician	[*stimulus: bib*] "What is this?"	Evoked trial
Child	"bi."	Omission of final /b/
Clinician	Pulls the stimulus toward her; records the response.	No corrective feedback
Clinician	[*stimulus: cub*] "What is this?"	The next evoked trial
Child	"cə."	Omission of final /b/
Clinician	Pulls the stimulus toward her; records the response.	No corrective feedback

Administer the modeled baserate trials only after completing the evoked trials on all 20 (or more) exemplars.

Scripts for Modeled Baserate Trial		Note
Clinician	[*stimulus: bib*] "What is this? Say, *bib*."	Modeled trial
Child	"Bib."	Correct response
Clinician	Pulls the stimulus toward her; records the response.	No reinforcement
Clinician	[*stimulus: cub*] "What is this? Say, *cub*."	The next modeled trial
Child	"cə."	Omission of final /b/
Clinician	Pulls the stimulus toward her; records the response	No corrective feedback

Use the recording sheet with exemplars shown on the next page to establish the baserates; print it from the CD.

/b/ in Word-Final Positions

Baserate Exemplars and Recording Sheet

Use stimuli from the **Stimulus Book,** *Volume 1.*

Print this page from the CD or photocopy this page for your clinical use.

Name/Age:	Date:
Goal: To establish the baserate production of /b/ in word-final positions.	Clinician:

Scoring: Correct: ✓   Incorrect or no response: X

/b/ in word-final positions	Evoked	Modeled
1. bib		
2. cub (lion)		
3. robe		
4. tub		
5. tube		
6. bathrobe		
7. light bulb		
8. ice cube		
9. wardrobe		
10. earlobe		
11. cube		
12. globe		
13. cab		
14. knob		
15. rib		
16. door knob		
17. taxi cab		
18. golden globe		
19. cobweb		
20. bath tub		
Percent correct baserate		

Replace or add new exemplars as you see fit for a given child. After establishing the baserates, begin production teaching. Follow the protocols given on the next page.

/b/ in Word-Final Positions

Treatment Protocols

Use stimuli from the **Stimulus Book,** *Volume 1.*

Teach 6 to 8 exemplars using the following script.

Place a relevant stimulus (an object, a picture, or a printed word) in front of the child and point to the stimulus as you ask an evoking question.

Scripts for Modeled Discrete Trial Training		Note
Clinician	[*stimulus: cub*] "What is this? Say, *cub.*"	Modeling; the target vocally emphasized
Child	"cə."	A wrong response
Clinician	"No. That's not correct. You said cə, but it's a *cub.*"	Corrective feedback
Clinician	[*the same stimulus*] "What is this? Say, *cub.* Don't forget the *b* at the end."	The next trial
Child	"Cub."	A correct response
Clinician	"Excellent! You didn't miss the *b* at the end of the word!"	Verbal praise

Repeat the trials until the child gives 5 consecutively correct, imitated responses.

When the child imitates 5 correct responses in sequence, fade the modeling.

Scripts for Fading the Modeling		Note
Clinician	[*stimulus: cub*] "What is this? Don't forget the *b* at the end."	Only a prompt
Child	"cə."	A wrong response
Clinician	"Gee, you forgot the *b* sound! It's a *cub,* not cə. Put the *b* at the end."	Corrective feedback
Clinician	[*the same stimulus*] "What is this? It ends with . . . " [*silently models the lip posture for the target sound.*]	The next trial; a partial modeling
Child	"Cub."	A correct response
Clinician	"You're right! You said *cub,* not cə."	Verbal praise
Clinician	[*the same stimulus*] "What is this?"	Typical question; evoked trial
Child	"Cub."	A correct response
Clinician	"Great job! You said it correctly!"	Verbal praise

If the wrong responses persist on 4 to 5 evoked trials, reinstate partial or full modeling for a few trials, again fade the modeling, and re-present the evoked trials.

When the child meets the tentative learning criterion of 10 consecutively correct, nonimitated responses for a given stimulus item, move on to the next stimulus item. With this procedure, teach 6 to 8 exemplars shown on the following recording sheet. Use different exemplars as you see fit for a given child.

/b/ in Word-Final Positions

Treatment Exemplars and Recording Sheet

*Use stimuli from the **Stimulus Book, Volume 1**.*

Print this page from CD or photocopy this page for your clinical use.

Name/Age:	Date:
Goal: Production of /b/ in word-final positions with 90% accuracy when asked an evoking question while showing a stimulus.	Clinician:

Scoring: Correct: ✓   Incorrect or no response: X

Target skills	Discrete Trials														
	1	2	3	4	5	6	7	8	9	10	11	12	13	14	15
1. bib															
2. cub (lion)															
3. robe															
4. tub															
5. tube															
6. bathrobe															
7. light bulb															
8. ice cube															

When the child has met the learning criterion of 10 consecutively correct evoked (nonimitated) responses for each of the 6 to 8 target exemplars, conduct a probe to see if the production has generalized to previously baserated but untrained exemplars.

If the probes do not meet the 90% correct criterion for untrained exemplars, teach additional exemplars and then probe again.

/b/ in Word-Final Positions

Probe Protocols and Recording Sheet

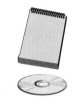

Use stimuli from the **Stimulus Book, Volume 1**.

Print this page from the CD or photocopy this page for your clinical use.

On the probes, present only the untrained exemplars (UT). When the child fails to meet the 90% correct probe criterion, either teach 2 to 4 new exemplars or give additional training trials on already trained stimuli. If needed, select new exemplars for probes. Probe at least 10 untrained exemplars. Alternate probes and treatment until the probe criterion is met.

Scripts for Probe Trials		Note
Clinician	[*untrained stimulus: wardrobe*] "What is this?"	No modeling or prompts.
Child	"Wardrobe."	A correct, generalized response
Clinician	Scores the response as correct.	No reinforcement
Clinician	[*untrained stimulus: earlobe*] "What is this?"	The second probe trial
Child	"earlo."	A wrong probe response
Clinician	Scores the response as incorrect.	No corrective feedback

Name:	Date:	Session #:
Age:	**Clinician:**	
Diagnosis: Articulation/Phonologic Disorder	**Word-final /b/ probe**	
Untrained Stimuli	**Score: + correct; – incorrect or no responses**	
1. wardrobe		
2. earlobe		
3. cube		
4. globe		
5. cab		
6. knob		
7. rib		
8. door knob		
9. taxi cab		
10. golden globe		
11. cobweb		
12. bath tub		
Percent correct: (Criterion: 90%)		

If the child does not meet the probe criterion, give additional training on already trained exemplars or teach a few new exemplars. Subsequently, readminister the probe trials. When the child meets the 90% correct probe criterion for the exemplars, shift training to the sentence or conversational level or to another phoneme.

/t/ in Word-Initial Positions

Baserate Protocols

Use stimuli from the **Stimulus Book,** *Volume 2.*

At the beginning of each trial, place a relevant stimulus (an object, a picture, or a printed word) in front of the child. Point to the stimulus as you ask an evoking question. Do not respond in any way to the child's correct, incorrect, or lack of responses.

Scripts for Evoked Baserate Trial		Note
Clinician	[*stimulus: tap*] "What is this?"	Evoked trial
Child	"æp."	Omission of initial /t/
Clinician	Pulls the stimulus toward her; records the response.	No corrective feedback
Clinician	[*stimulus: tape*] "What is this?"	The next evoked trial
Child	"ape."	Omission of initial /t/
Clinician	Pulls the stimulus toward her; records the response.	No corrective feedback

Administer the modeled baserate trials only after completing the evoked trials on all 20 (or more) exemplars.

Scripts for Modeled Baserate Trial		Note
Clinician	[*stimulus: tap*] "What is this? Say, *tap*."	Modeled trial
Child	"Tap."	Correct response
Clinician	Pulls the stimulus toward her; records the response.	No reinforcement
Clinician	[*stimulus: tape*] "What is this? Say, *tape*."	The next modeled trial
Child	"ape."	Omission of initial /t/
Clinician	Pulls the stimulus toward her; records the response.	No corrective feedback

Use the recording sheet with exemplars shown on the next page to establish the baserates; print it from the CD.

/t/ in Word-Initial Positions

Baserate Exemplars and Recording Sheet

Use stimuli from the **Stimulus Book, Volume 2**.

Print this page from the CD or photocopy this page for your clinical use.

Name/Age:	Date:
Goal: To establish the baserate production of /t/ in word-initial positions.	Clinician:

Scoring: Correct: ✓   Incorrect or no response: X

/t/ in word-initial positions	Evoked	Modeled
1. tap		
2. tape		
3. tin		
4. toy		
5. toes		
6. table		
7. tablet		
8. tomato		
9. toothbrush		
10. toaster		
11. tail		
12. tie		
13. tile		
14. taco		
15. toad		
16. teacher		
17. tennis		
18. tiger		
19. telephone		
20. toothpaste		
Percent correct baserate		

Replace or add new exemplars as you see fit for a given child. After establishing the baserates, begin production teaching. Follow the protocols given on the next page.

/t/ in Word-Initial Positions

Treatment Protocols

Use stimuli from the **Stimulus Book, Volume 2.**

Teach 6 to 8 exemplars using the following script.

Place a relevant stimulus in front of the child (an object, a picture, or a printed word) and ask a question as you point to the stimulus.

Scripts for Modeled Discrete Trial Training		Note
Clinician	[*stimulus: tap*] "What is this? Say, **tap**."	Modeling; the target vocally emphasized
Child	"æp."	A wrong response
Clinician	"No. That's not correct. You said æp, but it's a **tap**."	Corrective feedback
Clinician	[*the same stimulus*] "What is this? Say, **tap**. Don't forget the *t* at the beginning."	The next trial
Child	"Tap."	A correct response
Clinician	"Excellent! You didn't miss the *t* this time!"	Verbal praise

Repeat the trials until the child gives 5 consecutively correct, imitated responses.

When the child imitates 5 correct responses in sequence, fade the modeling.

Scripts for Fading the Modeling		Note
Clinician	[*stimulus: tap*] "What is this? Don't forget the *t* at the beginning."	Only a prompt
Child	"æp."	A wrong response
Clinician	"Gee, you forgot the *t* sound! It's a *tap*, not æp. Put the *t* at the beginning."	Corrective feedback
Clinician	[*the same stimulus*] "What is this? It starts with . . . " [*silently models the tongue posture for the target sound.*]	The next trial; a partial modeling
Child	"Tap."	A correct response
Clinician	"That's great! You said *tap*, not æp."	Verbal praise
Clinician	[*the same stimulus*] "What is this?"	Typical question; evoked trial
Child	"Tap."	A correct response
Clinician	"Great job! You said it correctly!"	Verbal praise

If the wrong responses persist on 4 to 5 evoked trials, reinstate partial or full modeling for a few trials, again fade the modeling, and re-present the evoked trials.

When the child meets the tentative learning criterion of 10 consecutively correct, nonimitated responses for a given stimulus item, move on to the next stimulus item. With this procedure, teach 6 to 8 exemplars shown on the following recording sheet. Use different exemplars as you see fit for a given child.

/t/ in Word-Initial Positions

Treatment Exemplars and Recording Sheet

Use stimuli from the **Stimulus Book, Volume 2**.

Print this page from CD or photocopy this page for your clinical use.

Name/Age:	Date:
Goal: Production of /t/ in word-initial positions with 90% accuracy when asked an evoking question while showing a stimulus.	Clinician:

Scoring: Correct: ✓   Incorrect or no response: X

Target skills	Discrete Trials														
	1	2	3	4	5	6	7	8	9	10	11	12	13	14	15
1. tap															
2. tape															
3. tin															
4. toy															
5. toes															
6. table															
7. tablet															
8. tomato															

When the child has met the learning criterion of 10 consecutively correct evoked (nonimitated) responses for each of the 6 to 8 target exemplars, conduct a probe to see if the production has generalized to previously baserated but untrained exemplars.

If the probes do not meet the 90% correct criterion for untrained exemplars, teach additional exemplars and then probe again.

/t/ in Word-Initial Positions

Probe Protocols and Recording Sheet

Use stimuli from the **Stimulus Book,** *Volume 2.*

Print this page from the CD or photocopy this page for your clinical use.

On the probes, present only the untrained exemplars (UT). When the child fails to meet the 90% correct probe criterion, either teach 2 to 4 new exemplars or give additional training trials on already trained stimuli. If needed, select new exemplars for probes. Probe at least 10 untrained exemplars. Alternate probes and treatment until the probe criterion is met.

Scripts for Probe Trials		Note
Clinician	[*untrained stimulus: toothbrush*] "What is this?"	No modeling or prompts
Child	"Toothbrush."	A correct, generalized response
Clinician	Scores the response as correct.	No reinforcement
Clinician	[*untrained stimulus: toaster*] "What is this?"	The second probe trial
Child	"oaster."	A wrong probe response
Clinician	Scores the response as incorrect.	No corrective feedback

Name:	Date:	Session #:
Age:	**Clinician:**	
Diagnosis: Articulation/Phonologic Disorder	**Word-initial /t/ probe**	
Untrained Stimuli	**Score: + correct; – incorrect or no responses**	
1. toothbrush		
2. toaster		
3. tail		
4. tie		
5. tile		
6. taco		
7. toad		
8. teacher		
9. tennis		
10. tiger		
11. telephone		
12. toothpaste		
Percent correct: (Criterion: 90%)		

If the child does not meet the probe criterion, give additional training on already trained exemplars or teach a few new exemplars. Subsequently, readminister the probe trials. When the child meets the 90% correct probe criterion for the exemplars, shift training to the sentence or conversational level or to another phoneme.

/t/ in Word-Final Positions

Baserate Protocols

Use stimuli from the **Stimulus Book,** *Volume 2.*

At the beginning of each trial, place a relevant stimulus (an object, a picture, or a printed word) in front of the child. Point to the stimulus as you ask an evoking question. Do not respond in any way to the child's correct, incorrect, or lack of responses.

Scripts for Evoked Baserate Trial		Note
Clinician	[*stimulus: bat*] "What is this?"	Evoked trial
Child	"bæ."	Omission of final /t/
Clinician	Pulls the stimulus toward her; records the response.	No corrective feedback
Clinician	[*stimulus: cat*] "What is this?"	The next evoked trial
Child	"cæ."	Omission of final /t/
Clinician	Pulls the stimulus toward her; records the response.	No corrective feedback

Administer the modeled baserate trials only after completing the evoked trials on all 20 (or more) exemplars.

Scripts for Modeled Baserate Trial		Note
Clinician	[*stimulus: bat*] "What is this? Say, *bat.*"	Modeled trial
Child	"Bat."	Correct response
Clinician	Pulls the stimulus toward her; records the response.	No reinforcement
Clinician	[*stimulus: cat*] "What is this? Say, *cat.*"	The next modeled trial
Child	"cæ."	Omission of final /t/
Clinician	Pulls the stimulus toward her; records the response.	No corrective feedback

Use the recording sheet with exemplars shown on the next page to establish the baserates; print it from the CD.

/t/ in Word-Final Positions

Baserate Exemplars and Recording Sheet

Use stimuli from the **Stimulus Book,** *Volume 2.*

Print this page from the CD or photocopy this page for your clinical use.

Name/Age:	Date:
Goal: To establish the baserate production of /t/ in word-final positions.	Clinician:

Scoring: Correct: ✓   Incorrect or no response: X

/t/ in word-final positions	Evoked	Modeled
1. bat		
2. cat		
3. hat		
4. mat		
5. feet		
6. chocolate		
7. rabbit		
8. coconut		
9. clarinet		
10. astronaut		
11. coat		
12. tent		
13. jet		
14. kite		
15. pot		
16. candlelight		
17. doughnut		
18. flashlight		
19. helmet		
20. rocket		
Percent correct baserate		

Replace or add new exemplars as you see fit for a given child. After establishing the baserates, begin production teaching. Follow the protocols given on the next page.

/t/ in Word-Final Positions

Treatment Protocols

Use stimuli from the **Stimulus Book, Volume 2**.

Teach 6 to 8 exemplars using the following script.

Place a relevant stimulus (an object, a picture, or a printed word) in front of the child and point to the stimulus as you ask an evoking question.

Scripts for Modeled Discrete Trial Training		Note
Clinician	[*stimulus: bat*] "What is this? Say, *ba**t**.*"	Modeling; the target vocally emphasized
Child	"bæ."	A wrong response
Clinician	"No. That's not correct. You said *bæ*, but it's a *ba**t**.*"	Corrective feedback
Clinician	[*the same stimulus*] "What is this? Say, *bat*. Don't forget the *t* at the end."	The next trial
Child	"Bat."	A correct response
Clinician	"Excellent! You didn't miss the *t* at the end of the word!"	Verbal praise

Repeat the trials until the child gives 5 consecutively correct, imitated responses.

When the child imitates 5 correct responses in sequence, fade the modeling.

Scripts for Fading the Modeling		Note
Clinician	[*stimulus: bat*] "What is this? Don't forget the *t* at the end."	Only a prompt
Child	"bæ."	A wrong response
Clinician	"Gee, you forgot the *t* sound! It's a *bat*, not *bæ*. Put the *t* at the end."	Corrective feedback
Clinician	[*the same stimulus*] "What is this? It ends with . . . " [*silently models the tongue posture for the target sound.*]	The next trial; a partial modeling
Child	"Bat."	A correct response
Clinician	"That's great! You said *bat*, not *bæ*."	Verbal praise
Clinician	[*the same stimulus*] "What is this?"	Typical question; evoked trial
Child	"Bat."	A correct response
Clinician	"I like it! You said it correctly!"	Verbal praise

If the wrong responses persist on 4 to 5 evoked trials, reinstate partial or full modeling for a few trials, again fade the modeling, and re-present the evoked trials.

When the child meets the tentative learning criterion of 10 consecutively correct, nonimitated responses for a given stimulus item, move on to the next stimulus item. With this procedure, teach 6 to 8 exemplars shown on the following recording sheet. Use different exemplars as you see fit for a given child.

/t/ in Word-Final Positions

Treatment Exemplars and Recording Sheet

Use stimuli from the **Stimulus Book,** *Volume 2.*

Print this page from CD or photocopy this page for your clinical use.

Name/Age:	Date:
Goal: Production of /t/ in word-final positions with 90% accuracy when asked an evoking question while showing a stimulus.	Clinician:

Scoring: Correct: ✓   Incorrect or no response: X

Target skills	Discrete Trials														
	1	2	3	4	5	6	7	8	9	10	11	12	13	14	15
1. bat															
2. cat															
3. hat															
4. mat															
5. feet															
6. chocolate															
7. rabbit															
8. coconut															

When the child has met the learning criterion of 10 consecutively correct evoked (nonimitated) responses for each of the 6 to 8 target exemplars, conduct a probe to see if the production has generalized to previously baserated but untrained exemplars.

If the probes do not meet the 90% correct criterion for untrained exemplars, teach additional exemplars and then probe again.

/t/ in Word-Final Positions

Probe Protocols and Recording Sheet

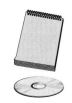

*Use stimuli from the **Stimulus Book, Volume 2**.*

Print this page from the CD or photocopy this page for your clinical use.

On the probes, present only the untrained exemplars (UT). When the child fails to meet the 90% correct probe criterion, either teach 2 to 4 new exemplars or give additional training trials on already trained stimuli. If needed, select new exemplars for probes. Probe at least 10 untrained exemplars. Alternate probes and treatment until the probe criterion is met.

Scripts for Probe Trials		Note
Clinician	[*untrained stimulus: clarinet*] "What is this?"	No modeling or prompts
Child	"Clarinet."	A correct, generalized response
Clinician	Scores the response as correct.	No reinforcement
Clinician	[*untrained stimulus: astronaut*] "What is this?"	The second probe trial
Child	"astronau."	A wrong probe response
Clinician	Scores the response as incorrect.	No corrective feedback

Name:	Date:	Session #:
Age:	**Clinician:**	
Diagnosis: Articulation/Phonologic Disorder	**Word-final /t/ probe**	
Untrained Stimuli	**Score: + correct; – incorrect or no responses**	
1. clarinet		
2. astronaut		
3. coat		
4. tent		
5. jet		
6. kite		
7. pot		
8. candlelight		
9. doughnut		
10. flashlight		
11. helmet		
12. rocket		
Percent correct: (Criterion: 90%)		

If the child does not meet the probe criterion, give additional training on already trained exemplars or teach a few new exemplars. Subsequently, readminister the probe trials. When the child meets the 90% correct probe criterion for the exemplars, shift training to the sentence or conversational level or to another phoneme.

/d/ in Word-Initial Positions

Baserate Protocols

Use stimuli from the **Stimulus Book, Volume 2**.

At the beginning of each trial, place a relevant stimulus (an object, a picture, or a printed word) in front of the child. Point to the stimulus as you ask an evoking question. Do not respond in any way to the child's correct, incorrect, or lack of responses.

Scripts for Evoked Baserate Trial		Note
Clinician	[*stimulus: deer*] "What is this?"	Evoked trial
Child	"eer."	Omission of initial /d/
Clinician	Pulls the stimulus toward her; records the response.	No corrective feedback
Clinician	[*stimulus: doll*] "What is this?"	The next evoked trial
Child	"oll."	Omission of initial /d/
Clinician	Pulls the stimulus toward her; records the response.	No corrective feedback

Administer the modeled baserate trials only after completing the evoked trials on all 20 (or more) exemplars.

Scripts for Modeled Baserate Trial		Note
Clinician	[*stimulus: deer*] "What is this? Say, *deer.*"	Modeled trial
Child	"Deer."	Correct response
Clinician	Pulls the stimulus toward her; records the response.	No reinforcement
Clinician	[*stimulus: doll*] "What is this? Say, *doll.*"	The next modeled trial
Child	"oll."	Omission of initial /d/
Clinician	Pulls the stimulus toward her; records the response.	No corrective feedback

Use the recording sheet with exemplars shown on the next page to establish the baserates; print it from the CD.

/d/ in Word-Initial Positions

Baserate Exemplars and Recording Sheet

Use stimuli from the **Stimulus Book,** *Volume 2*.

Print this page from the CD or photocopy this page for your clinical use.

Name/Age:	Date:
Goal: To establish the baserate production of /d/ in word-initial positions.	Clinician:

Scoring: Correct: ✓   Incorrect or no response: X

/d/ in word-initial positions	Evoked	Modeled
1. deer		
2. doll		
3. door		
4. duck		
5. dime		
6. dinosaur		
7. diamond		
8. dancing		
9. diving board		
10. dump truck		
11. desk		
12. dog		
13. daisy		
14. dollar		
15. disk		
16. dentist		
17. donkey		
18. daffodil		
19. dumbbell		
20. doorbell		
Percent correct baserate		

Replace or add new exemplars as you see fit for a given child. After establishing the baserates, begin production teaching. Follow the protocols given on the next page.

/d/ in Word-Initial Positions

Treatment Protocols

Use stimuli from the **Stimulus Book,** *Volume 2.*

Teach 6 to 8 exemplars using the following script.

Place a relevant stimulus in front of the child (an object, a picture, or a printed word) and ask a question as you point to the stimulus.

Scripts for Modeled Discrete Trial Training		Note
Clinician	[*stimulus: deer*] "What is this? Say, **deer.**"	Modeling; the target vocally emphasized
Child	"eer."	A wrong response
Clinician	"No. That's not correct. You said *eer*, but it's a **deer.**"	Corrective feedback
Clinician	[*the same stimulus*] "What is this? Say, **deer.** Don't forget the *d* at the beginning."	The next trial
Child	"Deer."	A correct response
Clinician	"Excellent! You didn't miss the *d* this time!"	Verbal praise

Repeat the trials until the child gives 5 consecutively correct, imitated responses.

When the child imitates 5 correct responses in sequence, fade the modeling.

Scripts for Fading the Modeling		Note
Clinician	[*stimulus: deer*] "What is this? Don't forget the *d* at the beginning."	Only a prompt
Child	"eer."	A wrong response
Clinician	"Gee, you forgot the *d* sound! It's a *deer*, not *eer*. Put the *d* at the beginning."	Corrective feedback
Clinician	[*the same stimulus*] "What is this? It starts with . . . " [*silently models the tongue posture for the target sound.*]	The next trial; a partial modeling
Child	"Deer."	A correct response
Clinician	"That's great! You said *deer*, not *eer*."	Verbal praise
Clinician	[*the same stimulus*] "What is this?"	Typical question; evoked trial
Child	"Deer."	A correct response
Clinician	"How nice! You said *deer* correctly!"	Verbal praise

If the wrong responses persist on 4 to 5 evoked trials, reinstate partial or full modeling for a few trials, again fade the modeling, and re-present the evoked trials.

When the child meets the tentative learning criterion of 10 consecutively correct, nonimitated responses for a given stimulus item, move on to the next stimulus item. With this procedure, teach 6 to 8 exemplars shown on the following recording sheet. Use different exemplars as you see fit for a given child.

/d/ in Word-Initial Positions

Treatment Exemplars and Recording Sheet

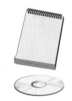

Use stimuli from the **Stimulus Book,** *Volume 2.*

Print this page from CD or photocopy this page for your clinical use.

Name/Age:	Date:
Goal: Production of /d/ in word-initial positions with 90% accuracy when asked an evoking question while showing a stimulus.	Clinician:

Scoring: Correct: ✓   Incorrect or no response: X

Target skills	Discrete Trials														
	1	2	3	4	5	6	7	8	9	10	11	12	13	14	15
1. deer															
2. doll															
3. door															
4. duck															
5. dime															
6. dinosaur															
7. diamond															
8. dancing															

When the child has met the learning criterion of 10 consecutively correct evoked (nonimitated) responses for each of the 6 to 8 target exemplars, conduct a probe to see if the production has generalized to previously baserated but untrained exemplars.

If the probes do not meet the 90% correct criterion for untrained exemplars, teach additional exemplars and then probe again.

/d/ in Word-Initial Positions

Probe Protocols and Recording Sheet

Use stimuli from the **Stimulus Book,** *Volume 2.*

Print this page from the CD or photocopy this page for your clinical use.

On the probes, present only the untrained exemplars (UT). When the child fails to meet the 90% correct probe criterion, either teach 2 to 4 new exemplars or give additional training trials on already trained stimuli. If needed, select new exemplars for probes. Probe at least 10 untrained exemplars. Alternate probes and treatment until the probe criterion is met.

Scripts for Probe Trials		Note
Clinician	[*untrained stimulus: diving board*] "What is this?"	No modeling or prompts
Child	"Diving board."	A correct, generalized response
Clinician	Scores the response as correct.	No reinforcement
Clinician	[*untrained stimulus: dump truck*] "What is this?"	The second probe trial
Child	"dump truck."	A wrong probe response
Clinician	Scores the response as incorrect.	No corrective feedback

Name:	Date:	Session #:
Age:	**Clinician:**	
Diagnosis: Articulation/Phonologic Disorder	**Word-initial /d/ probe**	
Untrained Stimuli	**Score: + correct; – incorrect or no responses**	
1. diving board		
2. dump truck		
3. desk		
4. dog		
5. daisy		
6. dollar		
7. disk		
8. dentist		
9. donkey		
10. daffodil		
11. dumbbell		
12. doorbell		
Percent correct: (Criterion: 90%)		

If the child does not meet the probe criterion, give additional training on already trained exemplars or teach a few new exemplars. Subsequently, readminister the probe trials. When the child meets the 90% correct probe criterion for the exemplars, shift training to the sentence or conversational level or to another phoneme.

/d/ in Word-Final Positions

Baserate Protocols

*Use stimuli from the **Stimulus Book, Volume 2**.*

At the beginning of each trial, place a relevant stimulus (an object, a picture, or a printed word) in front of the child. Point to the stimulus as you ask an evoking question. Do not respond in any way to the child's correct, incorrect, or lack of responses.

Scripts for Evoked Baserate Trial		Note
Clinician	[*stimulus: bed*] "What is this?"	Evoked trial
Child	"bɛ."	Omission of final /d/
Clinician	Pulls the stimulus toward her; records the response.	No corrective feedback
Clinician	[*stimulus: red*] "What color is this?"	The next evoked trial
Child	"rɛ."	Omission of final /d/
Clinician	Pulls the stimulus toward her; records the response.	No corrective feedback

Administer the modeled baserate trials only after completing the evoked trials on all 20 (or more) exemplars.

Scripts for Modeled Baserate Trial		Note
Clinician	[*stimulus: bed*] "What is this? Say, *bed*."	Modeled trial
Child	"Bed."	Correct response
Clinician	Pulls the stimulus toward her; records the response.	No reinforcement
Clinician	[*stimulus: red*] "What is this? Say, *red*."	The next modeled trial
Child	"rɛ."	Omission of final /d/
Clinician	Pulls the stimulus toward her; records the response	No corrective feedback

Use the recording sheet with exemplars shown on the next page to establish the baserates; print it from the CD.

/d/ in Word-Final Positions

Baserate Exemplars and Recording Sheet

Use stimuli from the **Stimulus Book, Volume 2.**

Print this page from the CD or photocopy this page for your clinical use.

Name/Age:	Date:
Goal: To establish the baserate production of /d/ in word-final positions.	Clinician:

Scoring: Correct: ✓   Incorrect or no response: X

/d/ in word-final positions	Evoked	Modeled
1. bed (any red object)		
2. red		
3. bead		
4. seed		
5. food		
6. salad		
7. railroad		
8. lemonade		
9. blackboard		
10. mermaid		
11. bud		
12. rod		
13. head		
14. hood		
15. lid		
16. dashboard		
17. bedspread		
18. checkerboard		
19. fishing rod		
20. arrowhead		
Percent correct baserate		

Replace or add new exemplars as you see fit for a given child. After establishing the baserates, begin production teaching. Follow the protocols given on the next page.

/d/ in Word-Final Positions

Treatment Protocols

Use stimuli from the **Stimulus Book,** *Volume 2.*

Teach 6 to 8 exemplars using the following script.

Place a relevant stimulus (an object, a picture, or a printed word) in front of the child and point to the stimulus as you ask an evoking question.

Scripts for Modeled Discrete Trial Training		Note
Clinician	[*stimulus: bed*] "What is this? Say, **bed**."	Modeling; the target vocally emphasized
Child	"bɛ."	A wrong response
Clinician	"No. That's not correct. You said *bɛ*, but it's a *bed*."	Corrective feedback
Clinician	[*the same stimulus*] "What is this? Say, **bed**. Don't forget the *d* at the end."	The next trial
Child	"Bed."	A correct response
Clinician	"You're super! You didn't miss the *d* at the end of the word!"	Verbal praise

Repeat the trials until the child gives 5 consecutively correct, imitated responses.

When the child imitates 5 correct responses in sequence, fade the modeling.

Scripts for Fading the Modeling		Note
Clinician	[*stimulus: bed*] "What is this? Don't forget the *d* at the end."	Only a prompt
Child	"bɛ."	A wrong response
Clinician	"Oops! you forgot the *d*! It's a *bed*, not *bɛ*. Put the *d* at the end."	Corrective feedback
Clinician	[*the same stimulus*] "What is this? It ends with . . . " [*silently models the tongue posture for the target sound.*]	The next trial; a partial modeling
Child	"Bed."	A correct response
Clinician	"That's great! You said *bed*, not *bɛ*."	Verbal praise
Clinician	[*the same stimulus*] "What is this?"	Typical question; evoked trial
Child	"Bed."	A correct response
Clinician	"I like it! You said it correctly!"	Verbal praise

If the wrong responses persist on 4 to 5 evoked trials, reinstate partial or full modeling for a few trials, again fade the modeling, and re-present the evoked trials.

When the child meets the tentative learning criterion of 10 consecutively correct, nonimitated responses for a given stimulus item, move on to the next stimulus item. With this procedure, teach 6 to 8 exemplars shown on the following recording sheet. Use different exemplars as you see fit for a given child.

/d/ in Word-Final Positions

Treatment Exemplars and Recording Sheet

Use stimuli from the **Stimulus Book,** *Volume 2.*

Print this page from CD or photocopy this page for your clinical use.

Name/Age:	Date:
Goal: Production of /d/ in word-final positions with 90% accuracy when asked an evoking question while showing a stimulus.	Clinician:

Scoring: Correct: ✓ Incorrect or no response: X

Target skills	Discrete Trials														
	1	2	3	4	5	6	7	8	9	10	11	12	13	14	15
1. bed															
2. red															
3. bead															
4. seed															
5. food															
6. salad															
7. railroad															
8. lemonade															

When the child has met the learning criterion of 10 consecutively correct evoked (nonimitated) responses for each of the 6 to 8 target exemplars, conduct a probe to see if the production has generalized to previously baserated but untrained exemplars.

If the probes do not meet the 90% correct criterion for untrained exemplars, teach additional exemplars and then probe again.

/d/ in Word-Final Positions

Probe Protocols and Recording Sheet

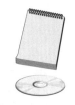

Use stimuli from the **Stimulus Book, Volume 2.**

Print this page from the CD or photocopy this page for your clinical use.

On the probes, present only the untrained exemplars (UT). When the child fails to meet the 90% correct probe criterion, either teach 2 to 4 new exemplars or give additional training trials on already trained stimuli. If needed, select new exemplars for probes. Probe at least 10 untrained exemplars. Alternate probes and treatment until the probe criterion is met.

Scripts for Probe Trials		Note
Clinician	[*untrained stimulus: blackboard*] "What is this?"	No modeling or prompts
Child	"Blackboard."	A correct, generalized response
Clinician	Scores the response as correct.	No reinforcement
Clinician	[*untrained stimulus: mermaid*] "What is this?"	The second probe trial
Child	"Mermay."	A wrong probe response
Clinician	Scores the response as incorrect.	No corrective feedback

Name:	Date:	Session #:
Age:	**Clinician:**	
Diagnosis: Articulation/Phonologic Disorder	**Word-final /d/probe**	
Untrained Stimuli	**Score: + correct; – incorrect or no responses**	
1. blackboard		
2. mermaid		
3. bud		
4. rod		
5. head		
6. hood		
7. lid		
8. dashboard		
9. bedspread		
10. checkerboard		
11. fishing rod		
12. arrowhead		
Percent correct: (Criterion: 90%)		

If the child does not meet the probe criterion, give additional training on already trained exemplars or teach a few new exemplars. Subsequently, readminister the probe trials. When the child meets the 90% correct probe criterion for the exemplars, shift training to the sentence or conversational level or to another phoneme.

/k/ in Word-Initial Positions

Baserate Protocols

Use stimuli from the **Stimulus Book, Volume 3**.

At the beginning of each trial, place a relevant stimulus (an object, a picture, or a printed word) in front of the child. Point to the stimulus as you ask an evoking question. Do not respond in any way to the child's correct, incorrect, or lack of responses.

Scripts for Evoked Baserate Trial		Note
Clinician	[*stimulus: king*] "What is this?"	Evoked trial
Child	"ing."	Omission of initial /k/
Clinician	Pulls the stimulus toward her; records the response.	No corrective feedback
Clinician	[*stimulus: kite*] "What is this?"	The next evoked trial
Child	"ite."	Omission of initial /k/
Clinician	Pulls the stimulus toward her; records the response.	No corrective feedback

Administer the modeled baserate trials only after completing the evoked trials on all 20 (or more) exemplars.

Scripts for Modeled Baserate Trial		Note
Clinician	[*stimulus: king*] "What is this? Say, *king.*"	Modeled trial
Child	"King."	Correct response
Clinician	Pulls the stimulus toward her; records the response.	No reinforcement
Clinician	[*stimulus: kite*] "What is this? Say, *kite.*"	The next modeled trial
Child	"ite."	Omission of initial /k/
Clinician	Pulls the stimulus toward her; records the response	No corrective feedback

Use the recording sheet with exemplars shown on the next page to establish the baserates; print it from the CD.

/k/ in Word-Initial Positions

Baserate Exemplars and Recording Sheet

Use stimuli from the **Stimulus Book,** *Volume 3.*

Print this page from the CD or photocopy this page for your clinical use.

Name/Age:	Date:
Goal: To establish the baserate production of /k/ in word-initial positions.	Clinician:

Scoring: Correct: ✓   Incorrect or no response: X

/k/ in word-initial positions	Evoked	Modeled
1. king		
2. kite		
3. key		
4. cake		
5. camel		
6. kangaroo		
7. caterpillar		
8. calendar		
9. cauliflower		
10. cucumber		
11. cap		
12. cage		
13. can		
14. car		
15. cup		
16. cabbage		
17. camera		
18. carpenter		
19. coyote		
20. computer		
Percent correct baserate		

Replace or add new exemplars as you see fit for a given child. After establishing the baserates, begin production teaching. Follow the protocols given on the next page.

/k/ in Word-Initial Positions

Treatment Protocols

Use stimuli from the **Stimulus Book,** *Volume 3.*

Teach 6 to 8 exemplars using the following script.

Place a relevant stimulus in front of the child (an object, a picture, or a printed word) and ask a question as you point to the stimulus.

Scripts for Modeled Discrete Trial Training		Note
Clinician	[*stimulus: king*] "What is this? Say, **king**."	Modeling; the target vocally emphasized
Child	"ing."	A wrong response
Clinician	"No. That's not correct. You said *ing*, but it's a **king**."	Corrective feedback
Clinician	[*the same stimulus*] "What is this? Say, **king**. Don't forget the *k* at the beginning."	The next trial
Child	"King."	A correct response
Clinician	"Excellent! You didn't miss the *k* this time!"	Verbal praise

Repeat the trials until the child gives 5 consecutively correct, imitated responses.

When the child imitates 5 correct responses in sequence, fade the modeling.

Scripts for Fading the Modeling		Note
Clinician	[*stimulus: king*] "What is this? Don't forget the *k* at the beginning."	Only a prompt
Child	"ing."	A wrong response
Clinician	"Gee, you forgot the *k* sound! It's a *king*, not *ing*. Put the *k* at the beginning."	Corrective feedback
Clinician	[*the same stimulus*] "What is this? It starts with . . . " [*silently models the tongue posture for the target sound.*]	The next trial; a partial modeling
Child	"King."	A correct response
Clinician	"That's great! You said *king*, not *ing*."	Verbal praise
Clinician	[*the same stimulus*] "What is this?"	Typical question; evoked trial
Child	"King."	A correct response
Clinician	"How nice! You said it correctly!"	Verbal praise

If the wrong responses persist on 4 to 5 evoked trials, reinstate partial or full modeling for a few trials, again fade the modeling, and re-present the evoked trials.

When the child meets the tentative learning criterion of 10 consecutively correct, nonimitated responses for a given stimulus item, move on to the next stimulus item. With this procedure, teach 6 to 8 exemplars shown on the following recording sheet. Use different exemplars as you see fit for a given child.

/k/ in Word-Initial Positions

Treatment Exemplars and Recording Sheet

Use stimuli from the **Stimulus Book, Volume 3**.

Print this page from CD or photocopy this page for your clinical use.

Name/Age:	Date:
Goal: Production of /k/ in word-initial positions with 90% accuracy when asked an evoking question while showing a stimulus.	Clinician:

Scoring: Correct: ✓   Incorrect or no response: X

Target skills	Discrete Trials														
	1	2	3	4	5	6	7	8	9	10	11	12	13	14	15
1. king															
2. kite															
3. key															
4. cake															
5. camel															
6. kangaroo															
7. caterpillar															
8. calendar															

When the child has met the learning criterion of 10 consecutively correct evoked (nonimitated) responses for each of the 6 to 8 target exemplars, conduct a probe to see if the production has generalized to previously baserated but untrained exemplars.

If the probes do not meet the 90% correct criterion for untrained exemplars, teach additional exemplars and then probe again.

/k/ in Word-Initial Positions

Probe Protocols and Recording Sheet

Use stimuli from the **Stimulus Book,** *Volume 3.*

Print this page from the CD or photocopy this page for your clinical use.

On the probes, present only the untrained exemplars (UT). When the child fails to meet the 90% correct probe criterion, either teach 2 to 4 new exemplars or give additional training trials on already trained stimuli. If needed, select new exemplars for probes. Probe at least 10 untrained exemplars. Alternate probes and treatment until the probe criterion is met.

Scripts for Probe Trials		Note
Clinician	[*untrained stimulus: cauliflower*] "What is this?"	No modeling or prompts
Child	"Cauliflower."	A correct, generalized response
Clinician	Scores the response as correct.	No reinforcement
Clinician	[*untrained stimulus: cucumber*] "What is this?"	The second probe trial
Child	"ucumber."	A wrong probe response
Clinician	Scores the response as incorrect.	No corrective feedback

Name:	Date:	Session #:
Age:	**Clinician:**	
Diagnosis: Articulation/Phonologic Disorder	**Word-initial /k/ probe**	
Untrained Stimuli	**Score: + correct; – incorrect or no responses**	
1. cauliflower		
2. cucumber		
3. cap		
4. cage		
5. can		
6. car		
7. cup		
8. cabbage		
9. camera		
10. carpenter		
11. coyote		
12. computer		
Percent correct: (Criterion: 90%)		

If the child does not meet the probe criterion, give additional training on already trained exemplars or teach a few new exemplars. Subsequently, readminister the probe trials. When the child meets the 90% correct probe criterion for the exemplars, shift training to the sentence or conversational level or to another phoneme.

/k/ in Word-Final Positions

Baserate Protocols

Use stimuli from the **Stimulus Book, Volume 3**.

At the beginning of each trial, place a relevant stimulus (an object, a picture, or a printed word) in front of the child. Point to the stimulus as you ask an evoking question. Do not respond in any way to the child's correct, incorrect, or lack of responses.

Scripts for Evoked Baserate Trial		Note
Clinician	[*stimulus: duck*] "What is this?"	Evoked trial
Child	"də."	Omission of final /k/
Clinician	Pulls the stimulus toward her; records the response.	No corrective feedback
Clinician	[*stimulus: sock*] "What is this?"	The next evoked trial
Child	"sɑ."	Omission of final /k/
Clinician	Pulls the stimulus toward her; records the response.	No corrective feedback

Administer the modeled baserate trials only after completing the evoked trials on all 20 (or more) exemplars.

Scripts for Modeled Baserate Trial		Note
Clinician	[*stimulus: duck*] "What is this? Say, *duck.*"	Modeled trial
Child	"Duck."	Correct response
Clinician	Pulls the stimulus toward her; records the response.	No reinforcement
Clinician	[*stimulus: sock*] "What is this? Say, *sock.*"	The next modeled trial
Child	"sɑ."	Omission of final /k/
Clinician	Pulls the stimulus toward her; records the response.	No corrective feedback

Use the recording sheet with exemplars shown on the next page to establish the baserates; print it from the CD.

/k/ in Word-Final Positions

Baserate Exemplars and Recording Sheet

Use stimuli from the **Stimulus Book, Volume 3**.

Print this page from the CD or photocopy this page for your clinical use.

Name/Age:	Date:
Goal: To establish the baserate production of /k/ in word-final positions.	Clinician:

Scoring: Correct: ✓   Incorrect or no response: X

/k/ in word-final positions	Evoked	Modeled
1. duck		
2. sock		
3. rock		
4. rake		
5. chalk		
6. rattlesnake		
7. broomstick		
8. artichoke		
9. candlestick		
10. peacock		
11. brick		
12. book		
13. bike		
14. block		
15. clock		
16. bike rack		
17. backpack		
18. snowflake		
19. lipstick		
20. chopstick		
Percent correct baserate		

Replace or add new exemplars as you see fit for a given child. After establishing the baserates, begin production teaching. Follow the protocols given on the next page.

/k/ in Word-Final Positions

Treatment Protocols

Use stimuli from the **Stimulus Book,** *Volume 3. #*

Teach 6 to 8 exemplars using the following script.

Place a relevant stimulus (an object, a picture, or a printed word) in front of the child and point to the stimulus as you ask an evoking question.

Scripts for Modeled Discrete Trial Training		Note
Clinician	[*stimulus: duck*] "What is this? Say, *du**ck**.*"	Modeling; the target vocally emphasized
Child	"də."	A wrong response
Clinician	"No. That's not correct. You said *də*, but it's a *duck.*"	Corrective feedback
Clinician	[*the same stimulus*] "What is this? Say, *duck*. Don't forget the *k* at the end."	The next trial
Child	"Duck."	A correct response
Clinician	"Excellent! You didn't miss the *k* at the end of the word!"	Verbal praise

Repeat the trials until the child gives 5 consecutively correct, imitated responses.

When the child imitates 5 correct responses in sequence, fade the modeling.

Scripts for Fading the Modeling		Note
Clinician	[*stimulus: duck*] "What is this? Don't forget the *k* at the end."	Only a prompt
Child	"də."	A wrong response
Clinician	"Gee, you forgot the *k* sound! It's a *duck*, not a *də*. Put the *k* at the end."	Corrective feedback
Clinician	[*the same stimulus*] "What is this? It ends with . . . " [*silently models the tongue posture for the target sound.*]	The next trial; a partial modeling
Child	"Duck."	A correct response
Clinician	"That's great! You said *duck*, not *də*."	Verbal praise
Clinician	[*the same stimulus*] "What is this?"	Typical question; evoked trial
Child	"Duck."	A correct response
Clinician	"I like it! You said it correctly!"	Verbal praise

If the wrong responses persist on 4 to 5 evoked trials, reinstate partial or full modeling for a few trials, again fade the modeling, and re-present the evoked trials.

When the child meets the tentative learning criterion of 10 consecutively correct, nonimitated responses for a given stimulus item, move on to the next stimulus item. With this procedure, teach 6 to 8 exemplars shown on the following recording sheet. Use different exemplars as you see fit for a given child.

/k/ in Word-Final Positions

Treatment Exemplars and Recording Sheet

Use stimuli from the **Stimulus Book,** *Volume 3.*

Print this page from CD or photocopy this page for your clinical use.

Name/Age:	Date:
Goal: Production of /k/ in word-final positions with 90% accuracy when asked an evoking question while showing a stimulus.	Clinician:

Scoring: Correct: ✓   Incorrect or no response: X

Target skills	Discrete Trials														
	1	2	3	4	5	6	7	8	9	10	11	12	13	14	15
1. duck															
2. sock															
3. rock															
4. rake															
5. chalk															
6. rattlesnake															
7. broomstick															
8. artichoke															

When the child has met the learning criterion of 10 consecutively correct evoked (nonimitated) responses for each of the 6 to 8 target exemplars, conduct a probe to see if the production has generalized to previously baserated but untrained exemplars.

If the probes do not meet the 90% correct criterion for untrained exemplars, teach additional exemplars and then probe again.

/k/ in Word-Final Positions

Probe Protocols and Recording Sheet

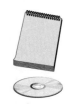

Use stimuli from the **Stimulus Book, Volume 3**.

Print this page from the CD or photocopy this page for your clinical use.

On the probes, present only the untrained exemplars (UT). When the child fails to meet the 90% correct probe criterion, either teach 2 to 4 new exemplars or give additional training trials on already trained stimuli. If needed, select new exemplars for probes. Probe at least 10 untrained exemplars. Alternate probes and treatment until the probe criterion is met.

Scripts for Probe Trials		Note
Clinician	[*untrained stimulus: candlestick*] "What is this?"	No modeling or prompts
Child	"Candlestick."	A correct, generalized response
Clinician	Scores the response as correct.	No reinforcement
Clinician	[*untrained stimulus: peacock*] "What is this?"	The second probe trial
Child	"Peaca."	A wrong probe response
Clinician	Scores the response as incorrect.	No corrective feedback

Name:	Date:	Session #:
Age:	**Clinician:**	
Diagnosis: Articulation/Phonologic Disorder	**Word-final /k/ probe**	
Untrained Stimuli	**Score: + correct; – incorrect or no responses**	
1. candlestick		
2. peacock		
3. brick		
4. book		
5. bike		
6. block		
7. clock		
8. bike rack		
9. backpack		
10. snowflake		
11. lipstick		
12. chopstick		
Percent correct: (Criterion: 90%)		

If the child does not meet the probe criterion, give additional training on already trained exemplars or teach a few new exemplars. Subsequently, readminister the probe trials. When the child meets the 90% correct probe criterion for the exemplars, shift training to the sentence or conversational level or to another phoneme.

/g/ in Word-Initial Positions

Baserate Protocols

Use stimuli from the **Stimulus Book, Volume 3**.

At the beginning of each trial, place a relevant stimulus (an object, a picture, or a printed word) in front of the child. Point to the stimulus as you ask an evoking question. Do not respond in any way to the child's correct, incorrect, or lack of responses.

Scripts for Evoked Baserate Trial		Note
Clinician	[*stimulus: gate*] "What is this?"	Evoked trial
Child	"ate."	Omission of initial /g/
Clinician	Pulls the stimulus toward her; records the response.	No corrective feedback
Clinician	[*stimulus: gift*] "What is this?"	The next evoked trial
Child	"ift."	Omission of initial /g/
Clinician	Pulls the stimulus toward her; records the response.	No corrective feedback

Administer the modeled baserate trials only after completing the evoked trials on all 20 (or more) exemplars.

Scripts for Modeled Baserate Trial		Note
Clinician	[*stimulus: gate*] "What is this? Say, *gate*."	Modeled trial
Child	"Gate."	Correct response
Clinician	Pulls the stimulus toward her; records the response.	No reinforcement
Clinician	[*stimulus: gift*] "What is this? Say, *gift*."	The next modeled trial
Child	"ift."	Omission of initial /g/
Clinician	Pulls the stimulus toward her; records the response.	No corrective feedback

Use the recording sheet with exemplars shown on the next page to establish the baserates; print it from the CD.

/g/ in Word-Initial Positions

Baserate Exemplars and Recording Sheet

Use stimuli from the **Stimulus Book, _Volume 3_**.

Print this page from the CD or photocopy this page for your clinical use.

Name/Age:	Date:
Goal: To establish the baserate production of /g/ in word-initial positions.	Clinician:

Scoring: Correct: ✓   Incorrect or no response: X

/g/ in word-initial positions	Evoked	Modeled
1. gate		
2. gift		
3. gum		
4. girl		
5. goose		
6. garage		
7. gorilla		
8. goldfish		
9. garden hose		
10. gardenia		
11. gold		
12. gecko		
13. gopher		
14. gazebo		
15. glove		
16. galaxy		
17. gardener		
18. giggling		
19. garbanzo		
20. gazelle		
Percent correct baserate		

Replace or add new exemplars as you see fit for a given child. After establishing the baserates, begin production teaching. Follow the protocols given on the next page.

/g/ in Word-Initial Positions
Treatment Protocols

Use stimuli from the **Stimulus Book,** *Volume 3.*

Teach 6 to 8 exemplars using the following script.

Place a relevant stimulus in front of the child (an object, a picture, or a printed word) and ask a question as you point to the stimulus.

Scripts for Modeled Discrete Trial Training		Note
Clinician	[*stimulus: gate*] "What is this? Say, *gate*."	Modeling; the target vocally emphasized
Child	"ate."	A wrong response
Clinician	"No. That's not correct. You said ate, but it's a *gate*."	Corrective feedback
Clinician	[*the same stimulus*] "What is this? Say, *gate*. Don't forget the *g* at the beginning."	The next trial
Child	"Gate."	A correct response
Clinician	"Excellent! You didn't miss the *g* this time!"	Verbal praise

Repeat the trials until the child gives 5 consecutively correct, imitated responses.

When the child imitates 5 correct responses in sequence, fade the modeling.

Scripts for Fading the Modeling		Note
Clinician	[*stimulus: gate*] "What is this? Don't forget the *g* at the beginning."	Only a prompt
Child	"ate."	A wrong response
Clinician	"Oh no! You forgot the *g* sound! It's a *gate*, not *ate*. Put the *g* sound at the beginning."	Corrective feedback
Clinician	[*the same stimulus*] "What is this? It starts with . . ." [*silently models the tongue posture for the target sound.*]	The next trial; a partial modeling
Child	"Gate."	A correct response
Clinician	"That's great! You said *gate*, not *ate*."	Verbal praise
Clinician	[*the same stimulus*] "What is this?"	Typical question; evoked trial
Child	"Gate."	A correct response
Clinician	"Great job! You said it correctly!"	Verbal praise

If the wrong responses persist on 4 to 5 evoked trials, reinstate partial or full modeling for a few trials, again fade the modeling, and re-present the evoked trials.

When the child meets the tentative learning criterion of 10 consecutively correct, nonimitated responses for a given stimulus item, move on to the next stimulus item. With this procedure, teach 6 to 8 exemplars shown on the following recording sheet. Use different exemplars as you see fit for a given child.

/g/ in Word-Initial Positions

Treatment Exemplars and Recording Sheet

Use stimuli from the **Stimulus Book,** *Volume 3.*

Print this page from CD or photocopy this page for your clinical use.

Name/Age:	Date:
Goal: Production of /g/ in word-initial positions with 90% accuracy when asked an evoking question while showing a stimulus.	Clinician:

Scoring: Correct: ✓   Incorrect or no response: X

Target skills	Discrete Trials														
	1	2	3	4	5	6	7	8	9	10	11	12	13	14	15
1. gate															
2. gift															
3. gum															
4. girl															
5. goose															
6. garage															
7. gorilla															
8. goldfish															

When the child has met the learning criterion of 10 consecutively correct evoked (nonimitated) responses for each of the 6 to 8 target exemplars, conduct a probe to see if the production has generalized to previously baserated but untrained exemplars.

If the probes do not meet the 90% correct criterion for untrained exemplars, teach additional exemplars and then probe again.

/g/ in Word-Initial Positions

Probe Protocols and Recording Sheet

Use stimuli from the **Stimulus Book, Volume 3.**

Print this page from the CD or photocopy this page for your clinical use.

On the probes, present only the untrained exemplars (UT). When the child fails to meet the 90% correct probe criterion, either teach 2 to 4 new exemplars or give additional training trials on already trained stimuli. If needed, select new exemplars for probes. Probe at least 10 untrained exemplars. Alternate probes and treatment until the probe criterion is met.

Scripts for Probe Trials		Note
Clinician	[*untrained stimulus: garden hose*] "What is this?"	No modeling or prompts
Child	"garden hose."	A correct, generalized response
Clinician	Scores the response as correct.	No reinforcement
Clinician	[*untrained stimulus: gardenia*] "What is this?"	The second probe trial
Child	"ardenia."	A wrong probe response
Clinician	Scores the response as incorrect.	No corrective feedback

Name:	Date:	Session #:
Age:	**Clinician:**	
Diagnosis: Articulation/Phonologic Disorder	**Word-initial /g/ probe**	
Untrained Stimuli	**Score: + correct; – incorrect or no responses**	
1. garden hose		
2. gardenia		
3. gold		
4. gecko		
5. gopher		
6. gazebo		
7. glove		
8. galaxy		
9. gardener		
10. giggling		
11. garbanzo		
12. gazelle		
Percent correct: (Criterion: 90%)		

If the child does not meet the probe criterion, give additional training on already trained exemplars or teach a few new exemplars. Subsequently, readminister the probe trials. When the child meets the 90% correct probe criterion for the exemplars, shift training to the sentence or conversational level or to another phoneme.

/g/ in Word-Final Positions

Baserate Protocols

Use stimuli from the **Stimulus Book,** *Volume 3.*

At the beginning of each trial, place a relevant stimulus (an object, a picture, or a printed word) in front of the child. Point to the stimulus as you ask an evoking question. Do not respond in any way to the child's correct, incorrect, or lack of responses.

Scripts for Evoked Baserate Trial		Note
Clinician	[*stimulus: dog*] "What is this?"	Evoked trial
Child	"dɑ."	Omission of final /g/
Clinician	Pulls the stimulus toward her; records the response.	No corrective feedback
Clinician	[*stimulus: flag*] "What is this?"	The next evoked trial
Child	"flæ."	Omission of final /g/
Clinician	Pulls the stimulus toward her; records the response.	No corrective feedback

Administer the modeled baserate trials only after completing the evoked trials on all 20 (or more) exemplars.

Scripts for Modeled Baserate Trial		Note
Clinician	[*stimulus: dog*] "What is this? Say, *dog.*"	Modeled trial
Child	"Dog."	Correct response
Clinician	Pulls the stimulus toward her; records the response.	No reinforcement
Clinician	[*stimulus: flag*] "What is this? Say, *flag.*"	The next modeled trial
Child	"flæ."	Omission of final /g/
Clinician	Pulls the stimulus toward her; records the response.	No corrective feedback

Use the recording sheet with exemplars shown on the next page to establish the baserates; print it from the CD.

/g/ in Word-Final Positions

Baserate Exemplars and Recording Sheet

Use stimuli from the **Stimulus Book,** *Volume 3*.

Print this page from the CD or photocopy this page for your clinical use.

Name/Age:		Date:	
Goal: To establish the baserate production of /g/ in word-final positions.		Clinician:	

Scoring: Correct: ✓   Incorrect or no response: X

/g/ in word-final positions	Evoked	Modeled
1. dog		
2. flag		
3. frog		
4. bag		
5. mug		
6. bulldog		
7. groundhog		
8. ladybug		
9. hotdog		
10. sleeping bag		
11. jug		
12. leg		
13. bug		
14. pig		
15. wig		
16. punching bag		
17. handbag		
18. bedbug		
19. litterbug		
20. bullfrog		
Percent correct baserate		

Replace or add new exemplars as you see fit for a given child. After establishing the baserates, begin production teaching. Follow the protocols given on the next page.

/g/ in Word-Final Positions

Treatment Protocols

Use stimuli from the **Stimulus Book,** *Volume 3*.

Teach 6 to 8 exemplars using the following script.

Place a relevant stimulus (an object, a picture, or a printed word) in front of the child and point to the stimulus as you ask an evoking question.

Scripts for Modeled Discrete Trial Training		Note
Clinician	[*stimulus: dog*] "What is this? Say, *dog*."	Modeling; the target vocally emphasized
Child	"da."	A wrong response
Clinician	"No. That's not correct. You said *da*, but it's *dog*."	Corrective feedback
Clinician	[*the same stimulus*] "What is this? Say, *dog*. Don't forget the *g* at the end."	The next trial
Child	"Dog."	A correct response
Clinician	"Excellent! You didn't miss the *g* at the end of the word!"	Verbal praise

Repeat the trials until the child gives 5 consecutively correct, imitated responses.

When the child imitates 5 correct responses in sequence, fade the modeling.

Scripts for Fading the Modeling		Note
Clinician	[*stimulus: dog*] "What is this? Don't forget the *g* at the end."	Only a prompt
Child	"da."	A wrong response
Clinician	"Gee, you forgot the *g* sound! It's a *dog*, not *da*. Put the *g* at the end."	Corrective feedback
Clinician	[*the same stimulus*] "What is this? It ends with . . . " [*silently models the tongue posture for the target sound.*]	The next trial; a partial modeling
Child	"Dog."	A correct response
Clinician	"That's great! You said *dog*, not *da*."	Verbal praise
Clinician	[*the same stimulus*] "What is this?"	Typical question; evoked trial
Child	"Dog."	A correct response
Clinician	"Wonderful! You said it correctly!"	Verbal praise

If the wrong responses persist on 4 to 5 evoked trials, reinstate partial or full modeling for a few trials, again fade the modeling, and re-present the evoked trials.

When the child meets the tentative learning criterion of 10 consecutively correct, nonimitated responses for a given stimulus item, move on to the next stimulus item. With this procedure, teach 6 to 8 exemplars shown on the following recording sheet. Use different exemplars as you see fit for a given child.

/g/ in Word-Final Positions

Treatment Exemplars and Recording Sheet

Use stimuli from the **Stimulus Book,** *Volume 3.*

Print this page from CD or photocopy this page for your clinical use.

Name/Age:	Date:
Goal: Production of /g/ in word-final positions with 90% accuracy when asked an evoking question while showing a stimulus.	Clinician:

Scoring: Correct: ✓   Incorrect or no response: X

Target skills	Discrete Trials														
	1	2	3	4	5	6	7	8	9	10	11	12	13	14	15
1. dog															
2. flag															
3. frog															
4. bag															
5. mug															
6. bulldog															
7. groundhog															
8. ladybug															

When the child has met the learning criterion of 10 consecutively correct evoked (nonimitated) responses for each of the 6 to 8 target exemplars, conduct a probe to see if the production has generalized to previously baserated but untrained exemplars.

If the probes do not meet the 90% correct criterion for untrained exemplars, teach additional exemplars and then probe again.

/g/ in Word-Final Positions

Probe Protocols and Recording Sheet

Use stimuli from the **Stimulus Book, Volume 3**.

Print this page from the CD or photocopy this page for your clinical use.

On the probes, present only the untrained exemplars (UT). When the child fails to meet the 90% correct probe criterion, either teach 2 to 4 new exemplars or give additional training trials on already trained stimuli. If needed, select new exemplars for probes. Probe at least 10 untrained exemplars. Alternate probes and treatment until the probe criterion is met.

Scripts for Probe Trials		Note
Clinician	[*untrained stimulus: hotdog*] "What is this?"	No modeling or prompts
Child	"Hotdog."	A correct, generalized response
Clinician	Scores the response as correct.	No reinforcement
Clinician	[*untrained stimulus: sleeping bag*] "What is this?"	The second probe trial
Child	"sleeping bæ."	A wrong probe response
Clinician	Scores the response as incorrect.	No corrective feedback

Name:	Date:	Session #:
Age:	**Clinician:**	
Diagnosis: Articulation/Phonologic Disorder	**Word-final /g/ probe**	
Untrained Stimuli	**Score: + correct; – incorrect or no responses**	
1. hotdog		
2. sleeping bag		
3. jug		
4. leg		
5. bug		
6. pig		
7. wig		
8. punching bag		
9. handbag		
10. bedbug		
11. litterbug		
12. bullfrog		
Percent correct: (Criterion: 90%)		

If the child does not meet the probe criterion, give additional training on already trained exemplars or teach a few new exemplars. Subsequently, readminister the probe trials. When the child meets the 90% correct probe criterion for the exemplars, shift training to the sentence or conversational level or to another phoneme.

/f/ in Word-Initial Positions

Baserate Protocols

Use stimuli from the **Stimulus Book, Volume 1**.

At the beginning of each trial, place a relevant stimulus (an object, a picture, or a printed word) in front of the child. Point to the stimulus as you ask an evoking question. Do not respond in any way to the child's correct, incorrect, or lack of responses.

Scripts for Evoked Baserate Trial		Note
Clinician	[*stimulus: fish*] "What is this?"	Evoked trial
Child	"ish."	Omission of initial /f/
Clinician	Pulls the stimulus toward her; records the response.	No corrective feedback
Clinician	[*stimulus: face*] "What do you call this?"	The next evoked trial
Child	"ace."	Omission of initial /f/
Clinician	Pulls the stimulus toward her; records the response.	No corrective feedback

Administer the modeled baserate trials only after completing the evoked trials on all 20 (or more) exemplars.

Scripts for Modeled Baserate Trial		Note
Clinician	[*stimulus: fish*] "What is this? Say, *fish.*"	Modeled trial
Child	"Fish."	Correct response
Clinician	Pulls the stimulus toward her; records the response.	No reinforcement
Clinician	[*stimulus: face*] "What is this? Say, *face.*"	The next modeled trial
Child	"ace."	Omission of initial /f/
Clinician	Pulls the stimulus toward her; records the response.	No corrective feedback

Use the recording sheet with exemplars shown on the next page to establish the baserates; print it from the CD.

/f/ in Word-Initial Positions

Baserate Exemplars and Recording Sheet

*Use stimuli from the **Stimulus Book, Volume 1**.*

Print this page from the CD or photocopy this page for your clinical use.

Name/Age:	Date:
Goal: To establish the baserate production of /f/ in word-initial positions.	Clinician:

Scoring: Correct: ✓ Incorrect or no response: X

/f/ in word-initial positions	Evoked	Modeled
1. fish		
2. face		
3. fan		
4. farm		
5. fence		
6. fireman		
7. fireplace		
8. fountain		
9. fisherman		
10. farmer		
11. fork		
12. fist		
13. foam		
14. fire		
15. phone		
16. fireworks		
17. forehead		
18. feather		
19. football		
20. photographer		
Percent correct baserate		

Replace or add new exemplars as you see fit for a given child. After establishing the baserates, begin production teaching. Follow the protocols given on the next page.

/f/ in Word-Initial Positions

Treatment Protocols

Use stimuli from the **Stimulus Book, Volume 1.**

Teach 6 to 8 exemplars using the following script.

Place a relevant stimulus in front of the child (an object, a picture, or a printed word) and ask a question as you point to the stimulus.

Scripts for Modeled Discrete Trial Training		Note
Clinician	[*stimulus: fish*] "What is this? Say, *fish.*"	Modeling; the target vocally emphasized
Child	"ish."	A wrong response
Clinician	"No. That's not correct. You said *ish*, but it's *fish.*"	Corrective feedback
Clinician	[*the same stimulus*] "What is this? Say, *fish.* Don't forget the *f* at the beginning."	The next trial
Child	"Fish."	A correct response
Clinician	"Excellent! You didn't miss the *f* this time!"	Verbal praise

Repeat the trials until the child gives 5 consecutively correct, imitated responses.

When the child imitates 5 correct responses in sequence, fade the modeling.

Scripts for Fading the Modeling		Note
Clinician	[*stimulus: fish*] "What is this? Don't forget the *f* at the beginning."	Only a prompt
Child	"ish."	A wrong response
Clinician	"Gee, you forgot the *f* sound! It's a *fish*, not *ish*. Put the *f* at the beginning."	Corrective feedback
Clinician	[*the same stimulus*] "What is this? It starts with . . . " [*silently models the lip-teeth posture for the target sound.*]	The next trial; a partial modeling
Child	"Fish."	A correct response
Clinician	"That's great! You said *fish*, not *ish.*"	Verbal praise
Clinician	[*the same stimulus*] "What is this?"	Typical question; evoked trial
Child	"Fish."	A correct response
Clinician	"Great job! You said it correctly!"	Verbal praise

If the wrong responses persist on 4 to 5 evoked trials, reinstate partial or full modeling for a few trials, again fade the modeling, and re-present the evoked trials.

When the child meets the tentative learning criterion of 10 consecutively correct, nonimitated responses for a given stimulus item, move on to the next stimulus item. With this procedure, teach 6 to 8 exemplars shown on the following recording sheet. Use different exemplars as you see fit for a given child.

/f/ in Word-Initial Positions

Treatment Exemplars and Recording Sheet

Use stimuli from the **Stimulus Book,** *Volume 1.*

Print this page from CD or photocopy this page for your clinical use.

Name/Age:	Date:
Goal: Production of /f/ in word-initial positions with 90% accuracy when asked an evoking question while showing a stimulus.	Clinician:

Scoring: Correct: ✓   Incorrect or no response: X

Target skills	Discrete Trials														
	1	2	3	4	5	6	7	8	9	10	11	12	13	14	15
1. fish															
2. face															
3. fan															
4. farm															
5. fence															
6. fireman															
7. fireplace															
8. fountain															

When the child has met the learning criterion of 10 consecutively correct evoked (nonimitated) responses for each of the 6 to 8 target exemplars, conduct a probe to see if the production has generalized to previously baserated but untrained exemplars.

If the probes do not meet the 90% correct criterion for untrained exemplars, teach additional exemplars and then probe again.

/f/ in Word-Initial Positions

Probe Protocols and Recording Sheet

Use stimuli from the **Stimulus Book, Volume 1**.

Print this page from the CD or photocopy this page for your clinical use.

On the probes, present only the untrained exemplars (UT). When the child fails to meet the 90% correct probe criterion, either teach 2 to 4 new exemplars or give additional training trials on already trained stimuli. If needed, select new exemplars for probes. Probe at least 10 untrained exemplars. Alternate probes and treatment until the probe criterion is met.

Scripts for Probe Trials		Note
Clinician	[*untrained stimulus: fisherman*] "Who is this?"	No modeling or prompts
Child	"Fisherman."	A correct, generalized response
Clinician	Scores the response as correct.	No reinforcement
Clinician	[*untrained stimulus: farmer*] "Who is this?"	The second probe trial
Child	"armer."	A wrong probe response
Clinician	Scores the response as incorrect.	No corrective feedback

Name:	Date:	Session #:
Age:	**Clinician:**	
Diagnosis: Articulation/Phonologic Disorder	**Word-initial /f/ probe**	
Untrained Stimuli	**Score: + correct; – incorrect or no responses**	
1. fisherman		
2. farmer		
3. fork		
4. fist		
5. foam		
6. fire		
7. phone		
8. fireworks		
9. forehead		
10. feather		
11. football		
12. photographer		
Percent correct: (Criterion: 90%)		

If the child does not meet the probe criterion, give additional training on already trained exemplars or teach a few new exemplars. Subsequently, readminister the probe trials. When the child meets the 90% correct probe criterion for the exemplars, shift training to the sentence or conversational level or to another phoneme.

/f/ in Word-Final Positions

Baserate Protocols

Use stimuli from the **Stimulus Book,** *Volume 1.*

At the beginning of each trial, place a relevant stimulus (an object, a picture, or a printed word) in front of the child. Point to the stimulus as you ask an evoking question. Do not respond in any way to the child's correct, incorrect, or lack of responses.

Scripts for Evoked Baserate Trial		Note
Clinician	[*stimulus: chef*] "Who is this?"	Evoked trial
Child	"chɛ."	Omission of final /f/
Clinician	Pulls the stimulus toward her; records the response.	No corrective feedback
Clinician	[*stimulus: calf*] "What is this?"	The next evoked trial
Child	"ca."	Omission of final /f/
Clinician	Pulls the stimulus toward her; records the response.	No corrective feedback

Administer the modeled baserate trials only after completing the evoked trials on all 20 (or more) exemplars.

Scripts for Modeled Baserate Trial		Note
Clinician	[*stimulus: chef*] "Who is this? Say, *chef.*"	Modeled trial
Child	"Chef."	Correct response
Clinician	Pulls the stimulus toward her; records the response.	No reinforcement
Clinician	[*stimulus: calf*] "What is this? Say, *calf.*"	The next modeled trial
Child	"ca."	Omission of final /f/
Clinician	Pulls the stimulus toward her; records the response	No corrective feedback

Use the recording sheet with exemplars shown on the next page to establish the baserates; print it from the CD.

/f/ in Word-Final Positions

Baserate Exemplars and Recording Sheet

Use stimuli from the **Stimulus Book,** *Volume 1.*

Print this page from the CD or photocopy this page for your clinical use.

Name/Age:	Date:
Goal: To establish the baserate production of /f/ in word-final positions.	Clinician:

Scoring: Correct: ✓   Incorrect or no response: X

/f/ in word-final positions	Evoked	Modeled
1. chef		
2. calf		
3. knife		
4. loaf		
5. giraffe		
6. handcuff		
7. bulletproof		
8. fire chief		
9. paragraph		
10. hunting knife		
11. beef		
12. thief		
13. roof		
14. sheriff		
15. leaf		
16. meatloaf		
17. powder puff		
18. handkerchief		
19. photograph		
20. telegraph		
Percent correct baserate		

Replace or add new exemplars as you see fit for a given child. After establishing the baserates, begin production teaching. Follow the protocols given on the next page.

/f/ in Word-Final Positions

Treatment Protocols

Use stimuli from the **Stimulus Book,** *Volume 1.*

Teach 6 to 8 exemplars using the following script.

Place a relevant stimulus (an object, a picture, or a printed word) in front of the child and point to the stimulus as you ask an evoking question.

Scripts for Modeled Discrete Trial Training		Note
Clinician	[*stimulus: chef*] "Who is this? Say, **ch***ef*."	Modeling; the target vocally emphasized
Child	"chε."	A wrong response
Clinician	"No. That's not correct. You said *chε*, but it's *chef*."	Corrective feedback
Clinician	[*the same stimulus*] "Who is this? Say, *chef*. Don't forget the *f* at the end."	The next trial
Child	"Chef."	A correct response
Clinician	"Excellent! You didn't miss the *f* at the end of the word!"	Verbal praise

Repeat the trials until the child gives 5 consecutively correct, imitated responses.

When the child imitates 5 correct responses in sequence, fade the modeling.

Scripts for Fading the Modeling		Note
Clinician	[*stimulus: chef*] "Who is this? Don't forget the *f* at the end."	Only a prompt
Child	"chε."	A wrong response
Clinician	"Oh no! you forgot the *f* sound! It's *chef*, not *chε*. Put the *f* at the end."	Corrective feedback
Clinician	[*the same stimulus*] "Who is this? It ends with . . ." [*silently models the teeth-lip posture for the target sound.*]	The next trial; a partial modeling
Child	"Chef."	A correct response
Clinician	"That's great! You said *chef*, not *chε*."	Verbal praise
Clinician	[*the same stimulus*] "Who is this?"	Typical question; evoked trial
Child	"Chef."	A correct response
Clinician	"I like it! You said it correctly!"	Verbal praise

If the wrong responses persist on 4 to 5 evoked trials, reinstate partial or full modeling for a few trials, again fade the modeling, and re-present the evoked trials.

When the child meets the tentative learning criterion of 10 consecutively correct, nonimitated responses for a given stimulus item, move on to the next stimulus item. With this procedure, teach 6 to 8 exemplars shown on the following recording sheet. Use different exemplars as you see fit for a given child.

/f/ in Word-Final Positions

Treatment Exemplars and Recording Sheet

Use stimuli from the **Stimulus Book,** *Volume 1.*

Print this page from CD or photocopy this page for your clinical use.

Name/Age:	Date:
Goal: Production of /f/ in word-final positions with 90% accuracy when asked an evoking question while showing a stimulus.	Clinician:

Scoring: Correct: ✓   Incorrect or no response: X

Target skills	Discrete Trials														
	1	2	3	4	5	6	7	8	9	10	11	12	13	14	15
1. chef															
2. calf															
3. knife															
4. loaf															
5. giraffe															
6. handcuff															
7. bulletproof															
8. fire chief															

When the child has met the learning criterion of 10 consecutively correct evoked (nonimitated) responses for each of the 6 to 8 target exemplars, conduct a probe to see if the production has generalized to previously baserated but untrained exemplars.

If the probes do not meet the 90% correct criterion for untrained exemplars, teach additional exemplars and then probe again.

/f/ in Word-Final Positions

Probe Protocols and Recording Sheet

Use stimuli from the **Stimulus Book,** *Volume 1.*

Print this page from the CD or photocopy this page for your clinical use.

On the probes, present only the untrained exemplars (UT). When the child fails to meet the 90% correct probe criterion, either teach 2 to 4 new exemplars or give additional training trials on already trained stimuli. If needed, select new exemplars for probes. Probe at least 10 untrained exemplars. Alternate probes and treatment until the probe criterion is met.

Scripts for Probe Trials		Note
Clinician	[*untrained stimulus: paragraph*] "When you see a bunch of sentences like this, what do you call it?"	No modeling or prompts
Child	"Paragraph."	A correct, generalized response
Clinician	Scores the response as correct.	No reinforcement
Clinician	[*untrained stimulus: hunting knife*] "What is this?"	The second probe trial
Child	"hunting nai." ["nai."]	A wrong probe response
Clinician	Scores the response as incorrect.	No corrective feedback

Name:	Date:	Session #:
Age:	**Clinician:**	
Diagnosis: Articulation/Phonologic Disorder	**Word-final /f/probe**	
Untrained Stimuli	**Score: + correct; – incorrect or no responses**	
1. paragraph		
2. hunting knife		
3. beef		
4. thief		
5. roof		
6. sheriff		
7. leaf		
8. meatloaf		
9. powder puff		
10. handkerchief		
11. photograph		
12. telegraph		
Percent correct: (Criterion: 90%)		

If the child does not meet the probe criterion, give additional training on already trained exemplars or teach a few new exemplars. Subsequently, readminister the probe trials. When the child meets the 90% correct probe criterion for the exemplars, shift training to the sentence or conversational level or to another phoneme.

/v/ in Word-Initial Positions

Baserate Protocols

Use stimuli from the **Stimulus Book, Volume 1.**

At the beginning of each trial, place a relevant stimulus (an object, a picture, or a printed word) in front of the child. Point to the stimulus as you ask an evoking question. Do not respond in any way to the child's correct, incorrect, or lack of responses.

Scripts for Evoked Baserate Trial		Note
Clinician	[*stimulus: vase*] "What is this?"	Evoked trial
Child	"ace."	Omission of initial /v/
Clinician	Pulls the stimulus toward her; records the response.	No corrective feedback
Clinician	[*stimulus: vest*] "What is this?"	The next evoked trial
Child	"est."	Omission of initial /v/
Clinician	Pulls the stimulus toward her; records the response.	No corrective feedback

Administer the modeled baserate trials only after completing the evoked trials on all 20 (or more) exemplars.

Scripts for Modeled Baserate Trial		Note
Clinician	[*stimulus: vase*] "What is this? Say, *vase.*"	Modeled trial
Child	"Vase."	Correct response
Clinician	Pulls the stimulus toward her; records the response.	No reinforcement
Clinician	[*stimulus: vest*] "What is this? Say, *vest.*"	The next modeled trial
Child	"est."	Omission of initial /v/
Clinician	Pulls the stimulus toward her; records the response.	No corrective feedback

Use the recording sheet with exemplars shown on the next page to establish the baserates; print it from the CD.

/v/ in Word-Initial Positions

Baserate Exemplars and Recording Sheet

Use stimuli from the **Stimulus Book,** *Volume 1.*

Print this page from the CD or photocopy this page for your clinical use.

Name/Age:	Date:
Goal: To establish the baserate production of /v/ in word-initial positions.	Clinician:

Scoring: Correct: ✓   Incorrect or no response: X

/v/ in word-initial positions	Evoked	Modeled
1. vase		
2. vest		
3. van		
4. vault		
5. veil		
6. vacuum cleaner		
7. violin		
8. vegetable		
9. Valentine's day		
10. Vaseline		
11. valve		
12. vent		
13. vine		
14. volcano		
15. violet		
16. vampire		
17. veterinarian		
18. ventriloquist		
19. vehicle		
20. violinist		
Percent correct baserate		

Replace or add new exemplars as you see fit for a given child. After establishing the baserates, begin production teaching. Follow the protocols given on the next page.

/v/ in Word-Initial Positions

Treatment Protocols

Use stimuli from the **Stimulus Book, Volume 1**.

Teach 6 to 8 exemplars using the following script.

Place a relevant stimulus in front of the child (an object, a picture, or a printed word) and ask a question as you point to the stimulus.

Scripts for Modeled Discrete Trial Training		Note
Clinician	[*stimulus: vase*] "What is this? Say, **vase**."	Modeling; the target vocally emphasized
Child	"ace."	A wrong response
Clinician	"No. That's not correct. You said *ace*, but it's **vase**."	Corrective feedback
Clinician	[*the same stimulus*] "What is this? Say, **vase**. Don't forget the *v* at the beginning."	The next trial
Child	"Vase."	A correct response
Clinician	"Excellent! You didn't miss the *v* this time!"	Verbal praise

Repeat the trials until the child gives 5 consecutively correct, imitated responses.

When the child imitates 5 correct responses in sequence, fade the modeling.

Scripts for Fading the Modeling		Note
Clinician	[*stimulus: vase*] "What is this? Don't forget the *v* at the beginning."	Only a prompt
Child	"ace."	A wrong response
Clinician	"Gee, you forgot the *v* sound! It's a *vase*, not *ace*. Put the v at the beginning."	Corrective feedback
Clinician	[*the same stimulus*] "What is this? It starts with . . . " [*silently models the upper teeth-lower lip posture for the target sound.*]	The next trial; a partial modeling
Child	"Vase."	A correct response
Clinician	"That's great! You said *vase*, not *ace*."	Verbal praise
Clinician	[*the same stimulus*] "What is this?"	Typical question; evoked trial
Child	"Vase."	A correct response
Clinician	"Fantastic! You again said it correctly!"	Verbal praise

If the wrong responses persist on 4 to 5 evoked trials, reinstate partial or full modeling for a few trials, again fade the modeling, and re-present the evoked trials.

When the child meets the tentative learning criterion of 10 consecutively correct, nonimitated responses for a given stimulus item, move on to the next stimulus item. With this procedure, teach 6 to 8 exemplars shown on the following recording sheet. Use different exemplars as you see fit for a given child.

/v/ in Word-Initial Positions

Treatment Exemplars and Recording Sheet

Use stimuli from the **Stimulus Book, *Volume 1***.

Print this page from CD or photocopy this page for your clinical use.

Name/Age:	Date:
Goal: Production of /v/ in word-initial positions with 90% accuracy when asked an evoking question while showing a stimulus.	Clinician:

Scoring: Correct: ✓   Incorrect or no response: X

Target skills	Discrete Trials														
	1	2	3	4	5	6	7	8	9	10	11	12	13	14	15
1. vase															
2. vest															
3. van															
4. vault															
5. veil															
6. vacuum cleaner															
7. violin															
8. vegetable															

When the child has met the learning criterion of 10 consecutively correct evoked (nonimitated) responses for each of the 6 to 8 target exemplars, conduct a probe to see if the production has generalized to previously baserated but untrained exemplars.

If the probes do not meet the 90% correct criterion for untrained exemplars, teach additional exemplars and then probe again.

/v/ in Word-Initial Positions

Probe Protocols and Recording Sheet

*Use stimuli from the **Stimulus Book, Volume 1**.*

Print this page from the CD or photocopy this page for your clinical use.

On the probes, present only the untrained exemplars (UT). When the child fails to meet the 90% correct probe criterion, either teach 2 to 4 new exemplars or give additional training trials on already trained stimuli. If needed, select new exemplars for probes. Probe at least 10 untrained exemplars. Alternate probes and treatment until the probe criterion is met.

Scripts for Probe Trials		Note
Clinician	[*untrained stimulus: Valentine's day*] "What day do you think is this?"	No modeling or prompts
Child	"Valentine's day."	A correct, generalized response
Clinician	Scores the response as correct.	No reinforcement
Clinician	[*untrained stimulus: vaseline*] "What is this?"	The second probe trial
Child	"æsaline."	A wrong probe response
Clinician	Scores the response as incorrect.	No corrective feedback

Name:	Date:	Session #:
Age:	**Clinician:**	
Diagnosis: Articulation/Phonologic Disorder	**Word-initial /v/ probe**	
Untrained Stimuli	**Score: + correct; – incorrect or no responses**	
1. Valentine's day		
2. Vaseline		
3. valve		
4. vent		
5. vine		
6. volcano		
7. violet		
8. vampire		
9. veterinarian		
10. ventriloquist		
11. vehicle		
12. violinist		
Percent correct: (Criterion: 90%)		

If the child does not meet the probe criterion, give additional training on already trained exemplars or teach a few new exemplars. Subsequently, readminister the probe trials. When the child meets the 90% correct probe criterion for the exemplars, shift training to the sentence or conversational level or to another phoneme.

/v/ in Word-Final Positions

Baserate Protocols

Use stimuli from the **Stimulus Book, Volume 1**.

At the beginning of each trial, place a relevant stimulus (an object, a picture, or a printed word) in front of the child. Point to the stimulus as you ask an evoking question. Do not respond in any way to the child's correct, incorrect, or lack of responses.

Scripts for Evoked Baserate Trial		Note
Clinician	[*stimulus: cave*] "What is this?"	Evoked trial
Child	"kay."	Omission of final /v/
Clinician	Pulls the stimulus toward her; records the response.	No corrective feedback
Clinician	[*stimulus: dove*] "What is this?"	The next evoked trial
Child	"də."	Omission of final /v/
Clinician	Pulls the stimulus toward her; records the response.	No corrective feedback

Administer the modeled baserate trials only after completing the evoked trials on all 20 (or more) exemplars.

Scripts for Modeled Baserate Trial		Note
Clinician	[*stimulus: cave*] "What is this? Say, *cave.*"	Modeled trial
Child	"Cave."	Correct response
Clinician	Pulls the stimulus toward her; records the response.	No reinforcement
Clinician	[*stimulus: dove*] "What is this? Say, *dove.*"	The next modeled trial
Child	"də."	Omission of final /v/
Clinician	Pulls the stimulus toward her; records the response.	No corrective feedback

Use the recording sheet with exemplars shown on the next page to establish the baserates; print it from the CD.

/v/ in Word-Final Positions

Baserate Exemplars and Recording Sheet

Use stimuli from the **Stimulus Book, Volume 1**.

Print this page from the CD or photocopy this page for your clinical use.

Name/Age:	Date:
Goal: To establish the baserate production of /v/ in word-final positions.	Clinician:

Scoring: Correct: ✓   Incorrect or no response: X

/v/ in word-final positions	Evoked	Modeled
1. cave		
2. dove		
3. five		
4. glove		
5. hive		
6. microwave		
7. adhesive		
8. skydive		
9. locomotive		
10. explosive		
11. grave		
12. sleeve		
13. wave		
14. olive		
15. save		
16. negative		
17. positive		
18. groove		
19. above		
20. alive		
Percent correct baserate		

Replace or add new exemplars as you see fit for a given child. After establishing the baserates, begin production teaching. Follow the protocols given on the next page.

/v/ in Word-Final Positions

Treatment Protocols

Use stimuli from the **Stimulus Book,** *Volume 1.*

Teach 6 to 8 exemplars using the following script.

Place a relevant stimulus (an object, a picture, or a printed word) in front of the child and point to the stimulus as you ask an evoking question.

Scripts for Modeled Discrete Trial Training		Note
Clinician	[*stimulus: cave*] "What is this? Say, *cave.*"	Modeling; the target vocally emphasized
Child	"kay."	A wrong response
Clinician	"No. That's not correct. You said *kay,* but it's *cave.*"	Corrective feedback
Clinician	[*the same stimulus*] "What is this? Say, *cave.* Don't forget the *v* at the end."	The next trial
Child	"Cave."	A correct response
Clinician	"Excellent! You didn't miss the *v* at the end of the word!"	Verbal praise

Repeat the trials until the child gives 5 consecutively correct, imitated responses.

When the child imitates 5 correct responses in sequence, fade the modeling.

Scripts for Fading the Modeling		Note
Clinician	[*stimulus: cave*] "What is this? Don't forget the *v* at the end."	Only a prompt
Child	"kay."	A wrong response
Clinician	"Oh no!, you forgot the *v* sound! It's a *cave,* not *kay.* Put the *v* at the end."	Corrective feedback
Clinician	[*the same stimulus*] "What is this? It ends with . . . " [*silently models the upper teeth-lower lip posture for the target sound.*]	The next trial; a partial modeling
Child	"Cave."	A correct response
Clinician	"That's great! You said *cave,* not *kay.*"	Verbal praise
Clinician	[*the same stimulus*] "What is this?"	Typical question; evoked trial
Child	"Cave."	A correct response
Clinician	"I like it! You said it correctly!"	Verbal praise

If the wrong responses persist on 4 to 5 evoked trials, reinstate partial or full modeling for a few trials, again fade the modeling, and re-present the evoked trials.

When the child meets the tentative learning criterion of 10 consecutively correct, nonimitated responses for a given stimulus item, move on to the next stimulus item. With this procedure, teach 6 to 8 exemplars shown on the following recording sheet: Use different exemplars as you see fit for a given child.

/v/ in Word-Final Positions

Treatment Exemplars and Recording Sheet

Use stimuli from the **Stimulus Book, Volume 1**.

Print this page from CD or photocopy this page for your clinical use.

Name/Age:	Date:
Goal: Production of /v/ in word-final positions with 90% accuracy when asked an evoking question while showing a stimulus.	Clinician:

Scoring: Correct: ✓   Incorrect or no response: X

Target skills	Discrete Trials														
	1	2	3	4	5	6	7	8	9	10	11	12	13	14	15
1. cave															
2. dove															
3. five															
4. glove															
5. hive															
6. microwave															
7. adhesive															
8. skydive															

When the child has met the learning criterion of 10 consecutively correct evoked (nonimitated) responses for each of the 6 to 8 target exemplars, conduct a probe to see if the production has generalized to previously baserated but untrained exemplars.

If the probes do not meet the 90% correct criterion for untrained exemplars, teach additional exemplars and then probe again.

/v/ in Word-Final Positions

Probe Protocols and Recording Sheet

Use stimuli from **Stimulus Book,** *Volume 1.*

Print this page from the CD or photocopy this page for your clinical use.

On the probes, present only the untrained exemplars (UT). When the child fails to meet the 90% correct probe criterion, either teach 2 to 4 new exemplars or give additional training trials on already trained stimuli. If needed, select new exemplars for probes. Probe at least 10 untrained exemplars. Alternate probes and treatment until the probe criterion is met.

Scripts for Probe Trials		Note
Clinician	[*untrained stimulus: locomotive*] "What is this?"	No modeling or prompts
Child	"Locomotive."	A correct, generalized response
Clinician	Scores the response as correct.	No reinforcement
Clinician	[*untrained stimulus: explosive*] "What is this?"	The second probe trial
Child	"explosi."	A wrong probe response
Clinician	Scores the response as incorrect.	No corrective feedback

Name:	Date:	Session #:
Age:	**Clinician:**	
Diagnosis: Articulation/Phonologic Disorder	**Word-final /v/probe**	
Untrained Stimuli	**Score: + correct; – incorrect or no responses**	
1. locomotive		
2. explosive		
3. grave		
4. sleeve		
5. wave		
6. olive		
7. save		
8. negative		
9. positive		
10. groove		
11. above		
12. alive		
Percent correct: (Criterion: 90%)		

If the child does not meet the probe criterion, give additional training on already trained exemplars or teach a few new exemplars. Subsequently, readminister the probe trials. When the child meets the 90% correct probe criterion for the exemplars, shift training to the sentence or conversational level or to another phoneme.

/θ/ in Word-Initial Positions

Baserate Protocols

Use stimuli from the **Stimulus Book, Volume 4**.

At the beginning of each trial, place a relevant stimulus (an object, a picture, or a printed word) in front of the child. Point to the stimulus as you ask an evoking question. Do not respond in any way to the child's correct, incorrect, or lack of responses.

Scripts for Evoked Baserate Trial		Note
Clinician	[*stimulus: a thick book*] "Is this book thick or thin?"	Evoked trial
Child	"ik."	Omission of initial /θ/
Clinician	Pulls the stimulus toward her; records the response.	No corrective feedback
Clinician	[*stimulus: a thin book*] "Is this book thick or thin?"	The next evoked trial
Child	"in."	Omission of initial /θ/
Clinician	Pulls the stimulus toward her; records the response.	No corrective feedback

Administer the modeled baserate trials only after completing the evoked trials on all 20 (or more) exemplars.

Scripts for Modeled Baserate Trial		Note
Clinician	[*stimulus: a thick book*] "Is this book thick or thin? Say, *thick*."	Modeled trial
Child	"Thick."	Correct response
Clinician	Pulls the stimulus toward her; records the response.	No reinforcement
Clinician	[*stimulus: a thin book*] "Is this book thick or thin? Say, *thin*."	The next modeled trial
Child	"in."	Omission of initial /θ/
Clinician	Pulls the stimulus toward her; records the response	No corrective feedback

Use the recording sheet with exemplars shown on the next page to establish the baserates; print it from the CD.

/θ/ in Word-Initial Positions

Baserate Exemplars and Recording Sheet

Use stimuli from the **Stimulus Book,** *Volume 4.*

Print this page from the CD or photocopy this page for your clinical use.

Name/Age:	Date:
Goal: To establish the baserate production of /θ/ in word-initial positions.	Clinician:

Scoring: Correct: ✓   Incorrect or no response: X

/θ/ in word-initial positions	Evoked	Modeled
1. thick		
2. thin		
3. thigh		
4. thumb		
5. thief		
6. thundershower		
7. thermos		
8. theater		
9. thanksgiving		
10. thumbtack		
11. thirty		
12. thorn		
13. thinking		
14. thong		
15. three		
16. thank you		
17. thousand		
18. thighbone		
19. thundercloud		
20. theme park		
Percent correct baserate		

Replace or add new exemplars as you see fit for a given child. After establishing the baserates, begin production teaching. Follow the protocols given on the next page.

/θ/ in Word-Initial Positions

Treatment Protocols

Use stimuli from the **Stimulus Book,** *Volume 4.*

Teach 6 to 8 exemplars using the following script.

Place a relevant stimulus in front of the child (an object, a picture, or a printed word) and ask a question as you point to the stimulus.

Scripts for Modeled Discrete Trial Training		Note
Clinician	[*stimulus: a thick book*] "Is this book thick or thin? Say, **thick**."	Modeling; the target vocally emphasized
Child	"ik."	A wrong response
Clinician	"No. That's not correct. You said *ik*, but it's **thick**."	Corrective feedback
Clinician	[*the same stimulus*] "Is this book thick or thin? Say, **thick**. Don't forget the θ at the beginning."	The next trial
Child	"Thick."	A correct response
Clinician	"Excellent! You didn't miss the θ this time!"	Verbal praise

Repeat the trials until the child gives 5 consecutively correct, imitated responses.

When the child imitates 5 correct responses in sequence, fade the modeling.

Scripts for Fading the Modeling		Note
Clinician	[*stimulus: a thick book*] "What is this? Don't forget the θ at the beginning."	Only a prompt
Child	"ik."	A wrong response
Clinician	"Gee, you forgot the θ! It's *thick*, not *ik*. Put the θ at the beginning."	Corrective feedback
Clinician	[*the same stimulus*] "What is this? It starts with . . . " [*silently models the tongue posture for the target sound.*]	The next trial; a partial modeling
Child	"Thick."	A correct response
Clinician	"That's great! You said *thick*, not *ik*."	Verbal praise
Clinician	[*the same stimulus*] "What is this?"	Typical question; evoked trial
Child	"Thick."	A correct response
Clinician	"Great job! You said it correctly!"	Verbal praise

If the wrong responses persist on 4 to 5 evoked trials, reinstate partial or full modeling for a few trials, again fade the modeling, and re-present the evoked trials.

When the child meets the tentative learning criterion of 10 consecutively correct, nonimitated responses for a given stimulus item, move on to the next stimulus item. With this procedure, teach 6 to 8 exemplars shown on the following recording sheet. Use different exemplars as you see fit for a given child.

/θ/ in Word-Initial Positions

Treatment Exemplars and Recording Sheet

Use stimuli from the **Stimulus Book,** *Volume 4.*

Print this page from CD or photocopy this page for your clinical use.

Name/Age:	Date:
Goal: Production of /θ/ in word-initial positions with 90% accuracy when asked an evoking question while showing a stimulus.	Clinician:

Scoring: Correct: ✓   Incorrect or no response: X

Target skills	Discrete Trials														
	1	2	3	4	5	6	7	8	9	10	11	12	13	14	15
1. thick															
2. thin															
3. thigh															
4. thumb															
5. thief															
6. thundershower															
7. thermos															
8. theater															

When the child has met the learning criterion of 10 consecutively correct evoked (nonimitated) responses for each of the 6 to 8 target exemplars, conduct a probe to see if the production has generalized to previously baserated but untrained exemplars.

If the probes do not meet the 90% correct criterion for untrained exemplars, teach additional exemplars and then probe again.

/θ/ in Word-Initial Positions

Probe Protocols and Recording Sheet

Use stimuli from the **Stimulus Book,** *Volume 4*.

Print this page from the CD or photocopy this page for your clinical use.

On the probes, present only the untrained exemplars (UT). When the child fails to meet the 90% correct probe criterion, either teach 2 to 4 new exemplars or give additional training trials on already trained stimuli. If needed, select new exemplars for probes. Probe at least 10 untrained exemplars. Alternate probes and treatment until the probe criterion is met.

Scripts for Probe Trials		Note
Clinician	[*untrained stimulus: Thanksgiving*] "They are enjoying a holiday here. What kind of holiday is this?"	No modeling or prompts
Child	"Thanksgiving."	A correct, generalized response
Clinician	Scores the response as correct.	No reinforcement
Clinician	[*untrained stimulus: thumbtack*] "What is this?"	The second probe trial
Child	"umbtack."	A wrong probe response
Clinician	Scores the response as incorrect.	No corrective feedback

Name:	Date:	Session #:
Age:	**Clinician:**	
Diagnosis: Articulation/Phonologic Disorder	**Word-initial /θ/ probe**	
Untrained Stimuli	**Score: + correct; – incorrect or no responses**	
1. Thanksgiving		
2. thumbtack		
3. thirty		
4. thorn		
5. thinking		
6. thong		
7. three		
8. thank you		
9. thousand		
10. thighbone		
11. thundercloud		
12. theme park		
Percent correct: (Criterion: 90%)		

If the child does not meet the probe criterion, give additional training on already trained exemplars or teach a few new exemplars. Subsequently, readminister the probe trials. When the child meets the 90% correct probe criterion for the exemplars, shift training to the sentence or conversational level or to another phoneme.

/θ/ in Word-Final Positions

Baserate Protocols

*Use stimuli from the **Stimulus Book, Volume 4**.*

At the beginning of each trial, place a relevant stimulus (an object, a picture, or a printed word) in front of the child. Point to the stimulus as you ask an evoking question. Do not respond in any way to the child's correct, incorrect, or lack of responses.

Scripts for Evoked Baserate Trial		Note
Clinician	[*stimulus: booth*] "What is this?"	Evoked trial
Child	"boo."	Omission of final /θ/
Clinician	Pulls the stimulus toward her; records the response.	No corrective feedback
Clinician	[*stimulus: mouth*] "What is this?"	The next evoked trial
Child	"mou."	Omission of final /θ/
Clinician	Pulls the stimulus toward her; records the response.	No corrective feedback

Administer the modeled baserate trials only after completing the evoked trials on all 20 (or more) exemplars.

Scripts for Modeled Baserate Trial		Note
Clinician	[*stimulus: booth*] "What is this? Say, *booth.*"	Modeled trial
Child	"Booth."	Correct response
Clinician	Pulls the stimulus toward her; records the response.	No reinforcement
Clinician	[*stimulus: mouth*] "What is this? Say, *mouth.*"	The next modeled trial
Child	"mou."	Omission of final /θ/
Clinician	Pulls the stimulus toward her; records the response.	No corrective feedback

Use the recording sheet with exemplars shown on the next page to establish the baserates; print it from the CD.

/θ/ in Word-Final Positions

Baserate Exemplars and Recording Sheet

Use stimuli from the **Stimulus Book,** *Volume 4*.

Print this page from the CD or photocopy this page for your clinical use.

Name/Age:	Date:
Goal: To establish the baserate production of /θ/ in word-final positions.	Clinician:

Scoring: Correct: ✓   Incorrect or no response: X

/θ/ in word-final positions	Evoked	Modeled
1. booth		
2. mouth		
3. bath		
4. moth		
5. teeth		
6. birdbath		
7. bubble bath		
8. bike path		
9. locksmith		
10. tablecloth		
11. south		
12. path		
13. tooth		
14. cloth		
15. earth		
16. phone booth		
17. underneath		
18. washcloth		
19. goldsmith		
20. sail cloth		
Percent correct baserate		

Replace or add new exemplars as you see fit for a given child. After establishing the baserates, begin production teaching. Follow the protocols given on the next page.

/θ/ in Word-Final Positions

Treatment Protocols

Use stimuli from the **Stimulus Book,** *Volume 4.*

Teach 6 to 8 exemplars using the following script.

Place a relevant stimulus (an object, a picture, or a printed word) in front of the child and point to the stimulus as you ask an evoking question.

Scripts for Modeled Discrete Trial Training		Note
Clinician	[*stimulus: booth*] "What is this? Say, *booth*."	Modeling; the target vocally emphasized
Child	"boo."	A wrong response
Clinician	"No. That's not correct. You said *boo*, but it's *booth*."	Corrective feedback
Clinician	[*the same stimulus*] "What is this? Say, *booth*. Don't forget the θ at the end."	The next trial
Child	"Booth."	A correct response
Clinician	"Excellent! You didn't miss the θ at the end of the word!"	Verbal praise

Repeat the trials until the child gives 5 consecutively correct, imitated responses.

When the child imitates 5 correct responses in sequence, fade the modeling.

Scripts for Fading the Modeling		Note
Clinician	[*stimulus: booth*] "What is this? Don't forget the θ at the end."	Only a prompt
Child	"boo."	A wrong response
Clinician	"Gee, you forgot the θ sound! It's a *booth*, not *boo*. Put the θ sound at the end."	Corrective feedback
Clinician	[*the same stimulus*] "What is this? It ends with . . . " [*silently models the tongue posture for the target sound.*]	The next trial; a partial modeling
Child	"Booth."	A correct response
Clinician	"That's great! You said *booth*, not *boo*."	Verbal praise
Clinician	[*the same stimulus*] "What is this?"	Typical question; evoked trial
Child	"Booth."	A correct response
Clinician	"Great job! You are working very hard!"	Verbal praise

If the wrong responses persist on 4 to 5 evoked trials, reinstate partial or full modeling for a few trials, again fade the modeling, and re-present the evoked trials.

When the child meets the tentative learning criterion of 10 consecutively correct, nonimitated responses for a given stimulus item, move on to the next stimulus item. With this procedure, teach 6 to 8 exemplars shown on the following recording sheet. Use different exemplars as you see fit for a given child.

/θ/ in Word-Final Positions

Treatment Exemplars and Recording Sheet

Use stimuli from the **Stimulus Book,** *Volume 4.*

Print this page from CD or photocopy this page for your clinical use.

Name/Age:	Date:
Goal: Production of /θ/ in word-final positions with 90% accuracy when asked an evoking question while showing a stimulus.	Clinician:

Scoring: Correct: ✓ Incorrect or no response: X

Target skills	Discrete Trials														
	1	2	3	4	5	6	7	8	9	10	11	12	13	14	15
1. booth															
2. mouth															
3. bath															
4. moth															
5. teeth															
6. birdbath															
7. bubble bath															
8. bike path															

When the child has met the learning criterion of 10 consecutively correct evoked (nonimitated) responses for each of the 6 to 8 target exemplars, conduct a probe to see if the production has generalized to previously baserated but untrained exemplars.

If the probes do not meet the 90% correct criterion for untrained exemplars, teach additional exemplars and then probe again.

/θ/ in Word-Final Positions

Probe Protocols and Recording Sheet

Use stimuli from the **Stimulus Book,** *Volume 4*.

Print this page from the CD or photocopy this page for your clinical use.

On the probes, present only the untrained exemplars (UT). When the child fails to meet the 90% correct probe criterion, either teach 2 to 4 new exemplars or give additional training trials on already trained stimuli. If needed, select new exemplars for probes. Probe at least 10 untrained exemplars. Alternate probes and treatment until the probe criterion is met.

Scripts for Probe Trials		Note
Clinician	[*untrained stimulus: locksmith*] "Who is this?"	No modeling or prompts
Child	"Locksmith."	A correct, generalized response
Clinician	Scores the response as correct.	No reinforcement
Clinician	[*untrained stimulus: tablecloth*] "What is this?"	The second probe trial
Child	"tablecla."	A wrong probe response
Clinician:	Scores the response as incorrect.	No corrective feedback

Name:	Date:	Session #:
Age:	**Clinician:**	
Diagnosis: Articulation/Phonologic Disorder	**Word-final /θ/probe**	
Untrained Stimuli	**Score: + correct; – incorrect or no responses**	
1. locksmith		
2. tablecloth		
3. south		
4. path		
5. tooth		
6. cloth		
7. earth		
8. phone booth		
9. underneath		
10. washcloth		
11. goldsmith		
12. sail cloth		
Percent correct: (Criterion: 90%)		

If the child does not meet the probe criterion, give additional training on already trained exemplars or teach a few new exemplars. Subsequently, readminister the probe trials. When the child meets the 90% correct probe criterion for the exemplars, shift training to the sentence or conversational level or to another phoneme.

/ð/ in Word-Initial Positions
Baserate Protocols

Use stimuli from the **Stimulus Book,** *Volume 4.*

Functional words that begin with /ð/ are few in English. Most are not picturable. For children who read, printed word stimuli are a practical means of evoking this sound. For children who do not read, the clinician names the printed stimulus and then asks the question.

At the beginning of each trial, place a relevant stimulus (an object, a picture, or a printed word) in front of the child. Point to the stimulus as you ask an evoking question. Do not respond in any way to the child's correct, incorrect, or lack of responses.

Scripts for Evoked Baserate Trial		Note
Clinician	[*stimulus:* printed word *than*] "Please read this word." [*for a nonreader*] "This word is *than*. What word is this?"	Evoked trial
Child	"an."	Omission of initial /ð/
Clinician	Pulls the stimulus toward her; records the response.	No corrective feedback
Clinician	[*stimulus:* printed word *that*] "Please read this word" [*for a nonreader*] "This word is *that*. What word is this?"	The next evoked trial
Child	"at."	Omission of initial /ð/
Clinician	Pulls the stimulus toward her; records the response.	No corrective feedback

Administer the modeled baserate trials only after completing the evoked trials on all 20 (or more) exemplars.

Scripts for Modeled Baserate Trial		Note
Clinician	[*stimulus:* printed word *than*] "This word is *than*. Say, *than*."	Modeled trial
Child	"Than."	Correct response
Clinician	Pulls the stimulus toward her; records the response.	No reinforcement
Clinician	[*stimulus:* printed word *that*] "This word is *that*. Say, that."	The next modeled trial
Child	"at."	Omission of initial /ð/
Clinician	Pulls the stimulus toward her; records the response.	No corrective feedback

Use the recording sheet with exemplars shown on the next page to establish the baserates; print it from the CD.

/ð/ in Word-Initial Positions

Baserate Exemplars and Recording Sheet

Use stimuli from the **Stimulus Book,** *Volume 4.*

Print this page from the CD or photocopy this page for your clinical use.

Name/Age:	Date:
Goal: To establish the baserate production of /ð/ in word-initial positions.	Clinician:

Scoring: Correct: ✓   Incorrect or no response: X

/ð/ in word-initial positions	Evoked	Modeled
1. than		
2. that		
3. this		
4. theirs		
5. these		
6. themselves		
7. therefore		
8. thereafter		
9. thereabout		
10. thereby		
11. they		
12. those		
13. there		
14. them		
15. then		
16. thus		
17. though		
18. thereupon		
19. thereafter		
20. thenceforth		
Percent correct baserate		

Replace or add new exemplars as you see fit for a given child. After establishing the baserates, begin production teaching. Follow the protocols given on the next page.

/ð/ in Word-Initial Positions

Treatment Protocols

Use stimuli from the **Stimulus Book,** *Volume 4..*

Teach 6 to 8 exemplars using the following script.

Place a relevant stimulus in front of the child (an object, a picture, or a printed word) and ask a question as you point to the stimulus.

Scripts for Modeled Discrete Trial Training		Note
Clinician	[*stimulus:* printed word *than*] "This word is *than.* Say, **th***an.*"	Modeling; the target vocally emphasized
Child	"an."	A wrong response
Clinician	"No. That's not correct. You said *an,* but it's **th***an.*"	Corrective feedback
Clinician	[*the same stimulus*] "This word is *than.* Say, *than.*" Don't forget the ð sound at the beginning."	The next trial
Child	"Than."	A correct response
Clinician	"Excellent! You didn't miss the ð sound this time!"	Verbal praise

Repeat the trials until the child gives 5 consecutively correct, imitated responses.

When the child imitates 5 correct responses in sequence, fade the modeling.

Scripts for Fading the Modeling		Note
Clinician	[*stimulus:* printed word *than*] "What word is this? Don't forget the ð sound at the beginning."	Only a prompt
Child	"an."	A wrong response
Clinician	"Gee, you forgot the ð sound! It's *than,* not *an.* Put the ð sound at the beginning."	Corrective feedback
Clinician	[*the same stimulus*] "What word is this? It starts with . . . " [*silently models the posture for the target sound.*]	The next trial; a partial modeling
Child	"Than."	A correct response
Clinician	"That's great! You said *than,* not *an.*"	Verbal praise
Clinician	[*the same stimulus*] "What word is this?"	Typical question; evoked trial
Child	"Than."	A correct response
Clinician	"Great job! You said it correctly!"	Verbal praise

If the wrong responses persist on 4 to 5 evoked trials, reinstate partial or full modeling for a few trials, again fade the modeling, and re-present the evoked trials.

When the child meets the tentative learning criterion of 10 consecutively correct, nonimitated responses for a given stimulus item, move on to the next stimulus item. With this procedure, teach 6 to 8 exemplars shown on the following recording sheet. Use different exemplars as you see fit for a given child.

/ð/ in Word-Initial Positions

Treatment Exemplars and Recording Sheet

Use stimuli from the **Stimulus Book, Volume 4.**

Print this page from CD or photocopy this page for your clinical use.

Name/Age:	Date:
Goal: Production of /ð/ in word-initial positions with 90% accuracy when asked an evoking question while showing a stimulus.	Clinician:

Scoring: Correct: ✓   Incorrect or no response: X

Target skills	Discrete Trials														
	1	2	3	4	5	6	7	8	9	10	11	12	13	14	15
1. than															
2. that															
3. this															
4. theirs															
5. these															
6. themselves															
7. therefore															
8. thereafter															

When the child has met the learning criterion of 10 consecutively correct evoked (nonimitated) responses for each of the 6 to 8 target exemplars, conduct a probe to see if the production has generalized to previously baserated but untrained exemplars.

If the probes do not meet the 90% correct criterion for untrained exemplars, teach additional exemplars and then probe again.

/ð/ in Word-Initial Positions

Probe Protocols and Recording Sheet

Use stimuli from the **Stimulus Book, Volume 4**.

Print this page from the CD or photocopy this page for your clinical use.

On the probes, present only the untrained exemplars (UT). When the child fails to meet the 90% correct probe criterion, either teach 2 to 4 new exemplars or give additional training trials on already trained stimuli. If needed, select new exemplars for probes. Probe at least 10 untrained exemplars. Alternate probes and treatment until the probe criterion is met.

Scripts for Probe Trials		Note
Clinician	[*untrained stimulus*: printed word *thereabout*] "What word is this?" [*for a nonreader*] "This word is *thereabout*. What word is this?"	No modeling or prompts
Child	"Thereabout."	A correct, generalized response
Clinician	Scores the response as correct.	No reinforcement
Clinician	[*untrained stimulus*: a printed word *thereby*] "What word is this?" [*for a nonreader*] "This word is *thereby*. What word is this?"	The second probe trial
Child	"erby."	A wrong probe response
Clinician	Scores the response as incorrect.	No corrective feedback

Name:	Date:	Session #:
Age:	Clinician:	
Diagnosis: Articulation/Phonologic Disorder	Word-initial /ð/ probe	
Untrained Stimuli	Score: + correct; – incorrect or no responses	
1. thereabout		
2. thereby		
3. they		
4. those		
5. there		
6. them		
7. then		
8. thus		
9. though		
10. thereupon		
11. thereafter		
12. thenceforth		
Percent correct: (Criterion: 90%)		

If the child does not meet the probe criterion, give additional training on already trained exemplars or teach a few new exemplars. Subsequently, readminister the probe trials. When the child meets the 90% correct probe criterion for the exemplars, shift training to the sentence or conversational level or to another phoneme.

/ð/ in Word-Final Positions

Baserate Protocols

Use stimuli from the **Stimulus Book,** *Volume 4.*

Functional words that end with /ð/ are few in English. Most are not picturable. For children who read, printed word stimuli are a practical means of evoking this sound. For children who do not read, the clinician names the printed stimulus and then asks the question.

At the beginning of each trial, place a relevant stimulus (an object, a picture, or a printed word) in front of the child. Point to the stimulus as you ask an evoking question. Do not respond in any way to the child's correct, incorrect, or lack of responses.

Scripts for Evoked Baserate Trial		Note
Clinician	[*stimulus:* breathe *for a child who reads*] "Please read this word." [*for a nonreader*] "This word is *breathe*. What word is this?"	Evoked trial
Child	"bree."	Omission of final /ð/
Clinician	Pulls the stimulus toward her; records the response.	No corrective feedback
Clinician	[*stimulus: smooth*] "Is this smooth or rough?"	The next evoked trial
Child	"smoo."	Omission of final/ð/
Clinician	Pulls the stimulus toward her; records the response.	No corrective feedback

Administer the modeled baserate trials only after completing the evoked trials on all 20 (or more) exemplars.

Scripts for Modeled Baserate Trial		Note
Clinician	[*stimulus: printed word* breathe] "This word is breathe. Say, *breathe*."	Modeled trial
Child	"Breathe."	Correct response
Clinician	Pulls the stimulus toward her; records the response.	No reinforcement
Clinician	[*stimulus: smooth*] "Is this smooth or rough? Say, *smooth*."	The next modeled trial
Child	"smoo."	Omission of final /ð/
Clinician	Pulls the stimulus toward her; records the response.	No corrective feedback

Use the recording sheet with exemplars shown on the next page to establish the baserates; print it from the CD.

/ð/ in Word-Final Positions

Baserate Exemplars and Recording Sheet

Use stimuli from the **Stimulus Book,** *Volume 4.*

Print this page from the CD or photocopy this page for your clinical use.

Name/Age:	Date:
Goal: To establish the baserate production of /ð/ in word-final positions.	Clinician:

Scoring: Correct: ✓   Incorrect or no response: X

/ð/ in word-final positions	Evoked	Modeled
1. breathe		
2. smooth		
3. loathe		
4. lathe		
5. clothe		
6. bathe		
7. seethe		
8. soothe		
9. teethe		
10. sunbathe		
11. scathe		
12. tithe		
13. scythe		
14. swathe		
15. sheathe		
16. wreathe		
17. writhe		
18. re-bathe		
19. unsheathe		
20. unswathe		
Percent correct baserate		

Replace or add new exemplars as you see fit for a given child. After establishing the baserates, begin production teaching. Follow the protocols given on the next page.

/ð/ in Word-Final Positions

Treatment Protocols

Use stimuli from the **Stimulus Book, Volume 4**.

Teach 6 to 8 exemplars using the following script.

Place a relevant stimulus (an object, a picture, or a printed word) in front of the child and point to the stimulus as you ask an evoking question. To teach and evoke a target word the child does not know, model it a few times while pointing to the picture or the printed word at the beginning of treatment trials.

Scripts for Modeled Discrete Trial Training		Note
Clinician	[*stimulus:* printed word *breathe*] "This word is *breathe*. Say, brea**the**."	Modeling; the target vocally emphasized
Child	"bree."	A wrong response
Clinician	"No. That's not correct. You said bree, but it's brea**the**."	Corrective feedback
Clinician	[*the same stimulus*] "What word is this? Say, brea**the**. Don't forget the ð sound at the end."	The next trial
Child	"Breathe."	A correct response
Clinician	"Excellent! You didn't miss the ð sound at the end of the word!"	Verbal praise

Repeat the trials until the child gives 5 consecutively correct, imitated responses.

When the child imitates 5 correct responses in sequence, fade the modeling.

Scripts for Fading the Modeling		Note
Clinician	[*stimulus:* printed word *breathe*] "What word is this? Don't forget the ð sound at the end."	Only a prompt
Child	"bree."	A wrong response
Clinician	"Oh no! you forgot the ð sound at the end! It's *breathe*, not *bree*. Put the ð sound at the end."	Corrective feedback
Clinician	[*the same stimulus*] "What word is this? It ends with . . . " [*silently models the tongue posture for the target sound.*]	The next trial; a partial modeling
Child	"Breathe."	A correct response
Clinician	"That's great! You said *breathe*, not *bree*."	Verbal praise
Clinician	[*the same stimulus*] "What is this?"	Typical question; evoked trial
Child	"Breathe."	A correct response
Clinician	"I like it! You said it correctly!"	Verbal praise

If the wrong responses persist on 4 to 5 evoked trials, reinstate partial or full modeling for a few trials, again fade the modeling, and re-present the evoked trials.

When the child meets the tentative learning criterion of 10 consecutively correct, nonimitated responses for a given stimulus item, move on to the next stimulus item. With this procedure, teach 6 to 8 exemplars shown on the following recording sheet. Use different exemplars as you see fit for a given child.

/ð/ in Word-Final Positions

Treatment Exemplars and Recording Sheet

*Use stimuli from the **Stimulus Book, Volume 4.***

Print this page from CD or photocopy this page for your clinical use.

Name/Age:	Date:
Goal: Production of /ð/ in word-final positions with 90% accuracy when asked an evoking question while showing a stimulus.	Clinician:

Scoring: Correct: ✓   Incorrect or no response: X

Target skills	Discrete Trials														
	1	2	3	4	5	6	7	8	9	10	11	12	13	14	15
1. breathe															
2. smooth															
3. loathe															
4. lathe															
5. clothe															
6. bathe															
7. seethe															
8. soothe															

When the child has met the learning criterion of 10 consecutively correct evoked (nonimitated) responses for each of the 6 to 8 target exemplars, conduct a probe to see if the production has generalized to previously baserated but untrained exemplars.

If the probes do not meet the 90% correct criterion for untrained exemplars, teach additional exemplars and then probe again.

/ð/ in Word-Final Positions

Probe Protocols and Recording Sheet

Use stimuli from the **Stimulus Book, Volume 4**.

Print this page from the CD or photocopy this page for your clinical use.

On the probes, present only the untrained exemplars (UT). When the child fails to meet the 90% correct probe criterion, either teach 2 to 4 new exemplars or give additional training trials on already trained stimuli. If needed, select new exemplars for probes. Probe at least 10 untrained exemplars. Alternate probes and treatment until the probe criterion is met.

Scripts for Probe Trials		Note
Clinician	[*untrained stimulus:* printed word *teethe*] "What word is this?" [*for a nonreader*] "This word is *teethe*. What word is this?"	No modeling or prompts
Child	"Teethe."	A correct, generalized response
Clinician	Scores the response as correct.	No reinforcement
Clinician	[*untrained stimulus:* printed word: *sunbathe*] "What word is this?" [*for a nonreader*] "This word is *sunbathe*. What word is this?"	The second probe trial
Child	"sunbɛ."	A wrong probe response
Clinician	Scores the response as incorrect.	No corrective feedback

Name:	Date:	Session #:
Age:	**Clinician:**	
Diagnosis: Articulation/Phonologic Disorder	**Word-final /ð/probe**	
Untrained Stimuli	**Score: + correct; – incorrect or no responses**	
1. teethe		
2. sunbathe		
3. scathe		
4. tithe		
5. scythe		
6. swathe		
7. sheathe		
8. wreathe		
9. writhe		
10. re-bathe		
11. unsheathe		
12. unswathe		
Percent correct: (Criterion: 90%)		

If the child does not meet the probe criterion, give additional training on already trained exemplars or teach a few new exemplars. Subsequently, readminister the probe trials. When the child meets the 90% correct probe criterion for the exemplars, shift training to the sentence or conversational level or to another phoneme.

/s/ in Word-Initial Positions

Baserate Protocols

Use stimuli from the **Stimulus Book, Volume 1**.

At the beginning of each trial, place a relevant stimulus (an object, a picture, or a printed word) in front of the child. Point to the stimulus as you ask an evoking question. Do not respond in any way to the child's correct, incorrect, or lack of responses.

Scripts for Evoked Baserate Trial		Note
Clinician	[*stimulus: sack*] "What is this?"	Evoked trial
Child	"æk."	Omission of initial /s/
Clinician	Pulls the stimulus toward her; records the response.	No corrective feedback
Clinician	[*stimulus: sand*] "What do you call this?"	The next evoked trial
Child	"and."	Omission of initial /s/
Clinician	Pulls the stimulus toward her; records the response	No corrective feedback

Administer the modeled baserate trials only after completing the evoked trials on all 20 (or more) exemplars.

Scripts for Modeled Baserate Trial		Note
Clinician	[*stimulus: sack*] "What is this? Say, *sack.*"	Modeled trial
Child	"Sack."	Correct response
Clinician	Pulls the stimulus toward her; records the response.	No reinforcement
Clinician	[*stimulus: sand*] "What is this? Say, *sand.*"	The next modeled trial
Child	"and."	Omission of initial /s/
Clinician	Pulls the stimulus toward her; records the response.	No corrective feedback

Use the recording sheet with exemplars shown on the next page to establish the baserates; print it from the CD.

/s/ in Word-Initial Positions

Baserate Exemplars and Recording Sheet

Use stimuli from the **Stimulus Book,** *Volume 1.*

Print this page from the CD or photocopy this page for your clinical use.

Name/Age:	Date:
Goal: To establish the baserate production of /s/ in word-initial positions.	Clinician:

Scoring: Correct: ✓   Incorrect or no response: X

/s/ in word-initial positions	Evoked	Modeled
1. sack		
2. sand		
3. seal		
4. sink		
5. sun		
6. sailboat		
7. sausage		
8. saddle		
9. sandpaper		
10. sandwich		
11. soup		
12. sock		
13. salt		
14. sofa		
15. six		
16. saxophone		
17. seaplane		
18. safari		
19. satellite		
20. sunflower		
Percent correct baserate		

Replace or add new exemplars as you see fit for a given child. After establishing the baserates, begin production teaching. Follow the protocols given on the next page.

/s/ in Word-Initial Positions

Treatment Protocols

Use stimuli from the **Stimulus Book, Volume 1**.

Teach 6 to 8 exemplars using the following script.

Place a relevant stimulus in front of the child (an object, a picture, or a printed word) and ask a question as you point to the stimulus.

Scripts for Modeled Discrete Trial Training		Note
Clinician	[*stimulus: sack*] "What is this? Say, **s**ack."	Modeling; the target vocally emphasized
Child	"æk."	A wrong response
Clinician	"No. That's not correct. You said *æk*, but it's **s**ack."	Corrective feedback
Clinician	[*the same stimulus*] "What is this? Say, **s**ack. Don't forget the *s* sound at the beginning."	The next trial
Child	"Sack."	A correct response
Clinician	"Excellent! You didn't miss the s this time!"	Verbal praise

Repeat the trials until the child gives 5 consecutively correct, imitated responses.

When the child imitates 5 correct responses in sequence, fade the modeling.

Scripts for Fading the Modeling		Note
Clinician	[*stimulus: sack*] "What is this? Don't forget the *s* sound at the beginning."	Only a prompt
Child	"æk."	A wrong response
Clinician	"Oh no! You forgot the *s* sound! It's a *sack*, not *æk*. Put the *s* sound at the beginning."	Corrective feedback
Clinician	[*the same stimulus*] "What is this? It starts with . . . " [*silently models the tongue posture for the target sound.*]	The next trial; a partial modeling
Child	"Sack."	A correct response
Clinician	"That's great! You said *sack*, not *æk*."	Verbal praise
Clinician	[*the same stimulus*] "What is this?"	Typical question; evoked trial
Child	"Sack."	A correct response
Clinician	"Great job! You are doing very well!"	Verbal praise

If the wrong responses persist on 4 to 5 evoked trials, reinstate partial or full modeling for a few trials, again fade the modeling, and re-present the evoked trials.

When the child meets the tentative learning criterion of 10 consecutively correct, nonimitated responses for a given stimulus item, move on to the next stimulus item. With this procedure, teach 6 to 8 exemplars shown on the following recording sheet. Use different exemplars as you see fit for a given child.

/s/ in Word-Initial Positions

Treatment Exemplars and Recording Sheet

*Use stimuli from the **Stimulus Book, Volume 1**.*

Print this page from CD or photocopy this page for your clinical use.

Name/Age:	Date:
Goal: Production of /s/ in word-initial positions with 90% accuracy when asked an evoking question while showing a stimulus.	Clinician:

Scoring: Correct: ✓   Incorrect or no response: X

Target skills	Discrete Trials														
	1	2	3	4	5	6	7	8	9	10	11	12	13	14	15
1. sack															
2. sand															
3. seal															
4. sink															
5. sun															
6. sailboat															
7. sausage															
8. saddle															

When the child has met the learning criterion of 10 consecutively correct evoked (nonimitated) responses for each of the 6 to 8 target exemplars, conduct a probe to see if the production has generalized to previously baserated but untrained exemplars.

If the probes do not meet the 90% correct criterion for untrained exemplars, teach additional exemplars and then probe again.

/s/ in Word-Initial Positions

Probe Protocols and Recording Sheet

Use stimuli from the **Stimulus Book,** *Volume 1.*

Print this page from the CD or photocopy this page for your clinical use.

On the probes, present only the untrained exemplars (UT). When the child fails to meet the 90% correct probe criterion, either teach 2 to 4 new exemplars or give additional training trials on already trained stimuli. If needed, select new exemplars for probes. Probe at least 10 untrained exemplars. Alternate probes and treatment until the probe criterion is met.

Scripts for Probe Trials		Note
Clinician	[*untrained stimulus: sandpaper*] "What is this?"	No modeling or prompts
Child	"Sandpaper."	A correct, generalized response
Clinician	Scores the response as correct.	No reinforcement
Clinician	[*untrained stimulus: sandwich*] "What is this?"	The second probe trial
Child	"andwich."	A wrong probe response
Clinician	Scores the response as incorrect.	No corrective feedback

Name:	Date:	Session #:
Age:	**Clinician:**	
Diagnosis: Articulation/Phonologic Disorder	**Word-initial /s/ probe**	
Untrained Stimuli	**Score: + correct; – incorrect or no responses**	
1. sandpaper		
2. sandwich		
3. soup		
4. sock		
5. salt		
6. sofa		
7. six		
8. saxophone		
9. seaplane		
10. safari		
11. satellite		
12. sunflower		
Percent correct: (Criterion: 90%)		

If the child does not meet the probe criterion, give additional training on already trained exemplars or teach a few new exemplars. Subsequently, readminister the probe trials. When the child meets the 90% correct probe criterion for the exemplars, shift training to the sentence or conversational level or to another phoneme.

/s/ in Word-Final Positions

Baserate Protocols

Use stimuli from the **Stimulus Book, *Volume 1***.

At the beginning of each trial, place a relevant stimulus (an object, a picture, or a printed word) in front of the child. Point to the stimulus as you ask an evoking question. Do not respond in any way to the child's correct, incorrect, or lack of responses.

Scripts for Evoked Baserate Trial		Note
Clinician	[*stimulus: bus*] "What is this?"	Evoked
Child	"bə."	Omission of final /s/
Clinician	Pulls the stimulus toward her; records the response.	No corrective feedback
Clinician	[*stimulus: goose*] "What is this?"	The next evoked trial
Child	"goo."	Omission of final/s/
Clinician	Pulls the stimulus toward her; records the response	No corrective feedback

Administer the modeled baserate trials only after completing the evoked trials on all 20 (or more) exemplars.

Scripts for Modeled Baserate Trial		Note
Clinician	[*stimulus: bus*] "What is this? Say, *bus.*"	Modeled trial
Child	"Bus."	Correct response
Clinician	Pulls the stimulus toward her; records the response.	No reinforcement
Clinician	[*stimulus: goose*] "What is this? Say, *goose.*"	The next modeled trial
Child	"goo."	Omission of final /s/
Clinician	Pulls the stimulus toward her; records the response.	No corrective feedback

Use the recording sheet with exemplars shown on the next page to establish the baserates; print it from the CD.

/s/ in Word-Final Positions

Baserate Exemplars and Recording Sheet

Use stimuli from the **Stimulus Book, Volume 1**.

Print this page from the CD or photocopy this page for your clinical use.

Name/Age:	Date:
Goal: To establish the baserate production of /s/ in word-final positions.	Clinician:

Scoring: Correct: ✓   Incorrect or no response: X

/s/ in word-final positions	Evoked	Modeled
1. bus		
2. goose		
3. dice		
4. lace		
5. mice		
6. lettuce		
7. necklace		
8. fireplace		
9. doghouse		
10. octopus		
11. face		
12. ice		
13. rice		
14. house		
15. ace		
16. hippopotamus		
17. lioness		
18. dangerous		
19. delicious		
20. asparagus		
Percent correct baserate		

Replace or add new exemplars as you see fit for a given child. After establishing the baserates, begin production teaching. Follow the protocols given on the next page.

/s/ in Word-Final Positions

Treatment Protocols

Use stimuli from the **Stimulus Book,** *Volume 1.*

Teach 6 to 8 exemplars using the following script.

Place a relevant stimulus (an object, a picture, or a printed word) in front of the child and point to the stimulus as you ask an evoking question.

Scripts for Modeled Discrete Trial Training		Note
Clinician	[*stimulus: bus*] "What is this? Say, *bus.*"	Modeling; the target vocally emphasized
Child	"bə."	A wrong response
Clinician	"No. That's not correct. You said bə, but it's a *bus.*"	Corrective feedback
Clinician	[*the same stimulus*] "What is this? Say, *bus.* Don't forget the *s* sound at the end."	The next trial
Child	"Bus."	A correct response
Clinician	"That's super! You didn't miss the *s* sound at the end of the word!"	Verbal praise

Repeat the trials until the child gives 5 consecutively correct, imitated responses.

When the child imitates 5 correct responses in sequence, fade the modeling.

Scripts for Fading the Modeling		Note
Clinician	[*stimulus: bus*] "What is this? Don't forget the *s* sound at the end."	Only a prompt
Child	"bə."	A wrong response
Clinician	"Gee, you forgot the *s* sound! It's a *bus*, not bə. Put the *s* at the end."	Corrective feedback
Clinician	[*the same stimulus*] "What is this? It ends with . . . " [*silently models the tongue posture for the target sound.*]	The next trial; a partial modeling
Child	"Bus."	A correct response
Clinician	"That's great! You said *bus*, not bə."	Verbal praise
Clinician	[*the same stimulus*] "What is this?"	Typical question; evoked trial
Child	"Bus."	A correct response
Clinician	"You are wonderful! You got it right!"	Verbal praise

If the wrong responses persist on 4 to 5 evoked trials, reinstate partial or full modeling for a few trials, again fade the modeling, and re-present the evoked trials.

When the child meets the tentative learning criterion of 10 consecutively correct, nonimitated responses for a given stimulus item, move on to the next stimulus item. With this procedure, teach 6 to 8 exemplars shown on the following recording sheet. Use different exemplars as you see fit for a given child.

/s/ in Word-Final Positions
Treatment Exemplars and Recording Sheet

*Use stimuli from the **Stimulus Book, Volume 1**.*

Print this page from CD or photocopy this page for your clinical use.

Name/Age:	Date:
Goal: Production of /s/ in word-final positions with 90% accuracy when asked an evoking question while showing a stimulus.	Clinician:

Scoring: Correct: ✓ Incorrect or no response: X

Target skills	Discrete Trials														
	1	2	3	4	5	6	7	8	9	10	11	12	13	14	15
1. bus															
2. goose															
3. dice															
4. lace															
5. mice															
6. lettuce															
7. necklace															
8. fireplace															

When the child has met the learning criterion of 10 consecutively correct evoked (nonimitated) responses for each of the 6 to 8 target exemplars, conduct a probe to see if the production has generalized to previously baserated but untrained exemplars.

If the probes do not meet the 90% correct criterion for untrained exemplars, teach additional exemplars and then probe again.

/s/ in Word-Final Positions

Probe Protocols and Recording Sheet

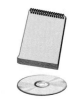

Use stimuli from the **Stimulus Book,** *Volume 1*.

Print this page from the CD or photocopy this page for your clinical use.

On the probes, present only the untrained exemplars (UT). When the child fails to meet the 90% correct probe criterion, either teach 2 to 4 new exemplars or give additional training trials on already trained stimuli. If needed, select new exemplars for probes. Probe at least 10 untrained exemplars. Alternate probes and treatment until the probe criterion is met.

Scripts for Probe Trials		Note
Clinician	[*untrained stimulus: doghouse*] "What is this?"	No modeling or prompts
Child	"Doghouse."	A correct, generalized response
Clinician	Scores the response as correct.	No reinforcement
Clinician	[*untrained stimulus: octopus*] "What is this?"	The second probe trial
Child	"octopə."	A wrong probe response
Clinician	Scores the response as incorrect.	No corrective feedback

Name:	Date:	Session #:
Age:	**Clinician:**	
Diagnosis: Articulation/Phonologic Disorder	**Word-final /s/probe**	
Untrained Stimuli	**Score: + correct; – incorrect or no responses**	
1. doghouse		
2. octopus		
3. face		
4. ice		
5. rice		
6. house		
7. ace		
8. hippopotamus		
9. lioness		
10. dangerous		
11. delicious		
12. asparagus		
Percent correct: (Criterion: 90%)		

If the child does not meet the probe criterion, give additional training on already trained exemplars or teach a few new exemplars. Subsequently, readminister the probe trials. When the child meets the 90% correct probe criterion for the exemplars, shift training to the sentence or conversational level or to another phoneme.

/z/ in Word-Initial Positions

Baserate Protocols

Use stimuli from the **Stimulus Book, Volume 1**.

At the beginning of each trial, place a relevant stimulus (an object, a picture, or a printed word) in front of the child. Point to the stimulus as you ask an evoking question. Do not respond in any way to the child's correct, incorrect, or lack of responses.

Scripts for Evoked Baserate Trial		Note
Clinician	[*stimulus: zoo*] "What is this?"	Evoked trial
Child	"oo."	Omission of initial /z/
Clinician	Pulls the stimulus toward her; records the response.	No corrective feedback
Clinician	[*stimulus: zebra*] "What is this?"	The next evoked trial
Child	"ebra."	Omission of initial /z/
Clinician	Pulls the stimulus toward her; records the response.	No corrective feedback

Administer the modeled baserate trials only after completing the evoked trials on all 20 (or more) exemplars.

Scripts for Modeled Baserate Trial		Note
Clinician	[*stimulus: zoo*] "What is this? Say, *zoo*."	Modeled trial
Child	"Zoo."	Correct response
Clinician	Pulls the stimulus toward her; records the response.	No reinforcement
Clinician	[*stimulus: zebra*] "What is this? Say, *zebra*."	The next modeled trial
Child	"ebra."	Omission of initial /z/
Clinician	Pulls the stimulus toward her; records the response.	No corrective feedback

Use the recording sheet with exemplars shown on the next page to establish the baserates; print it from the CD.

/z/ in Word-Initial Positions

Baserate Exemplars and Recording Sheet

Use stimuli from the **Stimulus Book,** *Volume 1.*

Print this page from the CD or photocopy this page for your clinical use.

Name/Age:	Date:
Goal: To establish the baserate production of /z/ in word-initial positions.	Clinician:

Scoring: Correct: ✓   Incorrect or no response: X

/z/ in word-initial positions	Evoked	Modeled
1. zoo		
2. zebra		
3. zero		
4. ziti		
5. zebu		
6. zigzag		
7. zinnia		
8. zipper		
9. zither		
10. zebrawood		
11. zee (alphabet)		
12. zany		
13. zori		
14. zone		
15. zeppelin		
16. zombie		
17. ZIP code		
18. zookeeper		
19. zucchini		
20. xylophone		
Percent correct baserate		

Replace or add new exemplars as you see fit for a given child. After establishing the baserates, begin production teaching. Follow the protocols given on the next page.

/z/ in Word-Initial Positions

Treatment Protocols

Use stimuli from the **Stimulus Book,** *Volume 1.*

Teach 6 to 8 exemplars using the following script.

Place a relevant stimulus in front of the child (an object, a picture, or a printed word) and ask a question as you point to the stimulus.

Scripts for Modeled Discrete Trial Training		Note
Clinician	[*stimulus: zoo*] "What is this? Say, **zoo**."	Modeling; the target vocally emphasized
Child	"oo."	A wrong response
Clinician	"No. That's not correct. You said *oo*, but it's a **zoo**."	Corrective feedback
Clinician	[*the same stimulus*] "What is this? Say, **zoo**. Don't forget the *z* sound at the beginning."	The next trial
Child	"Zoo."	A correct response
Clinician	"Excellent! You didn't miss the *z* this time!"	Verbal praise

Repeat the trials until the child gives 5 consecutively correct, imitated responses.

When the child imitates 5 correct responses in sequence, fade the modeling.

Scripts for Fading the Modeling		Note
Clinician	[*stimulus: zoo*] "What is this? Don't forget the *z* sound at the beginning."	Only a prompt
Child	"oo."	A wrong response
Clinician	"Gee, you forgot the *z* sound! It's a *zoo*, not *oo*. Put the *z* sound at the beginning."	Corrective feedback
Clinician	[*the same stimulus*] "What is this? It starts with . . . " [*silently models the articulatory posture for the target sound.*]	The next trial; a partial modeling
Child	"Zoo."	A correct response
Clinician	"That's great! You said *zoo*, not *oo*."	Verbal praise
Clinician	[*the same stimulus*] "What is this?"	Typical question; evoked trial
Child	"Zoo."	A correct response
Clinician	"Great job! You said it correctly!"	Verbal praise

If the wrong responses persist on 4 to 5 evoked trials, reinstate partial or full modeling for a few trials, again fade the modeling, and re-present the evoked trials.

When the child meets the tentative learning criterion of 10 consecutively correct, nonimitated responses for a given stimulus item, move on to the next stimulus item. With this procedure, teach 6 to 8 exemplars shown on the following recording sheet. Use different exemplars as you see fit for a given child.

/z/ in Word-Initial Positions

Treatment Exemplars and Recording Sheet

Use stimuli from the **Stimulus Book,** *Volume 1*.

Print this page from CD or photocopy this page for your clinical use.

Name/Age:	Date:
Goal: Production of /z/ in word-initial positions with 90% accuracy when asked an evoking question while showing a stimulus.	Clinician:

Scoring: Correct: ✓   Incorrect or no response: X

Target skills	Discrete Trials														
	1	2	3	4	5	6	7	8	9	10	11	12	13	14	15
1. zoo															
2. zebra															
3. zero															
4. ziti															
5. zebu															
6. zigzag															
7. zinnia															
8. zipper															

When the child has met the learning criterion of 10 consecutively correct evoked (nonimitated) responses for each of the 6 to 8 target exemplars, conduct a probe to see if the production has generalized to previously baserated but untrained exemplars.

If the probes do not meet the 90% correct criterion for untrained exemplars, teach additional exemplars and then probe again.

/z/ in Word-Initial Positions

Probe Protocols and Recording Sheet

Use stimuli from the **Stimulus Book, Volume 1**.

Print this page from the CD or photocopy this page for your clinical use.

On the probes, present only the untrained exemplars (UT). When the child fails to meet the 90% correct probe criterion, either teach 2 to 4 new exemplars or give additional training trials on already trained stimuli. If needed, select new exemplars for probes. Probe at least 10 untrained exemplars. Alternate probes and treatment until the probe criterion is met.

Scripts for Probe Trials		Note
Clinician	[*untrained stimulus: zither*] "This is called a zither. It's a musical instrument. What is this?"	No modeling or prompts
Child	"Zither."	A correct, generalized response
Clinician	Scores the response as correct.	No reinforcement
Clinician	[*untrained stimulus: zebrawood*] "This is called zebrawood. What is this?"	The second probe trial
Child	"ebrawood." [no response]	Both scored as incorrect
Clinician	Scores the response as incorrect.	No corrective feedback

Name:	Date:	Session #:
Age:	**Clinician:**	
Diagnosis: Articulation/Phonologic Disorder	**Word-initial /z/ probe**	
Untrained Stimuli	**Score: + correct; – incorrect or no responses**	
1. zither [a stringed musical instrument]		
2. zebrawood		
3. zee (the letter z)		
4. zany		
5. zori		
6. zone		
7. zeppelin		
8. zombie		
9. ZIP code		
10. zookeeper		
11. zucchini		
12. xylophone		
Percent correct: (Criterion: 90%)		

If the child does not meet the probe criterion, give additional training on already trained exemplars or teach a few new exemplars. Subsequently, readminister the probe trials. When the child meets the 90% correct probe criterion for the exemplars, shift training to the sentence or conversational level or to another phoneme.

/z/ in Word-Final Positions

Baserate Protocols

Use stimuli from the **Stimulus Book,** *Volume 1.*

At the beginning of each trial, place a relevant stimulus (an object, a picture, or a printed word) in front of the child. Point to the stimulus as you ask an evoking question. Do not respond in any way to the child's correct, incorrect, or lack of responses.

Scripts for Evoked Baserate Trial		Note
Clinician	[*stimulus: bees*] "What is this?"	Evoked trial
Child	"bee."	Omission of final /z/
Clinician	Pulls the stimulus toward her; records the response.	No corrective feedback
Clinician	[*stimulus: boys*] "What is this?"	The next evoked trial
Child	"boy."	Omission of final /z/
Clinician	Pulls the stimulus toward her; records the response.	No corrective feedback

Administer the modeled baserate trials only after completing the evoked trials on all 20 (or more) exemplars.

Scripts for Modeled Baserate Trial		Note
Clinician	[*stimulus: bees*] "What is this? Say, *bees.*"	Modeled trial
Child	"Bees."	Correct response
Clinician	Pulls the stimulus toward her; records the response.	No reinforcement
Clinician	[*stimulus: boys*] "What is this? Say, *boys.*"	The next modeled trial
Child	"boy."	Omission of final /z/
Clinician	Pulls the stimulus toward her; records the response	No corrective feedback

Use the recording sheet with exemplars shown on the next page to establish the baserates; print it from the CD.

/z/ in Word-Final Positions

Baserate Exemplars and Recording Sheet

Use stimuli from the **Stimulus Book,** *Volume 1*.

Print this page from the CD or photocopy this page for your clinical use.

Name/Age:	Date:
Goal: To establish the baserate production of /z/ in word-final positions.	Clinician:

Scoring: Correct: ✓   Incorrect or no response: X

/z/ in word-final positions	Evoked	Modeled
1. bees		
2. boys		
3. cheese		
4. hose		
5. rose		
6. exercise		
7. bananas		
8. batteries		
9. groceries		
10. strawberries		
11. guys		
12. dogs		
13. balls		
14. bags		
15. nose		
16. mayonnaise		
17. tomatoes		
18. factories		
19. bumblebees		
20. potatoes		
Percent correct baserate		

Replace or add new exemplars as you see fit for a given child. After establishing the baserates, begin production teaching. Follow the protocols given on the next page.

/z/ in Word-Final Positions

Treatment Protocols

Use stimuli from the **Stimulus Book, Volume 1.**

Teach 6 to 8 exemplars using the following script.

Place a relevant stimulus (an object, a picture, or a printed word) in front of the child and point to the stimulus as you ask an evoking question.

Scripts for Modeled Discrete Trial Training		Note
Clinician	[*stimulus: bees*] "What is this? Say, *bees.*"	Modeling; the target vocally emphasized
Child	"bee."	A wrong response
Clinician	"No. That's not correct. You said *bee*, but it's *bees.*"	Corrective feedback
Clinician	[*the same stimulus*] "What is this? Say, *bees.* Don't forget the *z* sound at the end."	The next trial
Child	"Bees."	A correct response
Clinician	"Excellent! You didn't miss the *z* sound at the end of the word!"	Verbal praise

Repeat the trials until the child gives 5 consecutively correct, imitated responses.

When the child imitates 5 correct responses in sequence, fade the modeling.

Scripts for Fading the Modeling		Note
Clinician	[*stimulus: bees*] "What is this? Don't forget the *z* at the end."	Only a prompt
Child	"bee."	A wrong response
Clinician	"Gee, you forgot the *z* sound! It's *bees*, not *bee*. Put the *z* at the end."	Corrective feedback
Clinician	[*the same stimulus*] "What is this? It ends with . . . " [*silently models the articulatory posture for the target sound.*]	The next trial; a partial modeling
Child	"bees."	A correct response
Clinician	"That's great! You said *bees*, not *bee*."	Verbal praise
Clinician	[*the same stimulus*] "What is this?"	Typical question; evoked trial
Child	"Bees."	A correct response
Clinician	"You are super! You said it correctly!"	Verbal praise

If the wrong responses persist on 4 to 5 evoked trials, reinstate partial or full modeling for a few trials, again fade the modeling, and re-present the evoked trials.

When the child meets the tentative learning criterion of 10 consecutively correct, nonimitated responses for a given stimulus item, move on to the next stimulus item. With this procedure, teach 6 to 8 exemplars shown on the following recording sheet. Use different exemplars as you see fit for a given child.

/z/ in Word-Final Positions

Treatment Exemplars and Recording Sheet

Use stimuli from the **Stimulus Book, *Volume 1***.

Print this page from CD or photocopy this page for your clinical use.

Name/Age:	Date:
Goal: Production of /z/ in word-final positions with 90% accuracy when asked an evoking question while showing a stimulus.	Clinician:

Scoring: Correct: ✓ Incorrect or no response: X

Target skills	Discrete Trials														
	1	2	3	4	5	6	7	8	9	10	11	12	13	14	15
1. bees															
2. boys															
3. cheese															
4. hose															
5. rose															
6. exercise															
7. bananas															
8. batteries															

When the child has met the learning criterion of 10 consecutively correct evoked (nonimitated) responses for each of the 6 to 8 target exemplars, conduct a probe to see if the production has generalized to previously baserated but untrained exemplars.

If the probes do not meet the 90% correct criterion for untrained exemplars, teach additional exemplars and then probe again.

/z/ in Word-Final Positions

Probe Protocols and Recording Sheet

Use stimuli from the **Stimulus Book, Volume 1**.

Print this page from the CD or photocopy this page for your clinical use.

On the probes, present only the untrained exemplars (UT). When the child fails to meet the 90% correct probe criterion, either teach 2 to 4 new exemplars or give additional training trials on already trained stimuli. If needed, select new exemplars for probes. Probe at least 10 untrained exemplars. Alternate probes and treatment until the probe criterion is met.

Scripts for Probe Trials		Note
Clinician	[untrained stimulus: groceries] "What are these?"	No modeling or prompts
Child	"Groceries."	A correct, generalized response
Clinician	Scores the response as correct.	No reinforcement
Clinician	[untrained stimulus: strawberries] "What are these?"	The second probe trial
Child	"Strawberry."	A wrong probe response
Clinician	Scores the response as incorrect.	No corrective feedback

Name:	Date:	Session #:
Age:	**Clinician:**	
Diagnosis: Articulation/Phonologic Disorder	**Word-final /z/ probe**	
Untrained Stimuli	**Score: + correct; – incorrect or no responses**	
1. groceries		
2. strawberries		
3. guys		
4. dogs		
5. balls		
6. bags		
7. nose		
8. mayonnaise		
9. tomatoes		
10. factories		
11. bumblebees		
12. potatoes		
Percent correct: (Criterion: 90%)		

If the child does not meet the probe criterion, give additional training on already trained exemplars or teach a few new exemplars. Subsequently, readminister the probe trials. When the child meets the 90% correct probe criterion for the exemplars, shift training to the sentence or conversational level or to another phoneme.

/ʃ/ in Word-Initial Positions

Baserate Protocols

Use stimuli from the **Stimulus Book,** *Volume 2.*

At the beginning of each trial, place a relevant stimulus (an object, a picture, or a printed word) in front of the child. Point to the stimulus as you ask an evoking question. Do not respond in any way to the child's correct, incorrect, or lack of responses.

Scripts for Evoked Baserate Trial		Note
Clinician	[*stimulus: sheep*] "What is this?"	Evoked trial
Child	"eep."	Omission of initial /ʃ/
Clinician	Pulls the stimulus toward her; records the response.	No corrective feedback
Clinician	[*stimulus: ship*] "What is this?"	The next evoked trial
Child	"ip."	Omission of initial /ʃ/
Clinician	Pulls the stimulus toward her; records the response.	No corrective feedback

Administer the modeled baserate trials only after completing the evoked trials on all 20 (or more) exemplars.

Scripts for Modeled Baserate Trial		Note
Clinician	[*stimulus: sheep*] "What is this? Say, *sheep.*"	Modeled trial
Child	"sheep."	Correct response
Clinician	Pulls the stimulus toward her; records the response.	No reinforcement
Clinician	[*stimulus: ship*] "What is this? Say, *ship.*"	The next modeled trial
Child	"ip."	Omission of initial /ʃ/
Clinician	Pulls the stimulus toward her; records the response	No corrective feedback

Use the recording sheet with exemplars shown on the next page to establish the baserates; print it from the CD.

/ʃ/ in Word-Initial Positions

Baserate Exemplars and Recording Sheet

Use stimuli from the **Stimulus Book,** *Volume 2.*

Print this page from the CD or photocopy this page for your clinical use.

Name/Age:	Date:
Goal: To establish the baserate production of /ʃ/ in word-initial positions.	Clinician:

Scoring: Correct: ✓   Incorrect or no response: X

/ʃ/ in word-initial positions	Evoked	Modeled
1. sheep		
2. ship		
3. shop		
4. shoe		
5. shade		
6. shampoo		
7. sharpener		
8. shoulder		
9. chandelier		
10. shoelace		
11. sugar		
12. shirt		
13. shovel		
14. shield		
15. shelf		
16. shopkeeper		
17. shoemaker		
18. shipmaster		
19. sheepskin		
20. shortening		
Percent correct baserate		

Replace or add new exemplars as you see fit for a given child. After establishing the baserates, begin production teaching. Follow the protocols given on the next page.

/ʃ/ in Word-Initial Positions

Treatment Protocols

*Use stimuli from the **Stimulus Book, Volume 2**.*

Teach 6 to 8 exemplars using the following script.

Place a relevant stimulus in front of the child (an object, a picture, or a printed word) and ask a question as you point to the stimulus.

Scripts for Modeled Discrete Trial Training		Note
Clinician	[*stimulus: sheep*] "What is this? Say, **sheep**."	Modeling; the target vocally emphasized
Child	"eep."	A wrong response
Clinician	"No. That's not correct. You said *eep*, but it's **sheep**."	Corrective feedback
Clinician	[*the same stimulus*] "What is this? Say, **sheep**. Don't forget the ʃ sound at the beginning."	The next trial
Child	"Sheep."	A correct response
Clinician	"Excellent! You didn't miss the ʃ sound this time!"	Verbal praise

Repeat the trials until the child gives 5 consecutively correct, imitated responses.

When the child imitates 5 correct responses in sequence, fade the modeling.

Scripts for Fading the Modeling		Note
Clinician	[*stimulus: sheep*] "What is this? Don't forget the ʃ sound at the beginning."	Only a prompt
Child	"eep."	A wrong response
Clinician	"Gee, you forgot the ʃ sound! It's *sheep*, not *eep*. Put the ʃ sound at the beginning."	Corrective feedback
Clinician	[*the same stimulus*] "What is this? It starts with . . . " [*silently models the articulatory posture for the target sound.*]	The next trial; a partial modeling
Child	"Sheep."	A correct response
Clinician	"That's great! You said *sheep*, not *eep*."	Verbal praise
Clinician	[*the same stimulus*] "What is this?"	Typical question; evoked trial
Child	"Sheep."	A correct response
Clinician	"Great job! You said it correctly!"	Verbal praise

If the wrong responses persist on 4 to 5 evoked trials, reinstate partial or full modeling for a few trials, again fade the modeling, and re-present the evoked trials.

When the child meets the tentative learning criterion of 10 consecutively correct, nonimitated responses for a given stimulus item, move on to the next stimulus item. With this procedure, teach 6 to 8 exemplars shown on the following recording sheet. Use different exemplars as you see fit for a given child.

/ʃ/ in Word-Initial Positions

Treatment Exemplars and Recording Sheet

Use stimuli from the **Stimulus Book,** *Volume 2.*

Print this page from CD or photocopy this page for your clinical use.

Name/Age:	Date:
Goal: Production of /ʃ/ in word-initial positions with 90% accuracy when asked an evoking question while showing a stimulus.	Clinician:

Scoring: Correct: ✓ Incorrect or no response: X

Target skills	Discrete Trials														
	1	2	3	4	5	6	7	8	9	10	11	12	13	14	15
1. sheep															
2. ship															
3. shop															
4. shoe															
5. shade															
6. shampoo															
7. sharpener															
8. shoulder															

When the child has met the learning criterion of 10 consecutively correct evoked (nonimitated) responses for each of the 6 to 8 target exemplars, conduct a probe to see if the production has generalized to previously baserated but untrained exemplars.

If the probes do not meet the 90% correct criterion for untrained exemplars, teach additional exemplars and then probe again.

/ʃ/ in Word-Initial Positions

Probe Protocols and Recording Sheet

Use stimuli from the **Stimulus Book, Volume 2**.

Print this page from the CD or photocopy this page for your clinical use.

On the probes, present only the untrained exemplars (UT). When the child fails to meet the 90% correct probe criterion, either teach 2 to 4 new exemplars or give additional training trials on already trained stimuli. If needed, select new exemplars for probes. Probe at least 10 untrained exemplars. Alternate probes and treatment until the probe criterion is met.

Scripts for Probe Trials		Note
Clinician	[*untrained stimulus: chandelier*] "What is this?"	No modeling or prompts
Child	"Chandelier."	A correct, generalized response
Clinician	Scores the response as correct.	No reinforcement
Clinician	[*untrained stimulus: shoelace*] "What is this?"	The second probe trial
Child	"oolace."	A wrong probe response
Clinician	Scores the response as incorrect.	No corrective feedback

Name:	Date:	Session #:
Age:	**Clinician:**	
Diagnosis: Articulation/Phonologic Disorder	**Word-initial /ʃ/ probe**	
Untrained Stimuli	**Score: + correct; – incorrect or no responses**	
1. chandelier		
2. shoelace		
3. sugar		
4. shirt		
5. shovel		
6. shield		
7. shelf		
8. shopkeeper		
9. shoemaker		
10. shipmaster		
11. sheepskin		
12. shortening		
Percent correct: (Criterion: 90%)		

If the child does not meet the probe criterion, give additional training on already trained exemplars or teach a few new exemplars. Subsequently, readminister the probe trials. When the child meets the 90% correct probe criterion for the exemplars, shift training to the sentence or conversational level or to another phoneme.

/ʃ/ in Word-Final Positions

Baserate Protocols

Use stimuli from the **Stimulus Book,** *Volume 2.*

At the beginning of each trial, place a relevant stimulus (an object, a picture, or a printed word) in front of the child. Point to the stimulus as you ask an evoking question. Do not respond in any way to the child's correct, incorrect, or lack of responses.

Scripts for Evoked Baserate Trial		Note
Clinician	[*stimulus: dish*] "What is this?"	Evoked trial
Child	"dee."	Omission of final /ʃ/
Clinician	Pulls the stimulus toward her; records	No corrective feedback
Clinician	[*stimulus: bush*] "What is this?"	The next evoked trial
Child	"boo."	Omission of /ʃ/
Clinician	Pulls the stimulus toward her; records the response.	No corrective feedback

Administer the modeled baserate trials only after completing the evoked trials on all 20 (or more) exemplars.

Scripts for Modeled Baserate Trial		Note
Clinician	[*stimulus: dish*] "What is this? Say, *dish.*"	Modeled trial
Child	"Dish."	Correct response
Clinician	Pulls the stimulus toward her; records the response.	No reinforcement
Clinician	[*stimulus: bush*] "What is this? Say, *bush.*"	The next modeled trial
Child	"boo."	Omission of final /ʃ/
Clinician	Pulls the stimulus toward her; records the response.	No corrective feedback

Use the recording sheet with exemplars shown on the next page to establish the baserates; print it from the CD.

/ʃ/ in Word-Final Positions

Baserate Exemplars and Recording Sheet

Use stimuli from the **Stimulus Book, Volume 2**.

Print this page from the CD or photocopy this page for your clinical use.

Name/Age:	Date:
Goal: To establish the baserate production of /ʃ/ in word-final positions.	Clinician:

Scoring: Correct: ✓   Incorrect or no response: X

/ʃ/ in word-final positions	Evoked	Modeled
1. dish		
2. bush		
3. fish		
4. trash		
5. wash		
6. eyelash		
7. mustache		
8. hairbrush		
9. mouthwash		
10. toothbrush		
11. leash		
12. catfish		
13. mesh		
14. rash		
15. cash		
16. rosebush		
17. shellfish		
18. horseradish		
19. whitewash		
20. paintbrush		
Percent correct baserate		

Replace or add new exemplars as you see fit for a given child. After establishing the baserates, begin production teaching. Follow the protocols given on the next page.

/ʃ/ in Word-Final Positions

Treatment Protocols

Use stimuli from the **Stimulus Book,** *Volume 2.*

Teach 6 to 8 exemplars using the following script.

Place a relevant stimulus (an object, a picture, or a printed word) in front of the child and point to the stimulus as you ask an evoking question.

Scripts for Modeled Discrete Trial Training		Note
Clinician	[*stimulus: dish*] "What is this? Say, **dish**."	Modeling; the target vocally emphasized
Child	"dee."	A wrong response
Clinician	"No. That's not correct. You said dee, but it's a **dish**."	Corrective feedback
Clinician	[*the same stimulus*] "What is this? Say, **dish**. Don't forget the ʃ sound at the end."	The next trial
Child	"Dish."	A correct response
Clinician	"Excellent! You didn't miss the ʃ at the end of the word!"	Verbal praise

Repeat the trials until the child gives 5 consecutively correct, imitated responses.

When the child imitates 5 correct responses in sequence, fade the modeling.

Scripts for Fading the Modeling		Note
Clinician	[*stimulus: dish*] "What is this? Don't forget the ʃ sound at the end."	Only a prompt
Child	"dee."	A wrong response
Clinician	"Gee, you forgot the ʃ sound! It's a *dish*, not *dee*. Put the ʃ at the end."	Corrective feedback
Clinician	[*the same stimulus*] "What is this? It ends with . . . " [*silently models the articulatory posture for the target sound.*]	The next trial; a partial modeling
Child	"Dish."	A correct response
Clinician	"That's great! You said *dish*, not *dee*."	Verbal praise
Clinician	[*the same stimulus*] "What is this?"	Typical question; evoked trial
Child	"Dish."	A correct response
Clinician	"I like it! You said it correctly!"	Verbal praise

If the wrong responses persist on 4 to 5 evoked trials, reinstate partial or full modeling for a few trials, again fade the modeling, and re-present the evoked trials.

When the child meets the tentative learning criterion of 10 consecutively correct, nonimitated responses for a given stimulus item, move on to the next stimulus item. With this procedure, teach 6 to 8 exemplars shown on the following recording sheet. Use different exemplars as you see fit for a given child.

/ʃ/ in Word-Final Positions

Treatment Exemplars and Recording Sheet

*Use stimuli from the **Stimulus Book, Volume 2**.*

Print this page from CD or photocopy this page for your clinical use.

Name/Age:	Date:
Goal: Production of /ʃ/ in word-final positions with 90% accuracy when asked an evoking question while showing a stimulus.	Clinician:

Scoring: Correct: ✓   Incorrect or no response: X

Target skills	Discrete Trials														
	1	2	3	4	5	6	7	8	9	10	11	12	13	14	15
1. dish															
2. bush															
3. fish															
4. trash															
5. wash															
6. eyelash															
7. mustache															
8. hairbrush															

When the child has met the learning criterion of 10 consecutively correct evoked (nonimitated) responses for each of the 6 to 8 target exemplars, conduct a probe to see if the production has generalized to previously baserated but untrained exemplars.

If the probes do not meet the 90% correct criterion for untrained exemplars, teach additional exemplars and then probe again.

/ʃ/ in Word-Final Positions

Probe Protocols and Recording Sheet

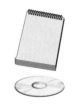

Use stimuli from the **Stimulus Book, Volume 2.**

Print this page from the CD or photocopy this page for your clinical use.

On the probes, present only the untrained exemplars (UT). When the child fails to meet the 90% correct probe criterion, either teach 2 to 4 new exemplars or give additional training trials on already trained stimuli. If needed, select new exemplars for probes. Probe at least 10 untrained exemplars. Alternate probes and treatment until the probe criterion is met.

Scripts for Probe Trials		Note
Clinician	[*untrained stimulus: mouthwash*] "What is this?"	No modeling or prompts
Child	"Mouthwash."	A correct, generalized response
Clinician	Scores the response as correct.	No reinforcement
Clinician	[*untrained stimulus: toothbrush*] "What is this?"	The second probe trial
Child	"toothbrə."	A wrong probe response
Clinician	Scores the response as incorrect.	No corrective feedback

Name:	Date:	Session #:
Age:	**Clinician:**	
Diagnosis: Articulation/Phonologic Disorder	**Word-final /ʃ/probe**	
Untrained Stimuli	**Score: + correct; – incorrect or no responses**	
1. mouthwash		
2. toothbrush		
3. leash		
4. catfish		
5. mesh		
6. rash		
7. cash		
8. rosebush		
9. shellfish		
10. horseradish		
11. whitewash		
12. paintbrush		
Percent correct: (Criterion: 90%)		

If the child does not meet the probe criterion, give additional training on already trained exemplars or teach a few new exemplars. Subsequently, readminister the probe trials. When the child meets the 90% correct probe criterion for the exemplars, shift training to the sentence or conversational level or to another phoneme.

/ʒ/ in Word-Final Positions

Baserate Protocols

Use stimuli from the **Stimulus Book, *Volume 2*.**

In English, /ʒ/ does not occur in initial positions; only a few functional words end with it.

At the beginning of each trial, place a relevant stimulus (an object, a picture, or a printed word) in front of the child. Point to the stimulus as you ask an evoking question. Do not respond in any way to the child's correct, incorrect, or lack of responses.

Scripts for Evoked Baserate Trial		Note
Clinician	[*stimulus: color beige*] "What color is this?"	Evoked trial
Child	"bei."	Omission of final /ʒ/
Clinician	Pulls the stimulus toward her; records the response.	No corrective feedback
Clinician	[*stimulus: garage*] "What is this?"	The next evoked trial
Child	"garɑ."	Omission of final /ʒ/
Clinician	Pulls the stimulus toward her; records the response.	No corrective feedback

Administer the modeled baserate trials only after completing the evoked trials on all 20 (or more) exemplars.

Scripts for Modeled Baserate Trial		Note
Clinician	[*stimulus: color beige*] "What color is this? Say, *beige*."	Modeled trial
Child	"Beige."	Correct response
Clinician	Pulls the stimulus toward her; records the response.	No reinforcement
Clinician	[*stimulus: garage*] "What is this? Say, *garage*."	The next modeled trial
Child	"garɑ."	Omission of final /ʒ/
Clinician	Pulls the stimulus toward her; records the response.	No corrective feedback

Use the recording sheet with exemplars shown on the next page to establish the baserates; print it from the CD.

/ʒ/ in Word-Final Positions

Baserate Exemplars and Recording Sheet

Use stimuli from the **Stimulus Book,** *Volume 2.*

Print this page from the CD or photocopy this page for your clinical use.

Name/Age:	Date:
Goal: To establish the baserate production of /ʒ/ in word-final positions.	Clinician:

Scoring: Correct: ✓   Incorrect or no response: X

/ʒ/ in word-final positions	Evoked	Modeled
1. beige		
2. garage		
3. rouge		
4. massage		
5. mirage		
6. corsage		
7. entourage		
8. collage		
9. barrage		
10. prestige		
11. luge		
12. decoupage		
13. dressage		
14. fuselage		
15. montage		
16. camouflage		
17. Baton Rouge		
18. concierge		
19. sabotage		
20. bon voyage		
Percent correct baserate		

Replace or add new exemplars as you see fit for a given child. After establishing the baserates, begin production teaching. Follow the protocols given on the next page.

/ʒ/ in Word-Final Positions

Treatment Protocols

Use stimuli from the **Stimulus Book,** *Volume 2.*

Teach 6 to 8 exemplars using the following script.

Place a relevant stimulus (an object, a picture, or a printed word) in front of the child and point to the stimulus as you ask an evoking question.

Scripts for Modeled Discrete Trial Training		Note
Clinician	[*stimulus: color beige*] "What color is this? *bei**ge**.*"	Modeling; the target vocally emphasized
Child	"bei."	A wrong response
Clinician	"No. That's not correct. You said *bei*, but it's *bei**ge**.*"	Corrective feedback
Clinician	[*the same stimulus*] "What color is this? Say, *bei**ge**. Don't forget the ʒ sound at the end."	The next trial
Child	"Beige."	A correct response
Clinician	"Excellent! You added the ʒ sound at the end of the word!"	Verbal praise

Repeat the trials until the child gives 5 consecutively correct, imitated responses.

When the child imitates 5 correct responses in sequence, fade the modeling.

Scripts for Fading the Modeling		Note
Clinician	[*stimulus: color beige*] "What color is this? Don't forget the ʒ sound at the end."	Only a prompt
Child	"bei."	A wrong response
Clinician	"Oh no! You forgot the ʒ sound at the end! It's *beige*, not *bei*. Put the ʒ sound at the end."	Corrective feedback
Clinician	[*the same stimulus*] "What is this? It ends with ʒ." [*silently models the articulatory posture for the target sound.*]	The next trial; a partial modeling
Child	"Beige."	A correct response
Clinician	"That's great! You said *beige*, not *bei*."	Verbal praise
Clinician	[*the same stimulus*] "What is this?"	Typical question; evoked trial
Child	"Beige."	A correct response
Clinician	"Wonderful! You said it correctly!"	Verbal praise

If the wrong responses persist on 4 to 5 evoked trials, reinstate partial or full modeling for a few trials, again fade the modeling, and re-present the evoked trials.

When the child meets the tentative learning criterion of 10 consecutively correct, nonimitated responses for a given stimulus item, move on to the next stimulus item. With this procedure, teach 4 to 6 exemplars shown on the following recording sheet. Use different exemplars as you see fit for a given child.

/ʒ/ in Word-Final Positions

Treatment Exemplars and Recording Sheet

*Use stimuli from the **Stimulus Book, Volume 2**.*

Print this page from CD or photocopy this page for your clinical use.

Name/Age:	Date:
Goal: Production of /ʒ/ in word-final positions with 90% accuracy when asked an evoking question while showing a stimulus.	Clinician:

Scoring: Correct: ✓   Incorrect or no response: X

Target skills	Discrete Trials														
	1	2	3	4	5	6	7	8	9	10	11	12	13	14	15
1. beige															
2. garage															
3. rouge															
4. massage															
5. mirage															
6. corsage															
7. entourage															
8. collage															

When the child has met the learning criterion of 10 consecutively correct evoked (nonimitated) responses for each of the 4 to 6 target exemplars, conduct a probe to see if the production has generalized to previously baserated but untrained exemplars.

If the probes do not meet the 90% correct criterion for untrained exemplars, teach additional exemplars and then probe again.

/ʒ/ in Word-Final Positions

Probe Protocols and Recording Sheet

Use stimuli from the **Stimulus Book, Volume 2**.

Print this page from the CD or photocopy this page for your clinical use.

On the probes, present only the untrained exemplars (UT). When the child fails to meet the 90% correct probe criterion, either teach 2 to 4 new exemplars or give additional training trials on already trained stimuli. If needed, select new exemplars for probes. Probe as many untrained exemplars as possible, although words ending in /ʒ/ are few. Alternate probes and treatment until the probe criterion is met.

Scripts for Probe Trials		Note
Clinician	[*untrained stimulus: printed word barrage*] "What is this word?" [*for a nonreader*] "This word is *barrage*. What is this word?"	No modeling or prompts
Child	"Barrage."	A correct, generalized response
Clinician	Scores the response as correct.	No reinforcement
Clinician	[*untrained stimulus: printed word prestige*] "What is this word?" [*for a nonreader*] "This word is *prestige*. What is this word?"	The second probe trial
Child	"prestee."	A wrong probe response
Clinician	Scores the response as incorrect.	No corrective feedback

Name:	Date:	Session #:
Age:	**Clinician:**	
Diagnosis: Articulation/Phonologic Disorder	**Word-final /ʒ/ probe**	
Untrained Stimuli	**Score: + correct; – incorrect or no responses**	
1. barrage		
2. prestige		
3. luge		
4. decoupage		
5. dressage		
6. fuselage		
7. montage		
8. camouflage		
9. Baton Rouge		
10. concierge		
11. sabotage		
12. bon voyage		
Percent correct: (Criterion: 90%)		

If the child does not meet the probe criterion, give additional training on already trained exemplars or teach a few new exemplars. Subsequently, readminister the probe trials. When the child meets the 90% correct probe criterion for the exemplars, shift training to the sentence or conversational level or to another phoneme.

/h/ in Word-Initial Positions

Baserate Protocols

Use stimuli from the **Stimulus Book,** *Volume 4*.

The English /h/ occurs only in word initial positions.

At the beginning of each trial, place a relevant stimulus (an object, a picture, or a printed word) in front of the child. Point to the stimulus as you ask an evoking question. Do not respond in any way to the child's correct, incorrect, or lack of responses.

Scripts for Evoked Baserate Trial		Note
Clinician	[*stimulus: hat*] "What is this?"	Evoked trial
Child	"æt."	Omission of initial /h/
Clinician	Pulls the stimulus toward her; records the response.	No corrective feedback
Clinician	[*stimulus: hay*] "What is this?"	The next evoked trial
Child	"ay."	Omission of initial /h/
Clinician	Pulls the stimulus toward her; records the response.	No corrective feedback

Administer the modeled baserate trials only after completing the evoked trials on all 20 (or more) exemplars.

Scripts for Modeled Baserate Trial		Note
Clinician	[*stimulus: hat*] "What is this? Say, *hat.*"	Modeled trial
Child	"Hat."	Correct response
Clinician	Pulls the stimulus toward her; records the response.	No reinforcement
Clinician	[*stimulus: hay*] "What is this? Say, *hay.*"	The next modeled trial
Child	"ay."	Omission of initial /h/
Clinician	Pulls the stimulus toward her; records the response.	No corrective feedback

Use the recording sheet with exemplars shown on the next page to establish the baserates; print it from the CD.

/h/ in Word-Initial Positions

Baserate Exemplars and Recording Sheet

Use stimuli from the **Stimulus Book,** *Volume 4.*

Print this page from the CD or photocopy this page for your clinical use.

Name/Age:	Date:
Goal: To establish the baserate production of /h/ in word-initial positions.	Clinician:

Scoring: Correct: ✓   Incorrect or no response: X

/h/ in word-initial positions	Evoked	Modeled
1. hat		
2. hay		
3. hand		
4. hoe		
5. head		
6. helmet		
7. hamburger		
8. harmonica		
9. helicopter		
10. honeycomb		
11. hill		
12. heart		
13. hog		
14. house		
15. hut		
16. highchair		
17. hibiscus		
18. hedgehog		
19. hummingbird		
20. hairdresser		
Percent correct baserate		

Replace or add new exemplars as you see fit for a given child. After establishing the baserates, begin production teaching. Follow the protocols given on the next page.

/h/ in Word-Initial Positions

Treatment Protocols

Use stimuli from the **Stimulus Book, *Volume 4***.

Teach 6 to 8 exemplars using the following script.

Place a relevant stimulus in front of the child (an object, a picture, or a printed word) and ask a question as you point to the stimulus.

Scripts for Modeled Discrete Trial Training		Note
Clinician	[*stimulus: hat*] "What is this? Say, **h***at*."	Modeling; the target vocally emphasized
Child	"æt."	A wrong response
Clinician	"No. That's not correct. You said æt, but it's **h***at*."	Corrective feedback
Clinician	[*the same stimulus*] "What is this? Say, **h***at*. Don't forget the *h* at the beginning."	The next trial
Child	"Hat."	A correct response
Clinician	"Excellent! You didn't miss the *h* sound this time!"	Verbal praise

Repeat the trials until the child gives 5 consecutively correct, imitated responses.

When the child imitates 5 correct responses in sequence, fade the modeling.

Scripts for Fading the Modeling		Note
Clinician	[*stimulus: hat*] "What is this? Don't forget the *h* at the beginning."	Only a prompt
Child	"æt."	A wrong response
Clinician	"Gee, you forgot the *h* sound! It's a *hat*, not æt. Put the *h* sound at the beginning."	Corrective feedback
Clinician	[*the same stimulus*] "What is this? It starts with . . . " [*silently models the articulatory posture for the target sound.*]	The next trial; a partial modeling
Child	"Hat."	A correct response
Clinician	"That's great! You said *hat*, not æt."	Verbal praise
Clinician	[*the same stimulus*] "What is this?"	Typical question; evoked trial
Child	"Hat."	A correct response
Clinician	"Great job! You said it correctly!"	Verbal praise

If the wrong responses persist on 4 to 5 evoked trials, reinstate partial or full modeling for a few trials, again fade the modeling, and re-present the evoked trials.

When the child meets the tentative learning criterion of 10 consecutively correct, nonimitated responses for a given stimulus item, move on to the next stimulus item. With this procedure, teach 6 to 8 exemplars shown on the following recording sheet. Use different exemplars as you see fit for a given child.

/h/ in Word-Initial Positions

Treatment Exemplars and Recording Sheet

Use stimuli from the **Stimulus Book, Volume 4**.

Print this page from CD or photocopy this page for your clinical use.

Name/Age:	Date:
Goal: Production of /h/ in word-initial positions with 90% accuracy when asked an evoking question while showing a stimulus.	Clinician:

Scoring: Correct: ✓ Incorrect or no response: X

Target skills	Discrete Trials														
	1	2	3	4	5	6	7	8	9	10	11	12	13	14	15
1. hat															
2. hay															
3. hand															
4. hoe															
5. head															
6. helmet															
7. hamburger															
8. harmonica															

When the child has met the learning criterion of 10 consecutively correct evoked (nonimitated) responses for each of the 6 to 8 target exemplars, conduct a probe to see if the production has generalized to previously baserated but untrained exemplars.

If the probes do not meet the 90% correct criterion for untrained exemplars, teach additional exemplars and then probe again.

/h/ in Word-Initial Positions

Probe Protocols and Recording Sheet

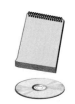

Use stimuli from the **Stimulus Book, *Volume 4***.

Print this page from the CD or photocopy this page for your clinical use.

On the probes, present only the untrained exemplars (UT). When the child fails to meet the 90% correct probe criterion, either teach 2 to 4 new exemplars or give additional training trials on already trained stimuli. If needed, select new exemplars for probes. Probe at least 10 untrained exemplars. Alternate probes and treatment until the probe criterion is met.

Scripts for Probe Trials		Note
Clinician	[*untrained stimulus: helicopter*] "What is this?"	No modeling or prompts
Child	"Helicopter."	A correct, generalized response
Clinician	Scores the response as correct.	No reinforcement
Clinician	[*untrained stimulus: honeycomb*] "What is this?"	The second probe trial
Child	"ənycomb."	A wrong probe response
Clinician	Scores the response as incorrect.	No corrective feedback

Name:	Date:	Session #:
Age:	**Clinician:**	
Diagnosis: Articulation/Phonologic Disorder	**Word-initial /h/ probe**	
Untrained Stimuli	**Score: + correct; – incorrect or no responses**	
1. helicopter		
2. honeycomb		
3. hill		
4. heart		
5. hog		
6. house		
7. hut		
8. highchair		
9. hibiscus		
10. hedgehog		
11. hummingbird		
12. hairdresser		
Percent correct: (Criterion: 90%)		

If the child does not meet the probe criterion, give additional training on already trained exemplars or teach a few new exemplars. Subsequently, readminister the probe trials. When the child meets the 90% correct probe criterion for the exemplars, shift training to the sentence or conversational level or to another phoneme.

/tʃ/ in Word-Initial Positions

Baserate Protocols

Use stimuli from the **Stimulus Book,** *Volume 2.*

At the beginning of each trial, place a relevant stimulus (an object, a picture, or a printed word) in front of the child. Point to the stimulus as you ask an evoking question. Do not respond in any way to the child's correct, incorrect, or lack of responses.

Scripts for Evoked Baserate Trial		Note
Clinician	[*stimulus: chain*] "What is this?"	Evoked trial
Child	"ain."	Omission of initial /tʃ/
Clinician	Pulls the stimulus toward her; records the response.	No corrective feedback
Clinician	[*stimulus: chair*] "What is this?"	The next evoked trial
Child	"air."	Omission of initial /tʃ/
Clinician	Pulls the stimulus toward her; records the response.	No corrective feedback

Administer the modeled baserate trials only after completing the evoked trials on all 20 (or more) exemplars.

Scripts for Modeled Baserate Trial		Note
Clinician	[*stimulus: chain*] "What is this? Say, *chain.*"	Modeled trial
Child	"Chain."	Correct response
Clinician	Pulls the stimulus toward her; records the response.	No reinforcement
Clinician	[*stimulus: chair*] "What is this? Say, *chair.*"	The next modeled trial
Child	"air."	Omission of initial /tʃ/
Clinician	Pulls the stimulus toward her; records the response.	No corrective feedback

Use the recording sheet with exemplars shown on the next page to establish the baserates; print it from the CD.

/tʃ/ in Word-Initial Positions

Baserate Exemplars and Recording Sheet

Use stimuli from the **Stimulus Book,** *Volume 2.*

Print this page from the CD or photocopy this page for your clinical use.

Name/Age:	Date:
Goal: To establish the baserate production of /tʃ/ in word-initial positions.	Clinician:

Scoring: Correct: ✓   Incorrect or no response: X

/tʃ/ in word-initial positions	Evoked	Modeled
1. chain		
2. chair		
3. chin		
4. chalk		
5. cheek		
6. chalkboard		
7. cheerleader		
8. chimpanzee		
9. chipmunk		
10. children		
11. chips		
12. chapel		
13. chicken		
14. chess		
15. cheese		
16. chocolate		
17. chewing gum		
18. chinchilla		
19. chili pepper		
20. Chihuahua		
Percent correct baserate		

Replace or add new exemplars as you see fit for a given child. After establishing the baserates, begin production teaching. Follow the protocols given on the next page.

/tʃ/ in Word-Initial Positions

Treatment Protocols

Use stimuli from the **Stimulus Book,** *Volume 2.*

Teach 6 to 8 exemplars using the following script.

Place a relevant stimulus in front of the child (an object, a picture, or a printed word) and ask a question as you point to the stimulus.

Scripts for Modeled Discrete Trial Training		Note
Clinician	[*stimulus: chain*] "What is this? Say, **ch**ain."	Modeling; the target vocally emphasized
Child	"ain."	A wrong response
Clinician	"No. That's not correct. You said *ain*, but it's a **ch**ain."	Corrective feedback
Clinician	[*the same stimulus*] "What is this? Say, **ch**ain. Don't forget the *ch* at the beginning."	The next trial
Child	"Chain."	A correct response
Clinician	"Excellent! You didn't miss the *ch* this time!"	Verbal praise

Repeat the trials until the child gives 5 consecutively correct, imitated responses.

When the child imitates 5 correct responses in sequence, fade the modeling.

Scripts for Fading the Modeling		Note
Clinician	[*stimulus: chain*] "What is this? Don't forget the *ch* at the beginning."	Only a prompt
Child	"ain."	A wrong response
Clinician	"Gee, you forgot the *ch* sound! It's a *chain*, not *ain*. Put the *ch* at the beginning."	Corrective feedback
Clinician	[*the same stimulus*] "What is this? It starts with . . . " [*silently models the articulatory posture for the target sound.*]	The next trial; a partial modeling
Child	"Chain."	A correct response
Clinician	"That's great! You said *chain*, not *ain*."	Verbal praise
Clinician	[*the same stimulus*] "What is this?"	Typical question; evoked trial
Child	"Chain."	A correct response
Clinician	"Great job! You said it correctly!"	Verbal praise

If the wrong responses persist on 4 to 5 evoked trials, reinstate partial or full modeling for a few trials, again fade the modeling, and re-present the evoked trials.

When the child meets the tentative learning criterion of 10 consecutively correct, nonimitated responses for a given stimulus item, move on to the next stimulus item. With this procedure, teach 6 to 8 exemplars shown on the following recording sheet. Use different exemplars as you see fit for a given child.

/tʃ/ in Word-Initial Positions

Treatment Exemplars and Recording Sheet

Use stimuli from the **Stimulus Book, Volume 2**.

Print this page from CD or photocopy this page for your clinical use.

Name/Age:	Date:
Goal: Production of /tʃ/ in word-initial positions with 90% accuracy when asked an evoking question while showing a stimulus.	Clinician:

Scoring: Correct: ✓   Incorrect or no response: X

Target skills	Discrete Trials														
	1	2	3	4	5	6	7	8	9	10	11	12	13	14	15
1. chain															
2. chair															
3. chin															
4. chalk															
5. cheek															
6. chalkboard															
7. cheerleader															
8. chimpanzee															

When the child has met the learning criterion of 10 consecutively correct evoked (nonimitated) responses for each of the 6 to 8 target exemplars, conduct a probe to see if the production has generalized to previously baserated but untrained exemplars.

If the probes do not meet the 90% correct criterion for untrained exemplars, teach additional exemplars and then probe again.

/tʃ/ in Word-Initial Positions

Probe Protocols and Recording Sheet

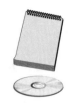

Use stimuli from the **Stimulus Book,** *Volume 2.*

Print this page from the CD or photocopy this page for your clinical use.

On the probes, present only the untrained exemplars (UT). When the child fails to meet the 90% correct probe criterion, either teach 2 to 4 new exemplars or give additional training trials on already trained stimuli. If needed, select new exemplars for probes. Probe at least 10 untrained exemplars. Alternate probes and treatment until the probe criterion is met.

Scripts for Probe Trials		Note
Clinician	[*untrained stimulus: chipmunk*] "What is this?"	No modeling or prompts
Child	"Chipmunk."	A correct, generalized response
Clinician	Scores the response as correct.	No reinforcement
Clinician	[*untrained stimulus: children*] "Who are these?"	The second probe trial
Child	"ildren."	A wrong probe response
Clinician	Scores the response as incorrect.	No corrective feedback

Name:	Date:	Session #:
Age:	**Clinician:**	
Diagnosis: Articulation/Phonologic Disorder	**Word-initial /tʃ/ probe**	
Untrained Stimuli	**Score: + correct; – incorrect or no responses**	
1. chipmunk		
2. children		
3. chips		
4. chapel		
5. chicken		
6. chess		
7. cheese		
8. chocolate		
9. chewing gum		
10. chinchilla		
11. chili pepper		
12. Chihuahua		
Percent correct: (Criterion: 90%)		

If the child does not meet the probe criterion, give additional training on already trained exemplars or teach a few new exemplars. Subsequently, readminister the probe trials. When the child meets the 90% correct probe criterion for the exemplars, shift training to the sentence or conversational level or to another phoneme.

/tʃ/ in Word-Final Positions

Baserate Protocols

Use stimuli from the **Stimulus Book,** *Volume 2.*

At the beginning of each trial, place a relevant stimulus (an object, a picture, or a printed word) in front of the child. Point to the stimulus as you ask an evoking question. Do not respond in any way to the child's correct, incorrect, or lack of responses.

Scripts for Evoked Baserate Trial		Note
Clinician	[*stimulus: beach*] "What is this?"	Evoked trial
Child	"bee."	Omission of final /tʃ/
Clinician	Pulls the stimulus toward her; records the response.	No corrective feedback
Clinician	[*stimulus: a bench*] "What is this?"	The next evoked trial
Child	"ben." ["bɛ"]	Omission of final /tʃ/
Clinician	Pulls the stimulus toward her; records the response.	No corrective feedback

Administer the modeled baserate trials only after completing the evoked trials on all 20 (or more) exemplars.

Scripts for Modeled Baserate Trial		Note
Clinician	[*stimulus: beach*] "What is this? Say, *beach.*"	Modeled trial
Child	"Beach."	Correct response
Clinician	Pulls the stimulus toward her; records the response.	No reinforcement
Clinician	[*stimulus: bench*] "What is this? Say, *bench.*"	The next modeled trial
Child	"ben." ["bɛ"]	Omission of final /tʃ/
Clinician	Pulls the stimulus toward her; records the response.	No corrective feedback

Use the recording sheet with exemplars shown on the next page to establish the baserates; print it from the CD.

/tʃ/ in Word-Final Positions

Baserate Exemplars and Recording Sheet

Use stimuli from the **Stimulus Book,** *Volume 2.*

Print this page from the CD or photocopy this page for your clinical use.

Name/Age:	Date:
Goal: To establish the baserate production of /tʃ/ in word-final positions.	Clinician:

Scoring: Correct: ✓   Incorrect or no response: X

/tʃ/ in word-final positions	Evoked	Modeled
1. beach		
2. bench		
3. couch		
4. watch		
5. match		
6. sandwich		
7. workbench		
8. ostrich		
9. hopscotch		
10. butterscotch		
11. wrench		
12. ranch		
13. peach		
14. branch		
15. ditch		
16. pumpkin patch		
17. featherstitch		
18. door latch		
19. pocket watch		
20. pony ranch		
Percent correct baserate		

Replace or add new exemplars as you see fit for a given child. After establishing the baserates, begin production teaching. Follow the protocols given on the next page.

/tʃ/ in Word-Final Positions

Treatment Protocols

Use stimuli from the **Stimulus Book,** *Volume 2.*

Teach 6 to 8 exemplars using the following script.

Place a relevant stimulus (an object, a picture, or a printed word) in front of the child and point to the stimulus as you ask an evoking question.

Scripts for Modeled Discrete Trial Training		Note
Clinician	[*stimulus: beach*] "What is this? Say, *bea**ch**.*"	Modeling; the target vocally emphasized
Child	"bee."	A wrong response
Clinician	"No. That's not correct. You said *bee*, but it's *bea**ch**.*"	Corrective feedback
Clinician	[*the same stimulus*] "What is this? Say, *bea**ch**. Don't forget the *ch* at the end."	The next trial
Child	"Beach."	A correct response
Clinician	"Excellent! You didn't miss the *ch* at the end of the word!"	Verbal praise

Repeat the trials until the child gives 5 consecutively correct, imitated responses.

When the child imitates 5 correct responses in sequence, fade the modeling.

Scripts for Fading the Modeling		Note
Clinician	[*stimulus: beach*] "What is this? Don't forget the *ch* at the end."	Only a prompt
Child	"Bee."	A wrong response
Clinician	"Gee, you forgot the *ch* sound! It's *beach*, not *bee*. Put the *ch* at the end."	Corrective feedback
Clinician	[*the same stimulus*] "What is this? It ends with . . . " [*silently models the articulatory posture for the target sound.*]	The next trial; a partial modeling
Child	"Beach."	A correct response
Clinician	"That's great! You said *beach*, not *bee*."	Verbal praise
Clinician	[*the same stimulus*] "What is this?"	Typical question; evoked trial
Child	"Beach."	A correct response
Clinician	"How nice! You said it correctly!"	Verbal praise

If the wrong responses persist on 4 to 5 evoked trials, reinstate partial or full modeling for a few trials, again fade the modeling, and re-present the evoked trials.

When the child meets the tentative learning criterion of 10 consecutively correct, nonimitated responses for a given stimulus item, move on to the next stimulus item. With this procedure, teach 6 to 8 exemplars shown on the following recording sheet. Use different exemplars as you see fit for a given child.

/tʃ/ in Word-Final Positions

Treatment Exemplars and Recording Sheet

*Use stimuli from the **Stimulus Book, Volume 2**.*

Print this page from CD or photocopy this page for your clinical use.

Name/Age:	Date:
Goal: Production of /tʃ/ in word-final positions with 90% accuracy when asked an evoking question while showing a stimulus.	Clinician:

Scoring: Correct: ✓   Incorrect or no response: X

Target skills	Discrete Trials														
	1	2	3	4	5	6	7	8	9	10	11	12	13	14	15
1. beach															
2. bench															
3. couch															
4. watch															
5. match															
6. sandwich															
7. workbench															
8. ostrich															

When the child has met the learning criterion of 10 consecutively correct evoked (nonimitated) responses for each of the 6 to 8 target exemplars, conduct a probe to see if the production has generalized to previously baserated but untrained exemplars.

If the probes do not meet the 90% correct criterion for untrained exemplars, teach additional exemplars and then probe again.

/tʃ/ in Word-Final Positions

Probe Protocols and Recording Sheet

Use stimuli from the **Stimulus Book, Volume 2.**

Print this page from the CD or photocopy this page for your clinical use.

On the probes, present only the untrained exemplars (UT). When the child fails to meet the 90% correct probe criterion, either teach 2 to 4 new exemplars or give additional training trials on already trained stimuli. If needed, select new exemplars for probes. Probe at least 10 untrained exemplars. Alternate probes and treatment until the probe criterion is met.

Scripts for Probe Trials		Note
Clinician	[*untrained stimulus: hopscotch*] "What is this?"	No modeling or prompts
Child	"Hopscotch."	A correct, generalized response
Clinician	Scores the response as correct.	No reinforcement
Clinician	[*untrained stimulus: butterscotch*] "What is this?"	The second probe trial
Child	"Buttersca."	A wrong probe response
Clinician	Scores the response as incorrect.	No corrective feedback

Name:	Date:	Session #:
Age:	**Clinician:**	
Diagnosis: Articulation/Phonologic Disorder	**Word-final /tʃ/ probe**	
Untrained Stimuli	**Score: + correct; – incorrect or no responses**	
1. hopscotch		
2. butterscotch		
3. wrench		
4. ranch		
5. peach		
6. branch		
7. ditch		
8. pumpkin patch		
9. featherstitch		
10. door latch		
11. pocket watch		
12. pony ranch		
Percent correct: (Criterion: 90%)		

If the child does not meet the probe criterion, give additional training on already trained exemplars or teach a few new exemplars. Subsequently, readminister the probe trials. When the child meets the 90% correct probe criterion for the exemplars, shift training to the sentence or conversational level or to another phoneme.

/dʒ/ in Word-Initial Positions

Baserate Protocols

Use stimuli from the **Stimulus Book, Volume 2**.

At the beginning of each trial, place a relevant stimulus (an object, a picture, or a printed word) in front of the child. Point to the stimulus as you ask an evoking question. Do not respond in any way to the child's correct, incorrect, or lack of responses.

Scripts for Evoked Baserate Trial		Note
Clinician	[*stimulus: jacket*] "What is this?"	Evoked trial
Child	"æket"	Omission of initial /dʒ/
Clinician	Pulls the stimulus toward her; records the response.	No corrective feedback
Clinician	[*stimulus: jar*] "What is this?"	The next evoked trial
Child	"ɑr."	Omission of initial /dʒ/
Clinician	Pulls the stimulus toward her; records the response.	No corrective feedback

Administer the modeled baserate trials only after completing the evoked trials on all 20 (or more) exemplars.

Scripts for Modeled Baserate Trial		Note
Clinician	[*stimulus: jacket*] "What is this? Say, *jacket.*"	Modeled trial
Child	"Jacket."	Correct response
Clinician	Pulls the stimulus toward her; records the response.	No reinforcement
Clinician	[*stimulus: jar*] "What is this? Say, *jar.*"	The next modeled trial
Child	"ɑr."	Omission of initial /dʒ/
Clinician	Pulls the stimulus toward her; records the response.	No corrective feedback

Use the recording sheet with exemplars shown on the next page to establish the baserates; print it from the CD.

/dʒ/ in Word-Initial Positions

Baserate Exemplars and Recording Sheet

*Use stimuli from the **Stimulus Book, Volume 2**.*

Print this page from the CD or photocopy this page for your clinical use.

Name/Age:	Date:
Goal: To establish the baserate production of /dʒ/ in word-initial positions.	Clinician:

Scoring: Correct: ✓   Incorrect or no response: X

/dʒ/ in word-initial positions	Evoked	Modeled
1. jacket		
2. jar		
3. jam		
4. jet		
5. jug		
6. jumping		
7. jungle		
8. juggler		
9. junkyard		
10. jaguar		
11. jaw		
12. juice		
13. jade		
14. jail		
15. jackal		
16. janitor		
17. jogging		
18. jellyfish		
19. jellybean		
20. jukebox		
Percent correct baserate		

Replace or add new exemplars as you see fit for a given child. After establishing the baserates, begin production teaching. Follow the protocols given on the next page.

/dʒ/ in Word-Initial Positions

Treatment Protocols

Use stimuli from the **Stimulus Book,** *Volume 2.*

Teach 6 to 8 exemplars using the following script.

Place a relevant stimulus in front of the child (an object, a picture, or a printed word) and ask a question as you point to the stimulus.

Scripts for Modeled Discrete Trial Training		Note
Clinician	[*stimulus: jacket*] "What is this? Say, **ja**cket."	Modeling; the target vocally emphasized
Child	"æket."	A wrong response
Clinician	"No. That's not correct. You said æket, but it's a **ja**cket."	Corrective feedback
Clinician	[*the same stimulus*] "What is this? Say, **ja**cket. Don't forget the *dʒ* sound at the beginning."	The next trial
Child	"Jacket."	A correct response
Clinician	"Excellent! You didn't miss the *dʒ* sound this time!"	Verbal praise

Repeat the trials until the child gives 5 consecutively correct, imitated responses.

When the child imitates 5 correct responses in sequence, fade the modeling.

Scripts for Fading the Modeling		Note
Clinician	[*stimulus: jacket*] "What is this? Don't forget the *dʒ* sound at the beginning."	Only a prompt
Child	"æket."	A wrong response
Clinician	"Gee, you forgot the *dʒ* sound! It's a *jacket*, not æket. Put the *dʒ* sound at the beginning."	Corrective feedback
Clinician	[*the same stimulus*] "What is this? It starts with . . . " [*silently models the articulatory posture for the target sound.*]	The next trial; a partial modeling
Child	"Jacket."	A correct response
Clinician	"That's great! You said *jacket*, not *æket*."	Verbal praise
Clinician	[*the same stimulus*] "What is this?"	Typical question; evoked trial
Child	"Jacket."	A correct response
Clinician	"Great job! You said it correctly!"	Verbal praise

If the wrong responses persist on 4 to 5 evoked trials, reinstate partial or full modeling for a few trials, again fade the modeling, and re-present the evoked trials.

When the child meets the tentative learning criterion of 10 consecutively correct, nonimitated responses for a given stimulus item, move on to the next stimulus item. With this procedure, teach 6 to 8 exemplars shown on the following recording sheet. Use different exemplars as you see fit for a given child.

/dʒ/ in Word-Initial Positions

Treatment Exemplars and Recording Sheet

Use stimuli from the **Stimulus Book,** *Volume 2.*

Print this page from CD or photocopy this page for your clinical use.

Name/Age:	Date:
Goal: Production of /dʒ/ in word-initial positions with 90% accuracy when asked an evoking question while showing a stimulus.	Clinician:

Scoring: Correct: ✓   Incorrect or no response: X

Target skills	Discrete Trials														
	1	2	3	4	5	6	7	8	9	10	11	12	13	14	15
1. jacket															
2. jar															
3. jam															
4. jet															
5. jug															
6. jumping															
7. jungle															
8. juggler															

When the child has met the learning criterion of 10 consecutively correct evoked (nonimitated) responses for each of the 6 to 8 target exemplars, conduct a probe to see if the production has generalized to previously baserated but untrained exemplars.

If the probes do not meet the 90% correct criterion for untrained exemplars, teach additional exemplars and then probe again.

/dʒ/ in Word-Initial Positions

Probe Protocols and Recording Sheet

Use stimuli from the **Stimulus Book,** *Volume 2.*

Print this page from the CD or photocopy this page for your clinical use.

On the probes, present only the untrained exemplars (UT). When the child fails to meet the 90% correct probe criterion, either teach 2 to 4 new exemplars or give additional training trials on already trained stimuli. If needed, select new exemplars for probes. Probe at least 10 untrained exemplars. Alternate probes and treatment until the probe criterion is met.

Scripts for Probe Trials		Note
Clinician	[*untrained stimulus: junkyard*] "What is this?"	No modeling or prompts
Child	"Junkyard."	A correct, generalized response
Clinician	Scores the response as correct.	No reinforcement
Clinician	[*untrained stimulus: jaguar*] "What is this?"	The second probe trial
Child	"aguar."	A wrong probe response
Clinician	Scores the response as incorrect.	No corrective feedback

Name:	Date:	Session #:
Age:	**Clinician:**	
Diagnosis: Articulation/Phonologic Disorder	**Word-initial /dʒ/ probe**	
Untrained Stimuli	**Score: + correct; – incorrect or no responses**	
1. junkyard		
2. jaguar		
3. jaw		
4. juice		
5. jade		
6. jail		
7. jackal		
8. janitor		
9. jogging		
10. jellyfish		
11. jellybean		
12. jukebox		
Percent correct: (Criterion: 90%)		

If the child does not meet the probe criterion, give additional training on already trained exemplars or teach a few new exemplars. Subsequently, readminister the probe trials. When the child meets the 90% correct probe criterion for the exemplars, shift training to the sentence or conversational level or to another phoneme.

/dʒ/ in Word-Final Positions

Baserate Protocols

Use stimuli from the **Stimulus Book, *Volume 2***.

At the beginning of each trial, place a relevant stimulus (an object, a picture, or a printed word) in front of the child. Point to the stimulus as you ask an evoking question. Do not respond in any way to the child's correct, incorrect, or lack of responses.

Scripts for Evoked Baserate Trial		Note
Clinician	[*stimulus: badge*] "What is this?"	Evoked trial
Child	"bæ."	Omission of final /dʒ/
Clinician	Pulls the stimulus toward her; records the response.	No corrective feedback
Clinician	[*stimulus: cage*] "What is this?"	The next evoked trial
Child	"cɛ."	Omission of final /dʒ/
Clinician	Pulls the stimulus toward her; records the response.	No corrective feedback

Administer the modeled baserate trials only after completing the evoked trials on all 20 (or more) exemplars.

Scripts for Modeled Baserate Trial		Note
Clinician	[*stimulus: badge*] "What is this? Say, *badge*."	Modeled trial
Child	"Badge."	Correct response
Clinician	Pulls the stimulus toward her; records the response.	No reinforcement
Clinician	[*stimulus: cage*] "What is this? Say, *cage*."	The next modeled trial
Child	"cɛ."	Omission of final /dʒ/
Clinician	Pulls the stimulus toward her; records the response.	No corrective feedback

Use the recording sheet with exemplars shown on the next page to establish the baserates; print it from the CD.

/dʒ/ in Word-Final Positions

Baserate Exemplars and Recording Sheet

*Use stimuli from the **Stimulus Book, Volume 2**.*

Print this page from the CD or photocopy this page for your clinical use.

Name/Age:	Date:
Goal: To establish the baserate production of /dʒ/ in word-final positions.	Clinician:

Scoring: Correct: ✓   Incorrect or no response: X

/dʒ/ in word-final positions	Evoked	Modeled
1. badge		
2. cage		
3. page		
4. fudge		
5. hedge		
6. luggage		
7. garbage		
8. package		
9. cabbage		
10. bandage		
11. bridge		
12. ridge		
13. stage		
14. lodge		
15. judge		
16. carriage		
17. sausage		
18. beverage		
19. village		
20. college		
Percent correct baserate		

Replace or add new exemplars as you see fit for a given child. After establishing the baserates, begin production teaching. Follow the protocols given on the next page.

/dʒ/ in Word-Final Positions

Treatment Protocols

Use stimuli from the **Stimulus Book,** *Volume 2.*

Teach 6 to 8 exemplars using the following script.

Place a relevant stimulus (an object, a picture, or a printed word) in front of the child and point to the stimulus as you ask an evoking question.

Scripts for Modeled Discrete Trial Training		Note
Clinician	[*stimulus: badge*] "What is this? Say, *ba**dge***."	Modeling; the target vocally emphasized
Child	"bæ."	A wrong response
Clinician	"No. That's not correct. You said *bæ*, but it's a *ba**dge**.*"	Corrective feedback
Clinician	[*the same stimulus*] "What is this? Say, *ba**dge**. Don't forget the *dʒ* sound at the end."	The next trial
Child	"Badge."	A correct response
Clinician	"Excellent! You didn't miss the *dʒ* sound at the end of the word!"	Verbal praise

Repeat the trials until the child gives 5 consecutively correct, imitated responses.

When the child imitates 5 correct responses in sequence, fade the modeling.

Scripts for Fading the Modeling		Note
Clinician	[*stimulus: badge*] "What is this? Don't forget the *dʒ* sound at the end."	Only a prompt
Child	"bæ."	A wrong response
Clinician	"Didn't you forget the *dʒ*? It's a *badge*, not *bæ*. Remember to say *dʒ* sound at the end."	Corrective feedback
Clinician	[*the same stimulus*] "What is this? It ends with . . . " [*silently models the articulatory posture for the target sound.*]	The next trial; a partial modeling
Child	"Badge."	A correct response
Clinician	"That's great! You said *badge*, not *bæ*."	Verbal praise
Clinician	[*the same stimulus*] "What is this?"	Typical question; evoked trial
Child	"Badge."	A correct response
Clinician	"I like it! You said it correctly!"	Verbal praise

If the wrong responses persist on 4 to 5 evoked trials, reinstate partial or full modeling for a few trials, again fade the modeling, and re-present the evoked trials.

When the child meets the tentative learning criterion of 10 consecutively correct, nonimitated responses for a given stimulus item, move on to the next stimulus item. With this procedure, teach 6 to 8 exemplars shown on the following recording sheet. Use different exemplars as you see fit for a given child.

/dʒ/ in Word-Final Positions

Treatment Exemplars and Recording Sheet

Use stimuli from the **Stimulus Book,** *Volume 2.*

Print this page from CD or photocopy this page for your clinical use.

Name/Age:		Date:
Goal: Production of /dʒ/ in word-final positions with 90% accuracy when asked an evoking question while showing a stimulus.		Clinician:

Scoring: Correct: ✓   Incorrect or no response: X

Target skills	Discrete Trials														
	1	2	3	4	5	6	7	8	9	10	11	12	13	14	15
1. badge															
2. cage															
3. page															
4. fudge															
5. hedge															
6. luggage															
7. garbage															
8. package															

When the child has met the learning criterion of 10 consecutively correct evoked (nonimitated) responses for each of the 6 to 8 target exemplars, conduct a probe to see if the production has generalized to previously baserated but untrained exemplars.

If the probes do not meet the 90% correct criterion for untrained exemplars, teach additional exemplars and then probe again.

/dʒ/ in Word-Final Positions

Probe Protocols and Recording Sheet

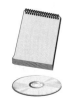

Use stimuli from the **Stimulus Book, Volume 2**.

Print this page from the CD or photocopy this page for your clinical use.

On the probes, present only the untrained exemplars (UT). When the child fails to meet the 90% correct probe criterion, either teach 2 to 4 new exemplars or give additional training trials on already trained stimuli. If needed, select new exemplars for probes. Probe at least 10 untrained exemplars. Alternate probes and treatment until the probe criterion is met.

Scripts for Probe Trials		Note
Clinician	[*untrained stimulus: cabbage*] "What is this?"	No modeling or prompts
Child	"Cabbage."	A correct, generalized response
Clinician	Scores the response as correct.	No reinforcement
Clinician	[*untrained stimulus: bandage*] "What is this?"	The second probe trial
Child	"Bandɛ."	A wrong probe response
Clinician	Scores the response as incorrect.	No corrective feedback

Name:	Date:	Session #:
Age:	**Clinician:**	
Diagnosis: Articulation/Phonologic Disorder	**Word-final /dʒ/ probe**	
Untrained Stimuli	**Score: + correct; – incorrect or no responses**	
1. cabbage		
2. bandage		
3. bridge		
4. ridge		
5. stage		
6. lodge		
7. judge		
8. carriage		
9. sausage		
10. beverage		
11. village		
12. college		
Percent correct: (Criterion: 90%)		

If the child does not meet the probe criterion, give additional training on already trained exemplars or teach a few new exemplars. Subsequently, readminister the probe trials. When the child meets the 90% correct probe criterion for the exemplars, shift training to the sentence or conversational level or to another phoneme.

/w/ in Word-Initial Positions

Baserate Protocols

Use stimuli from the **Stimulus Book,** *Volume 4.*

The English /w/ does not occur in word-final positions.

At the beginning of each trial, place a relevant stimulus (an object, a picture, or a printed word) in front of the child. Point to the stimulus as you ask an evoking question. Do not respond in any way to the child's correct, incorrect, or lack of responses.

Scripts for Evoked Baserate Trial		Note
Clinician	[*stimulus: wall*] "What is this?"	Evoked trial
Child	"all."	Omission of initial /w/
Clinician	Pulls the stimulus toward her; records the response.	No corrective feedback
Clinician	[*stimulus: wagon*] "What is this?"	The next evoked trial
Child	"ægon."	Omission of initial /w/
Clinician	Pulls the stimulus toward her; records the response.	No corrective feedback

Administer the modeled baserate trials only after completing the evoked trials on all 20 (or more) exemplars.

Scripts for Modeled Baserate Trial		Note
Clinician	[*stimulus: wall*] "What is this? Say, *wall.*"	Modeled trial
Child	"Wall."	Correct response
Clinician	Pulls the stimulus toward her; records the response.	No reinforcement
Clinician	[*stimulus: wagon*] "What is this? Say, *wagon.*"	The next modeled trial
Child	"ægon."	Omission of initial /w/
Clinician	Pulls the stimulus toward her; records the response.	No corrective feedback

Use the recording sheet with exemplars shown on the next page to establish the baserates; print it from the CD.

/w/ in Word-Initial Positions

Baserate Exemplars and Recording Sheet

Use stimuli from the **Stimulus Book,** *Volume 4.*

Print this page from the CD or photocopy this page for your clinical use.

Name/Age:	Date:
Goal: To establish the baserate production of /w/ in word-initial positions.	Clinician:

Scoring: Correct: ✓   Incorrect or no response: X

/w/ in word-initial positions	Evoked	Modeled
1. wall		
2. wagon		
3. wallet		
4. wand		
5. wood		
6. waitress		
7. wardrobe		
8. watermelon		
9. woodpecker		
10. woman		
11. web		
12. worm		
13. wolf		
14. wok		
15. weed		
16. watchtower		
17. wallaby		
18. windmill		
19. walkie-talkie		
20. wolverine		
Percent correct baserate		

Replace or add new exemplars as you see fit for a given child. After establishing the baserates, begin production teaching. Follow the protocols given on the next page.

/w/ in Word-Initial Positions

Treatment Protocols

Use stimuli from the **Stimulus Book, Volume 4.**

Teach 6 to 8 exemplars using the following script.

Place a relevant stimulus in front of the child (an object, a picture, or a printed word) and ask a question as you point to the stimulus.

Scripts for Modeled Discrete Trial Training		Note
Clinician	[*stimulus: wall*] "What is this? Say, **wa**ll."	Modeling; the target vocally emphasized
Child	"all."	A wrong response
Clinician	"No. That's not correct. You said *all*, but it's a **wa**ll."	Corrective feedback
Clinician	[*the same stimulus*] "What is this? Say, **wa**ll. Don't forget the *wə* sound at the beginning."	The next trial
Child	"Wall."	A correct response
Clinician	"Excellent! You didn't miss the *w* sound this time!"	Verbal praise

Repeat the trials until the child gives 5 consecutively correct, imitated responses.

When the child imitates 5 correct responses in sequence, fade the modeling.

Scripts for Fading the Modeling		Note
Clinician	[*stimulus: wall*] "What is this? Don't forget the *wə* sound at the beginning."	Only a prompt
Child	"all."	A wrong response
Clinician	"Gee, you forgot the *wə* sound! It's a *wall*, not *all*. Put the *w* at the beginning."	Corrective feedback
Clinician	[*the same stimulus*] "What is this? It starts with . . . " [*silently models the articulatory posture for the target sound.*]	The next trial; a partial modeling
Child	"Wall."	A correct response
Clinician	"That's great! You correctly said wall, not all."	Verbal praise
Clinician	[*the same stimulus*] "What is this?"	Typical question; evoked trial
Child	"Wall."	A correct response
Clinician	"Great job! You are doing very well!"	Verbal praise

If the wrong responses persist on 4 to 5 evoked trials, reinstate partial or full modeling for a few trials, again fade the modeling, and re-present the evoked trials.

When the child meets the tentative learning criterion of 10 consecutively correct, nonimitated responses for a given stimulus item, move on to the next stimulus item. With this procedure, teach 6 to 8 exemplars shown on the following recording sheet. Use different exemplars as you see fit for a given child.

/w/ in Word-Initial Positions

Treatment Exemplars and Recording Sheet

Use stimuli from the **Stimulus Book, *Volume 4***.

Print this page from CD or photocopy this page for your clinical use.

Name/Age:	Date:
Goal: Production of /w/ in word-initial positions with 90% accuracy when asked an evoking question while showing a stimulus.	Clinician:

Scoring: Correct: ✓ Incorrect or no response: X

Target skills	Discrete Trials														
	1	2	3	4	5	6	7	8	9	10	11	12	13	14	15
1. wall															
2. wagon															
3. wallet															
4. wand															
5. wood															
6. waitress															
7. wardrobe															
8. watermelon															

When the child has met the learning criterion of 10 consecutively correct evoked (nonimitated) responses for each of the 6 to 8 target exemplars, conduct a probe to see if the production has generalized to previously baserated but untrained exemplars.

If the probes do not meet the 90% correct criterion for untrained exemplars, teach additional exemplars and then probe again.

/w/ in Word-Initial Positions

Probe Protocols and Recording Sheet

Use stimuli from the **Stimulus Book,** *Volume 4.*

Print this page from the CD or photocopy this page for your clinical use.

On the probes, present only the untrained exemplars (UT). When the child fails to meet the 90% correct probe criterion, either teach 2 to 4 new exemplars or give additional training trials on already trained stimuli. If needed, select new exemplars for probes. Probe at least 10 untrained exemplars. Alternate probes and treatment until the probe criterion is met.

Scripts for Probe Trials		
Clinician	[*untrained stimulus: woodpecker*] "What do they call this bird?"	No modeling or prompts
Child	"Woodpecker."	A correct, generalized response
Clinician	Scores the response as correct.	No reinforcement
Clinician	[*untrained stimulus: woman*] "Who is this?"	The second probe trial
Child	"oman."	A wrong probe response
Clinician	Scores the response as incorrect.	No corrective feedback

Name:	Date:	Session #:
Age:	**Clinician:**	
Diagnosis: Articulation/Phonologic Disorder	**Word-initial /w/ probe**	
Untrained Stimuli	**Score: + correct; – incorrect or no responses**	
1. woodpecker		
2. woman		
3. web		
4. worm		
5. wolf		
6. wok		
7. weed		
8. watchtower		
9. wallaby		
10. windmill		
11. walkie-talkie		
12. wolverine		
Percent correct: (Criterion: 90%)		

If the child does not meet the probe criterion, give additional training on already trained exemplars or teach a few new exemplars. Subsequently, readminister the probe trials. When the child meets the 90% correct probe criterion for the exemplars, shift training to the sentence or conversational level or to another phoneme.

/j/ in Word-Initial Positions

Baserate Protocols

Use stimuli from the **Stimulus Book,** *Volume 4.*

English words do not end in /j/.

At the beginning of each trial, place a relevant stimulus (an object, a picture, or a printed word) in front of the child. Point to the stimulus as you ask an evoking question. Do not respond in any way to the child's correct, incorrect, or lack of responses.

Scripts for Evoked Baserate Trial		Note
Clinician	[*stimulus: color yellow*] "What color is this?"	Evoked trial
Child	"ellow."	Omission of initial /j/
Clinician	Pulls the stimulus toward her; records the response.	No corrective feedback
Clinician	[*stimulus: yak*] "What is this?"	The next evoked trial
Child	"æk."	Omission of initial /j/
Clinician	Pulls the stimulus toward her; records the response.	No corrective feedback

Administer the modeled baserate trials only after completing the evoked trials on all 20 (or more) exemplars.

Scripts for Modeled Baserate Trial		Note
Clinician	[*stimulus: color yellow*] "What color is this? Say, *yellow.*"	Modeled trial
Child	"Yellow."	Correct response
Clinician	Pulls the stimulus toward her; records the response.	No reinforcement
Clinician	[*stimulus: yak*] "What is this? Say, *yak.*"	The next modeled trial
Child	"æk."	Omission of initial /j/
Clinician	Pulls the stimulus toward her; records the response.	No corrective feedback

Use the recording sheet with exemplars shown on the next page to establish the baserates; print it from the CD.

/j/ in Word-Initial Positions

Baserate Exemplars and Recording Sheet

Use stimuli from the **Stimulus Book,** *Volume 4.*

Print this page from the CD or photocopy this page for your clinical use.

Name/Age:	Date:
Goal: To establish the baserate production of /j/ in word-initial positions.	Clinician:

Scoring: Correct: ✓   Incorrect or no response: X

/j/ in word-initial positions	Evoked	Modeled
1. yellow		
2. yak		
3. yam		
4. yard		
5. yoke		
6. unicorn		
7. uniform		
8. yellowbird		
9. unicycle		
10. ukulele		
11. yacht		
12. yarn		
13. yogurt		
14. yolk		
15. yew		
16. utensil		
17. uvula		
18. yellow jacket		
19. Yellowstone		
20. Yankee Doodle		
Percent correct baserate		

Replace or add new exemplars as you see fit for a given child. After establishing the baserates, begin production teaching. Follow the protocols given on the next page.

/j/ in Word-Initial Positions

Treatment Protocols

Use stimuli from the **Stimulus Book, Volume 4**.

Teach 6 to 8 exemplars using the following script.

Place a relevant stimulus in front of the child (an object, a picture, or a printed word) and ask a question as you point to the stimulus.

Scripts for Modeled Discrete Trial Training		Note
Clinician	[*stimulus: color yellow*] "What color is this? Say, **ye**llow."	Modeling; the target vocally emphasized
Child	"ellow."	A wrong response
Clinician	"No. That's not correct. You said *ellow*, but it's **ye**llow."	Corrective feedback
Clinician	[*the same stimulus*] "What color is this? Say, **ye**llow. Don't forget the *j* sound at the beginning."	The next trial
Child	"Yellow."	A correct response
Clinician	"Excellent! You remembered the *j* sound this time!"	Verbal praise

Repeat the trials until the child gives 5 consecutively correct, imitated responses.

When the child imitates 5 correct responses in sequence, fade the modeling.

Scripts for Fading the Modeling		Note
Clinician	[*stimulus: color yellow*] "What color is this? Don't forget the *j* sound at the beginning."	Only a prompt
Child	"ellow."	A wrong response
Clinician	"Did you forget something? The *j* sound! It's *yellow*, not *ellow*. Put the *j* sound at the beginning."	Corrective feedback
Clinician	[*the same stimulus*] "What color is this? It starts with . . . " [*silently models the articulatory posture for the target sound.*]	The next trial; a partial modeling
Child	"Yellow."	A correct response
Clinician	"That's great! You said *yellow*, not *ellow*."	Verbal praise
Clinician	[*the same stimulus*] "What color is this?"	Typical question; evoked trial
Child	"Yellow."	A correct response
Clinician	"Great job! You are very smart!"	Verbal praise

If the wrong responses persist on 4 to 5 evoked trials, reinstate partial or full modeling for a few trials, again fade the modeling, and re-present the evoked trials.

When the child meets the tentative learning criterion of 10 consecutively correct, nonimitated responses for a given stimulus item, move on to the next stimulus item. With this procedure, teach 6 to 8 exemplars shown on the following recording sheet. Use different exemplars as you see fit for a given child.

/j/ in Word-Initial Positions

Treatment Exemplars and Recording Sheet

Use stimuli from the **Stimulus Book,** *Volume 4.*

Print this page from CD or photocopy this page for your clinical use.

Name/Age:	Date:
Goal: Production of /j/ in word-initial positions with 90% accuracy when asked an evoking question while showing a stimulus.	Clinician:

Scoring: Correct: ✓   Incorrect or no response: X

Target skills	Discrete Trials														
	1	2	3	4	5	6	7	8	9	10	11	12	13	14	15
1. yellow															
2. yak															
3. yam															
4. yard															
5. yoke															
6. unicorn															
7. uniform															
8. yellowbird															

When the child has met the learning criterion of 10 consecutively correct evoked (nonimitated) responses for each of the 6 to 8 target exemplars, conduct a probe to see if the production has generalized to previously baserated but untrained exemplars.

If the probes do not meet the 90% correct criterion for untrained exemplars, teach additional exemplars and then probe again.

/j/ in Word-Initial Positions

Probe Protocols and Recording Sheet

Use stimuli from the **Stimulus Book, Volume 4**.

Print this page from the CD or photocopy this page for your clinical use.

On the probes, present only the untrained exemplars (UT). When the child fails to meet the 90% correct probe criterion, either teach 2 to 4 new exemplars or give additional training trials on already trained stimuli. If needed, select new exemplars for probes. Probe at least 10 untrained exemplars. Alternate probes and treatment until the probe criterion is met.

Scripts for Probe Trials		Note
Clinician	[untrained stimulus: unicycle] "What do you call this?"	No modeling or prompts
Child	"Unicycle."	A correct, generalized response
Clinician	Scores the response as correct.	No reinforcement
Clinician	[untrained stimulus: ukulele] "What is this?"	The second probe trial
Child	"kəlele."	A wrong probe response
Clinician	Scores the response as incorrect.	No corrective feedback

Name:	Date:	Session #:
Age:	**Clinician:**	
Diagnosis: Articulation/Phonologic Disorder	**Word-initial /j/ probe**	
Untrained Stimuli	**Score: + correct; – incorrect or no responses**	
1. unicycle		
2. ukulele		
3. yacht		
4. yarn		
5. yogurt		
6. yolk		
7. yew		
8. utensil		
9. uvula		
10. yellow jacket		
11. Yellowstone		
12. Yankee Doodle		
Percent correct: (Criterion: 90%)		

If the child does not meet the probe criterion, give additional training on already trained exemplars or teach a few new exemplars. Subsequently, readminister the probe trials. When the child meets the 90% correct probe criterion for the exemplars, shift training to the sentence or conversational level or to another phoneme.

/l/ in Word-Initial Positions

Baserate Protocols

Use stimuli from the **Stimulus Book,** *Volume 3.*

At the beginning of each trial, place a relevant stimulus (an object, a picture, or a printed word) in front of the child. Point to the stimulus as you ask an evoking question. Do not respond in any way to the child's correct, incorrect, or lack of responses.

Scripts for Evoked Baserate Trial		Note
Clinician	[*stimulus: lake*] "What is this?"	Evoked trial
Child	"ake."	Omission of initial /l/
Clinician	Pulls the stimulus toward her; records the response.	No corrective feedback
Clinician	[*stimulus: lamb*] "What is this?"	The next evoked trial
Child	"æmb."	Omission of initial /l/
Clinician	Pulls the stimulus toward her; records the response.	No corrective feedback

Administer the modeled baserate trials only after completing the evoked trials on all 20 (or more) exemplars.

Scripts for Modeled Baserate Trial		Note
Clinician	[*stimulus: lake*] "What is this? Say, *lake.*"	Modeled trial
Child	"Lake."	Correct response
Clinician	Pulls the stimulus toward her; records the response.	No reinforcement
Clinician	[*stimulus: lamb*] "What is this? Say, *lamb.*"	The next modeled trial
Child	"æmb."	Omission of initial /l/
Clinician	Pulls the stimulus toward her; records the response.	No corrective feedback

Use the recording sheet with exemplars shown on the next page to establish the baserates; print it from the CD.

/l/ in Word-Initial Positions

Baserate Exemplars and Recording Sheet

Use stimuli from the **Stimulus Book,** *Volume 3.*

Print this page from the CD or photocopy this page for your clinical use.

Name/Age:	Date:
Goal: To establish the baserate production of /l/ in word-initial positions.	Clinician:

Scoring: Correct: ✓   Incorrect or no response: X

/l/ in word-initial positions	Evoked	Modeled
1. lake		
2. lamb		
3. lamp		
4. lid		
5. lock		
6. loudspeaker		
7. launch pad		
8. lightning bug		
9. lemonade		
10. lawn mower		
11. lace		
12. leaf		
13. light		
14. lime		
15. lung		
16. leatherback		
17. leopard		
18. library		
19. lighthouse		
20. laboratory		
Percent correct baserate		

Replace or add new exemplars as you see fit for a given child. After establishing the baserates, begin production teaching. Follow the protocols given on the next page.

/l/ in Word-Initial Positions

Treatment Protocols

Use stimuli from the **Stimulus Book,** *Volume 3.*

Teach 6 to 8 exemplars using the following script.

Place a relevant stimulus in front of the child (an object, a picture, or a printed word) and ask a question as you point to the stimulus.

Scripts for Modeled Discrete Trial Training		Note
Clinician	[*stimulus: lake*] "What is this? Say, **la**ke."	Modeling; the target vocally emphasized
Child	"ake."	A wrong response
Clinician	"No. That's not correct. You said *ake*, but it's a **la**ke."	Corrective feedback
Clinician	[*the same stimulus*] "What is this? Say, **la**ke. Don't forget the *l* sound at the beginning."	The next trial
Child	"Lake."	A correct response
Clinician	"Excellent! You didn't miss the *l* sound this time!"	Verbal praise

Repeat the trials until the child gives 5 consecutively correct, imitated responses.

When the child imitates 5 correct responses in sequence, fade the modeling.

Scripts for Fading the Modeling		Note
Clinician	[*stimulus: lake*] "What is this? Don't forget the *l* sound at the beginning."	Only a prompt
Child	"ake."	A wrong response
Clinician	"Oh no! You forgot the *l* sound! It's a *lake*, not *ake*. Put the l at the beginning."	Corrective feedback
Clinician	[*the same stimulus*] "What is this? It starts with . . . " [*silently models the tongue posture for the target sound.*]	The next trial; a partial modeling
Child	"Lake."	A correct response
Clinician	"That's great! It is a *lake* as you correctly said, not *ake*!"	Verbal praise
Clinician	[*the same stimulus*] "What is this?"	Typical question; evoked trial
Child	"Lake."	A correct response
Clinician	"Great job! You are correct again!"	Verbal praise

If the wrong responses persist on 4 to 5 evoked trials, reinstate partial or full modeling for a few trials, again fade the modeling, and re-present the evoked trials.

When the child meets the tentative learning criterion of 10 consecutively correct, nonimitated responses for a given stimulus item, move on to the next stimulus item. With this procedure, teach 6 to 8 exemplars shown on the following recording sheet. Use different exemplars as you see fit for a given child.

/l/ in Word-Initial Positions

Treatment Exemplars and Recording Sheet

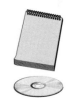

Use stimuli from the **Stimulus Book,** *Volume 3.*

Print this page from CD or photocopy this page for your clinical use.

Name/Age:	Date:
Goal: Production of /l/ in word-initial positions with 90% accuracy when asked an evoking question while showing a stimulus.	Clinician:

Scoring: Correct: ✓   Incorrect or no response: X

Target skills	Discrete Trials														
	1	2	3	4	5	6	7	8	9	10	11	12	13	14	15
1. lake															
2. lamb															
3. lamp															
4. lid															
5. lock															
6. loudspeaker															
7. launch pad															
8. lightning bug															

When the child has met the learning criterion of 10 consecutively correct evoked (nonimitated) responses for each of the 6 to 8 target exemplars, conduct a probe to see if the production has generalized to previously baserated but untrained exemplars.

If the probes do not meet the 90% correct criterion for untrained exemplars, teach additional exemplars and then probe again.

/l/ in Word-Initial Positions

Probe Protocols and Recording Sheet

Use stimuli from the **Stimulus Book, Volume 3**.

Print this page from the CD or photocopy this page for your clinical use.

On the probes, present only the untrained exemplars (UT). When the child fails to meet the 90% correct probe criterion, either teach 2 to 4 new exemplars or give additional training trials on already trained stimuli. If needed, select new exemplars for probes. Probe at least 10 untrained exemplars. Alternate probes and treatment until the probe criterion is met.

Scripts for Probe Trials		Note
Clinician	[*untrained stimulus: lemonade*] "What is this?"	No modeling or prompts
Child	"Lemonade."	A correct, generalized response
Clinician	Scores the response as correct.	No reinforcement
Clinician	[*untrained stimulus: lawn mower*] "What is this?"	The second probe trial
Child	"awn mower."	A wrong probe response
Clinician	Scores the response as incorrect.	No corrective feedback

Name:	Date:	Session #:
Age:	**Clinician:**	
Diagnosis: Articulation/Phonologic Disorder	**Word-initial /l/ probe**	
Untrained Stimuli	**Score: + correct; – incorrect or no responses**	
1. lemonade		
2. lawn mower		
3. lace		
4. leaf		
5. light		
6. lime		
7. lung		
8. leatherback		
9. leopard		
10. library		
11. lighthouse		
12. laboratory		
Percent correct: (Criterion: 90%)		

If the child does not meet the probe criterion, give additional training on already trained exemplars or teach a few new exemplars. Subsequently, readminister the probe trials. When the child meets the 90% correct probe criterion for the exemplars, shift training to the sentence or conversational level or to another phoneme.

/l/ in Word-Final Positions

Baserate Protocols

Use stimuli from the **Stimulus Book,** *Volume 3.*

At the beginning of each trial, place a relevant stimulus (an object, a picture, or a printed word) in front of the child. Point to the stimulus as you ask an evoking question. Do not respond in any way to the child's correct, incorrect, or lack of responses.

Scripts for Evoked Baserate Trial		Note
Clinician	[*stimulus: doll*] "What is this?"	Evoked trial
Child	"dɑ."	Omission of final /l/
Clinician	Pulls the stimulus toward her; records the response.	No corrective feedback
Clinician	[*stimulus: ball*] "What is this?"	The next evoked trial
Child	"bɑ."	Omission of /l/
Clinician	Pulls the stimulus toward her; records the response.	No corrective feedback

Administer the modeled baserate trials only after completing the evoked trials on all 20 (or more) exemplars.

Scripts for Modeled Baserate Trial		Note
Clinician	[*stimulus: doll*] "What is this? Say, *doll.*"	Modeled trial
Child	"Doll."	Correct response
Clinician	Pulls the stimulus toward her; records the response.	No reinforcement
Clinician	[*stimulus: ball*] "What is this? Say, *ball.*"	The next modeled trial
Child	"bɑ."	Omission of final /l/
Clinician	Pulls the stimulus toward her; records the response.	No corrective feedback

Use the recording sheet with exemplars shown on the next page to establish the baserates; print it from the CD.

/l/ in Word-Final Positions

Baserate Exemplars and Recording Sheet

Use stimuli from the **Stimulus Book,** *Volume 3.*

Print this page from the CD or photocopy this page for your clinical use.

Name/Age:	Date:
Goal: To establish the baserate production of /l/ in word-final positions.	Clinician:

Scoring: Correct: ✓   Incorrect or no response: X

/l/ in word-final positions	Evoked	Modeled
1. doll		
2. ball		
3. bell		
4. bowl		
5. bull		
6. basketball		
7. carousel		
8. ponytail		
9. nightingale		
10. automobile		
11. nail		
12. owl		
13. peal		
14. pool		
15. tail		
16. treadmill		
17. racquetball		
18. snowmobile		
19. garage sale		
20. waterwheel		
Percent correct baserate		

Replace or add new exemplars as you see fit for a given child. After establishing the baserates, begin production teaching. Follow the protocols given on the next page.

/l/ in Word-Final Positions

Treatment Protocols

Use stimuli from the **Stimulus Book,** *Volume 3.*

Teach 6 to 8 exemplars using the following script.

Place a relevant stimulus (an object, a picture, or a printed word) in front of the child and point to the stimulus as you ask an evoking question.

Scripts for Modeled Discrete Trial Training		Note
Clinician	[*stimulus: doll*] "What is this? Say, *doll.*"	Modeling; the target vocally emphasized
Child	"da."	A wrong response
Clinician	"No. That's not correct. You said *da*, but it's a *doll.*"	Corrective feedback
Clinician	[*the same stimulus*] "What is this? Say, *doll*. Don't forget the *l* sound at the end."	The next trial
Child	"Doll."	A correct response
Clinician	"Excellent! You did say the *l* sound at the end of the word!"	Verbal praise

Repeat the trials until the child gives 5 consecutively correct, imitated responses.

When the child imitates 5 correct responses in sequence, fade the modeling.

Scripts for Fading the Modeling		Note
Clinician	[*stimulus: doll*] "What is this? Don't forget the *l* at the end."	Only a prompt
Child	"da."	A wrong response
Clinician	"Oh no! I didn't hear the *l* sound! It's a *doll*, not *da*. Say the *l* at the end."	Corrective feedback
Clinician	[*the same stimulus*] "What is this? It ends with . . . " [*silently models the tongue posture for the target sound.*]	The next trial; a partial modeling
Child	"Doll."	A correct response
Clinician	"That's great! You said *doll*, not *da*."	Verbal praise
Clinician	[*the same stimulus*] "What is this?"	Typical question; evoked trial
Child	"Doll."	A correct response
Clinician	"That's great! I head the *l* sound this time!"	Verbal praise

If the wrong responses persist on 4 to 5 evoked trials, reinstate partial or full modeling for a few trials, again fade the modeling, and re-present the evoked trials.

When the child meets the tentative learning criterion of 10 consecutively correct, nonimitated responses for a given stimulus item, move on to the next stimulus item. With this procedure, teach 6 to 8 exemplars shown on the following recording sheet. Use different exemplars as you see fit for a given child.

/l/ in Word-Final Positions

Treatment Exemplars and Recording Sheet

Use stimuli from the **Stimulus Book, Volume 3.**

Print this page from CD or photocopy this page for your clinical use.

Name/Age:	Date:
Goal: Production of /l/ in word-final positions with 90% accuracy when asked an evoking question while showing a stimulus.	Clinician:

Scoring: Correct: ✓ Incorrect or no response: X

Target skills	Discrete Trials														
	1	2	3	4	5	6	7	8	9	10	11	12	13	14	15
1. doll															
2. ball															
3. bell															
4. bowl															
5. bull															
6. basketball															
7. carousel															
8. ponytail															

When the child has met the learning criterion of 10 consecutively correct evoked (nonimitated) responses for each of the 6 to 8 target exemplars, conduct a probe to see if the production has generalized to previously baserated but untrained exemplars.

If the probes do not meet the 90% correct criterion for untrained exemplars, teach additional exemplars and then probe again.

/l/ in Word-Final Positions

Probe Protocols and Recording Sheet

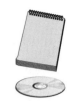

Use stimuli from the **Stimulus Book,** *Volume 3.*

Print this page from the CD or photocopy this page for your clinical use.

On the probes, present only the untrained exemplars (UT). When the child fails to meet the 90% correct probe criterion, either teach 2 to 4 new exemplars or give additional training trials on already trained stimuli. If needed, select new exemplars for probes. Probe at least 10 untrained exemplars. Alternate probes and treatment until the probe criterion is met.

Scripts for Probe Trials		Note
Clinician	[*untrained stimulus: nightingale*] "What is this bird called?"	No modeling or prompts
Child	"Nightingale."	A correct, generalized response
Clinician	Scores the response as correct.	No reinforcement
Clinician	[*untrained stimulus: automobile*] "What is this? It begins like *automo* . . . "	The second probe trial
Child	"automobi."	A wrong probe response
Clinician	Scores the response as incorrect.	No corrective feedback

Name:	Date:	Session #:
Age:	Clinician:	
Diagnosis: Articulation/Phonologic Disorder	**Word-final /l/ probe**	
Untrained Stimuli	**Score: + correct; – incorrect or no responses**	
1. nightingale		
2. automobile		
3. nail		
4. owl		
5. peal		
6. pool		
7. tail		
8. treadmill		
9. racquetball		
10. snowmobile		
11. garage sale		
12. waterwheel		
Percent correct: (Criterion: 90%)		

If the child does not meet the probe criterion, give additional training on already trained exemplars or teach a few new exemplars. Subsequently, readminister the probe trials. When the child meets the 90% correct probe criterion for the exemplars, shift training to the sentence or conversational level or to another phoneme.

/r/ in Word-Initial Positions

Baserate Protocols

Use stimuli from the **Stimulus Book, Volume 4**.

At the beginning of each trial, place a relevant stimulus (an object, a picture, or a printed word if the child can read) in front of the child. Point to the stimulus as you ask an evoking question. Do not respond in any way to the child's correct, incorrect, or lack of responses.

Scripts for Evoked Baserate Trial		Note
Clinician	[*stimulus: rock*] "What is this?"	Evoked trial
Child	"A wock."	Substitution of w for r
Clinician	Pulls the stimulus toward her; records the response.	No corrective feedback
Clinician	[*stimulus: red*] "What color is this?"	The next evoked trial
Child	"wed."	Substitution of w for r
Clinician	Pulls the stimulus toward her; records the response.	No corrective feedback

Administer the modeled baserate trials only after completing the evoked trials on all 20 (or more) exemplars.

Scripts for Modeled Baserate Trial		Note
Clinician	[*stimulus: rock*] "What is this? Say, *rock.*"	Modeled trial
Child	"wock."	Substitution of w for r
Clinician	Pulls the stimulus toward her; records the response.	No corrective feedback
Clinician	[*stimulus: red*] "What color is this? Say, *red.*"	The next modeled trial
Child	"wed."	Substitution of w for r
Clinician	Pulls the stimulus toward her; records the response.	No corrective feedback

Use the recording sheet with exemplars shown on the next page to establish the baserates; print it from the CD.

/r/ in Word-Initial Positions

Baserate Exemplars and Recording Sheet

Use stimuli from the **Stimulus Book,** *Volume 4.*

Print this page from the CD or photocopy this page for your clinical use.

Name/Age:	Date:
Goal: To establish the baserate production of /r/ in word-initial positions.	Clinician:

Scoring: Correct: ✓   Incorrect or no response: X

/r/ in word-initial positions	Evoked	Modeled
1. rock		
2. red		
3. wrist		
4. rake		
5. rib		
6. rabbit		
7. remote		
8. relish		
9. rainbow		
10. raisin		
11. raft		
12. rice		
13. rag		
14. rat		
15. robe		
16. raccoon		
17. rainfall		
18. rowboat		
19. relaxing		
20. reptile		
Percent correct baserate		

Replace or add new exemplars as you see fit for a given child. After establishing the baserates, begin production teaching. Follow the protocols given on the next page.

/r/ in Word-Initial Positions

Treatment Protocols

Use stimuli from the **Stimulus Book,** *Volume 4.*

Teach 6 to 8 exemplars using the following script.

Place a relevant stimulus in front of the child (an object, a picture, or a printed word if the child can read) and ask a question as you point to the stimulus.

Scripts for Modeled Discrete Trial Training		Note
Clinician	[*stimulus: rock*] "What is this? Say, *rock*."	Modeling; the target vocally emphasized
Child	"wock."	A wrong response
Clinician	"No. That's not correct. You said *wock*, but it's a *rock*. You need to say the **r** sound instead of the *w* sound at the beginning"	Corrective feedback
Clinician	[*the same stimulus*] "What is this? Say, *rock*. Don't forget the *r* at the beginning, *rock*."	The next trial
Child	"Rock."	A correct response
Clinician	"Marvelous! You didn't miss the *r* this time!"	Verbal praise

Repeat the trials until the child gives 5 consecutively correct, imitated responses.

When the child imitates 5 correct responses in sequence, fade the modeling.

Scripts for Fading the Modeling		Note
Clinician	[*stimulus: rock*] "What is this? Don't forget to say the *r* sound instead of the *w* sound at the beginning."	Only a prompt
Child	"wock."	A wrong response
Clinician	"Oops, you said the *w* sound instead of the *r* sound! It's a *rock*, not *wock*. Put the *r* at the beginning."	Corrective feedback
Clinician	[*the same stimulus*] "What is this? It starts with . . . " [*silently models the articulatory posture for initial /r/.*]	The next trial; a partial modeling
Child	"Rock."	A correct response
Clinician	"Fantastic job! You said *rock*, not *wock*."	Verbal praise
Clinician	[*the same stimulus*] "What is this?"	Typical question; evoked trial
Child	"Rock."	A correct response
Clinician	"Way to go! You said it correctly! Keep up the good work."	Verbal praise

If the wrong responses persist on 4 to 5 evoked trials, reinstate partial or full modeling for a few trials, again fade the modeling, and re-present the evoked trials.

When the child meets the tentative learning criterion of 10 consecutively correct, nonimitated responses for a given stimulus item, move on to the next stimulus item. With this procedure, teach 6 to 8 exemplars shown on the following recording sheet. Use different exemplars as you see fit for a given child.

/r/ in Word-Initial Positions

Treatment Exemplars and Recording Sheet

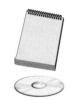

Use stimuli from the **Stimulus Book,** *Volume 4.*

Print this page from CD or photocopy this page for your clinical use.

Name/Age:	Date:
Goal: Production of /r/ in word-initial positions with 90% accuracy when asked an evoking question while showing a stimulus.	Clinician:

Scoring: Correct: ✓   Incorrect or no response: X

Target skills	Discrete Trials														
	1	2	3	4	5	6	7	8	9	10	11	12	13	14	15
1. rock															
2. red															
3. wrist															
4. rake															
5. rib															
6. rabbit															
7. remote															
8. relish															

When the child has met the learning criterion of 10 consecutively correct evoked (nonimitated) responses for each of the 6 to 8 target exemplars, conduct a probe to see if the production has generalized to previously baserated but untrained exemplars.

If the probes do not meet the 90% correct criterion for untrained exemplars, teach additional exemplars and then probe again.

/r/ in Word-Initial Positions

Probe Protocols and Recording Sheet

*Use stimuli from the **Stimulus Book, Volume 4**.*

Print this page from the CD or photocopy this page for your clinical use.

On the probes, present only the untrained exemplars (UT). When the child fails to meet the 90% correct probe criterion, either teach 2 to 4 new exemplars or give additional training trials on already trained stimuli. If needed, select new exemplars for probes. Probe at least 10 untrained exemplars. Alternate probes and treatment until the probe criterion is met.

Scripts for Probe Trials		Note
Clinician	[*untrained stimulus: rainbow*] "What is this?"	No modeling or prompts
Child	"Rainbow."	A correct, generalized response
Clinician	Scores the response as correct.	No reinforcement
Clinician	[*untrained stimulus: raisin*] "What is this?"	The second probe trial
Child	"waisin."	A wrong probe response
Clinician	Scores the response as incorrect.	No corrective feedback

Name:	Date:	Session #:
Age:	**Clinician:**	
Diagnosis: Articulation/Phonologic Disorder	**Word-initial /r/ probe**	
Untrained Stimuli	**Score: + correct; – incorrect or no responses**	
1. rainbow		
2. raisin		
3. raft		
4. rice		
5. rag		
6. rat		
7. robe		
8. raccoon		
9. rainfall		
10. rowboat		
11. relaxing		
12. reptile		
Percent correct: (Criterion: 90%)		

If the child does not meet the probe criterion, give additional training on already trained exemplars or teach a few new exemplars. Subsequently, readminister the probe trials. When the child meets the 90% correct probe criterion for the exemplars, shift training to the sentence or conversational level or to another phoneme.

/r/ in Word-Final Positions

Baserate Protocols

Use stimuli from the **Stimulus Book,** *Volume 4.*

At the beginning of each trial, place a relevant stimulus (an object, a picture, or a printed word if the child can read) in front of the child. Point to the stimulus as you ask an evoking question. Do not respond in any way to the child's correct, incorrect, or lack of responses.

Scripts for Evoked Baserate Trial		Note
Clinician	[*stimulus: door*] "What is this?"	Evoked trial
Child	"doə."	Vowelization of final /r/
Clinician	Pulls the stimulus toward her; records the response.	No corrective feedback
Clinician	[*stimulus: bear*] "What is this?"	The next evoked trial
Child	"beə."	Vowelization of final /r/
Clinician	Pulls the stimulus toward her; records the response.	No corrective feedback

Administer the modeled baserate trials only after completing the evoked trials on all 20 (or more) exemplars.

Scripts for Modeled Baserate Trial		Note
Clinician	[*stimulus: door*] "What is this? Say, *door.*"	Modeled trial
Child	"Door."	Correct response
Clinician	Pulls the stimulus toward her; records the response.	No reinforcement
Clinician	[*stimulus: bear*] "What is this? Say, *bear.*"	The next modeled trial
Child	"beə."	Vowelization of final /r/
Clinician	Pulls the stimulus toward her; records the response.	No corrective feedback

Use the recording sheet with exemplars shown on the next page to establish the baserates; print it from the CD.

/r/ in Word-Final Positions

Baserate Exemplars and Recording Sheet

Use stimuli from the **Stimulus Book,** *Volume 4.*

Print this page from the CD or photocopy this page for your clinical use.

Name/Age:	Date:
Goal: To establish the baserate production of /r/ in word-final positions.	Clinician:

Scoring: Correct: ✓ Incorrect or no response: X

/r/ in word-final positions	Evoked	Modeled
1. door		
2. bear		
3. deer		
4. tire		
5. pear		
6. bookstore		
7. jaguar		
8. sapphire		
9. dinosaur		
10. guitar		
11. scar		
12. jar		
13. four		
14. hair		
15. ear		
16. campfire		
17. seashore		
18. umpire		
19. cashier		
20. handlebar		
Percent correct baserate		

Replace or add new exemplars as you see fit for a given child. After establishing the baserates, begin production teaching. Follow the protocols given on the next page.

/r/ in Word-Final Positions

Treatment Protocols

Use stimuli from the **Stimulus Book,** *Volume 4.*

Teach 6 to 8 exemplars using the following script.

Place a relevant stimulus (an object, a picture, or a printed word if the child can read) in front of the child and point to the stimulus as you ask an evoking question.

Scripts for Modeled Discrete Trial Training		Note
Clinician	[*stimulus: door*] "What is this? Say, *door.*"	Modeling; the target vocally emphasized
Child	"doə."	A wrong response
Clinician	"No. That's not correct. You said *doə*, but it's a *door*. You need to say the *r* sound at the end of the word."	Corrective feedback
Clinician	[*the same stimulus*] "What is this? Say, *door*. Don't forget the *r* at the end."	The next trial
Child	"Door."	A correct response
Clinician	"Fantastic! You didn't miss the *r* at the end of the word!"	Verbal praise

Repeat the trials until the child gives 5 consecutively correct, imitated responses.

When the child imitates 5 correct responses in sequence, fade the modeling.

Scripts for Fading the Modeling		Note
Clinician	[*stimulus: door*] "What is this? Don't forget the *r* at the end."	Only a prompt
Child	"doə."	A wrong response
Clinician	"Uh, oh, you forgot the *r*! It's a *door*, not *doə*. Put the *r* at the end."	Corrective feedback
Clinician	[*the same stimulus*] "What is this? It ends with . . . " [*silently models the articulatory posture for final /r/.*]	The next trial; a partial modeling
Child	"Door."	A correct response
Clinician	"Brilliant! You said *door*, not *doə*."	Verbal praise
Clinician	[*the same stimulus*] "What is this?"	Typical question; evoked trial
Child	"Door."	A correct response
Clinician	"Good for you! You said it correctly!"	Verbal praise

If the wrong responses persist on 4 to 5 evoked trials, reinstate partial or full modeling for a few trials, again fade the modeling, and re-present the evoked trials.

When the child meets the tentative learning criterion of 10 consecutively correct, nonimitated responses for a given stimulus item, move on to the next stimulus item. With this procedure, teach 6 to 8 exemplars shown on the following recording sheet. Use different exemplars as you see fit for a given child.

/r/ in Word-Final Positions

Treatment Exemplars and Recording Sheet

Use stimuli from the **Stimulus Book, Volume 4**.

Print this page from CD or photocopy this page for your clinical use.

Name/Age:	Date:
Goal: Production of /r/ in word-final positions with 90% accuracy when asked an evoking question while showing a stimulus.	Clinician:

Scoring: Correct: ✓ Incorrect or no response: X

Target skills	Discrete Trials														
	1	2	3	4	5	6	7	8	9	10	11	12	13	14	15
1. door															
2. bear															
3. dear															
4. tire															
5. pear															
6. bookstore															
7. jaguar															
8. sapphire															

When the child has met the learning criterion of 10 consecutively correct evoked (nonimitated) responses for each of the 6 to 8 target exemplars, conduct a probe to see if the production has generalized to previously baserated but untrained exemplars.

If the probes do not meet the 90% correct criterion for untrained exemplars, teach additional exemplars and then probe again.

/r/ in Word-Final Positions

Probe Protocols and Recording Sheet

Use stimuli from the **Stimulus Book,** *Volume 4.*

Print this page from the CD or photocopy this page for your clinical use.

On the probes, present only the untrained exemplars (UT). When the child fails to meet the 90% correct probe criterion, either teach 2 to 4 new exemplars or give additional training trials on already trained stimuli. If needed, select new exemplars for probes. Probe at least 10 untrained exemplars. Alternate probes and treatment until the probe criterion is met.

Scripts for Probe Trials		Note
Clinician	[*untrained stimulus: dinosaur*] "What is this?"	No modeling or prompts
Child	"Dinosaur."	A correct, generalized response
Clinician	Scores the response as correct.	No reinforcement
Clinician	[*untrained stimulus: guitar*] "What is this?"	The second probe trial
Child	"Guitar."	A correct, generalized response
Clinician	Scores the response as correct.	No reinforcement

Name:	Date:	Session #:
Age:	**Clinician:**	
Diagnosis: Articulation/Phonologic Disorder	**Word-initial /r/probe**	
Untrained Stimuli	**Score: + correct; – incorrect or no responses**	
1. dinosaur		
2. guitar		
3. scar		
4. jar		
5. four		
6. scare		
7. ear		
8. campfire		
9. seashore		
10. umpire		
11. cashier		
12. handlebar		
Percent correct: (Criterion: 90%)		

If the child does not meet the probe criterion, give additional training on already trained exemplars or teach a few new exemplars. Subsequently, readminister the probe trials. When the child meets the 90% correct probe criterion for the exemplars, shift training to the sentence or conversational level or to another phoneme.

/ɚ/ in Word-Final Positions

Baserate Protocols

Use stimuli from the **Stimulus Book,** *Volume 4.*

At the beginning of each trial, place a relevant stimulus (an object, a picture, or a printed word if the child can read) in front of the child. Point to the stimulus as you ask an evoking question. Do not respond in any way to the child's correct, incorrect, or lack of responses.

Scripts for Evoked Baserate Trial		Note
Clinician	[*stimulus: hammer*] "What is this?"	Evoked trial
Child	"hammoe."	Vowelization of /ɚ/
Clinician	Pulls the stimulus toward her; records the response.	No corrective feedback
Clinician	[*stimulus: tiger*] "What is this?"	The next evoked trial
Child	"tiego."	Vowelization of /ɚ/
Clinician	Pulls the stimulus toward her; records the response.	No corrective feedback

Administer the modeled baserate trials only after completing the evoked trials on all 20 (or more) exemplars.

Scripts for Modeled Baserate Trial		Note
Clinician	[*stimulus: hammer*] "What is this? Say, *hammer.*"	Modeled trial
Child	"Hammer."	Correct response
Clinician	Pulls the stimulus toward her; records the response.	No reinforcement
Clinician	[*stimulus: tiger*] "What is this? Say, *tiger.*"	The next modeled trial
Child	"Tiger."	Correct response
Clinician	Pulls the stimulus toward her; records the response.	No reinforcement

Use the recording sheet with exemplars shown on the next page to establish the baserates; print it from the CD.

/ɚ/ in Word-Final Positions

Baserate Exemplars and Recording Sheet

Use stimuli from the **Stimulus Book,** *Volume 4.*

Print this page from the CD or photocopy this page for your clinical use.

Name/Age:	Date:
Goal: To establish the baserate production of /ɚ/ in word-final positions.	Clinician:

Scoring: Correct: ✓   Incorrect or no response: X

/ɚ/ in word-final positions	Evoked	Modeled
1. hammer		
2. tiger		
3. father		
4. toaster		
5. washer		
6. number		
7. spider		
8. picture		
9. flower		
10. jaguar		
11. beaver		
12. shower		
13. soccer		
14. gopher		
15. golfer		
16. anchor		
17. player		
18. soldier		
19. teacher		
20. finger		
Percent correct baserate		

Replace or add new exemplars as you see fit for a given child. After establishing the baserates, begin production teaching. Follow the protocols given on the next page.

/ɚ/ in Word-Final Positions

Treatment Protocols

Use stimuli from the **Stimulus Book,** *Volume 4.*

Teach 6 to 8 exemplars using the following script.

Place a relevant stimulus (an object, a picture, or a printed word if the child can read) in front of the child and point to the stimulus as you ask an evoking question.

Scripts for Modeled Discrete Trial Training		Note
Clinician	[*stimulus: hammer*] "What is this? Say, *hamm**er**.*"	Modeling; the target vocally emphasized
Child	"hammoe."	A wrong response
Clinician	"No. That's not correct. You said hammoe, but it's a *hamm**er**.* You need to say the /ɚ/ sound instead of the *o* sound at the end of the word."	Corrective feedback
Clinician	[*the same stimulus*] "What is this? Say, *hamm**er**.* Don't forget the /ɚ/ at the end. Put your tongue up and back."	The next trial
Child	"Hammer."	A correct response
Clinician	"Excellent! You didn't miss the /ɚ/ at the end of the word!"	Verbal praise

Repeat the trials until the child gives 5 consecutively correct, imitated responses.

When the child imitates 5 correct responses in sequence, fade the modeling.

Scripts for Fading the Modeling		Note
Clinician	[*stimulus: hammer*] "What is this? Don't forget the /ɚ/ at the end."	Only a prompt
Child	"hammoe."	A wrong response
Clinician	"Oops, you forgot the /ɚ/! It's a *hammer*, not *hammoe*. Put the /ɚ/ instead of the *o* at the end."	Corrective feedback
Clinician	[*the same stimulus*] "What is this? It ends with . . . " [*silently models the articulatory posture for the /ɚ/ sound.*]	The next trial; a partial modeling
Child	"Hammer."	A correct response
Clinician	"That's outstanding! You said *hammer*, not *hammoe*."	Verbal praise
Clinician	[*the same stimulus*] "What is this?"	Typical question; evoked trial
Child	"Hammer."	A correct response
Clinician	"Super job! You said it right! I knew you had it in you."	Verbal praise

If the wrong responses persist on 4 to 5 evoked trials, reinstate partial or full modeling for a few trials, again fade the modeling, and re-present the evoked trials.

When the child meets the tentative learning criterion of 10 consecutively correct, nonimitated responses for a given stimulus item, move on to the next stimulus item. With this procedure, teach 6 to 8 exemplars shown on the following recording sheet. Use different exemplars as you see fit for a given child.

/ɚ/ in Word-Final Positions

Treatment Exemplars and Recording Sheet

Use stimuli from the **Stimulus Book, *Volume 4***.

Print this page from CD or photocopy this page for your clinical use.

Name/Age:	Date:
Goal: Production of /ɚ/ in word-final positions with 90% accuracy when asked an evoking question while showing a stimulus.	Clinician:

Scoring: Correct: ✓   Incorrect or no response: X

Target skills	Discrete Trials														
	1	2	3	4	5	6	7	8	9	10	11	12	13	14	15
1. hammer															
2. tiger															
3. father															
4. toaster															
5. washer															
6. number															
7. spider															
8. picture															

When the child has met the learning criterion of 10 consecutively correct evoked (nonimitated) responses for each of the 6 to 8 target exemplars, conduct a probe to see if the production has generalized to previously baserated but untrained exemplars.

If the probes do not meet the 90% correct criterion for untrained exemplars, teach additional exemplars and then probe again.

/ɚ/ in Word-Final Positions

Probe Protocols and Recording Sheet

Use stimuli from the **Stimulus Book, Volume 4**.

Print this page from the CD or photocopy this page for your clinical use.

On the probes, present only the untrained exemplars (UT). When the child fails to meet the 90% correct probe criterion, either teach 2 to 4 new exemplars or give additional training trials on already trained stimuli. If needed, select new exemplars for probes. Probe at least 10 untrained exemplars. Alternate probes and treatment until the probe criterion is met.

Scripts for Probe Trials		Note
Clinician	[*untrained stimulus: flower*] "What is this?"	No modeling or prompts
Child	"flowa."	A wrong probe response
Clinician	Scores the response as incorrect.	No corrective feedback
Clinician	[*untrained stimulus: jaguar*] "What is this?"	The second probe trial
Child	"Jaguar."	A correct generalized response
Clinician	Scores the response as correct.	No reinforcement

Name:	Date:	Session #:
Age:	**Clinician:**	
Diagnosis: Articulation/Phonologic Disorder	**Word-final /ɚ/probe**	
Untrained Stimuli	**Score: + correct; – incorrect or no responses**	
1. flower		
2. jaguar		
3. beaver		
4. shower		
5. soccer		
6. gopher		
7. golfer		
8. anchor		
9. player		
10. soldier		
11. teacher		
12. finger		
Percent correct: (Criterion: 90%)		

If the child does not meet the probe criterion, give additional training on already trained exemplars or teach a few new exemplars. Subsequently, readminister the probe trials. When the child meets the 90% correct probe criterion for the exemplars, shift training to the sentence or conversational level or to another phoneme.

/ɚ/ in Word-Medial Positions

Baserate Protocols

Use stimuli from the **Stimulus Book,** *Volume 4.*

At the beginning of each trial, place a relevant stimulus (an object, a picture, or a printed word if the child can read) in front of the child. Point to the stimulus as you ask an evoking question. Do not respond in any way to the child's correct, incorrect, or lack of responses.

Scripts for Evoked Baserate Trial		Note
Clinician	[*stimulus: butterfly*] "What is this?"	Evoked trial
Child	"buttofly."	Vowelization of medial /ɚ/
Clinician	Pulls the stimulus toward her; records the response.	No corrective feedback
Clinician	[*stimulus: overalls*] "What is this?"	The next evoked trial
Child	"ovəalls."	Vowelization of medial /ɚ/
Clinician	Pulls the stimulus toward her; records the response.	No corrective feedback

Administer the modeled baserate trials only after completing the evoked trials on all 20 (or more) exemplars.

Scripts for Modeled Baserate Trial		Note
Clinician	[*stimulus: butterfly*] "What is this? Say, *butterfly.*"	Modeled trial
Child	"buttofly."	Vowelization of medial /ɚ/
Clinician	Pulls the stimulus toward her; records the response.	No corrective feedback
Clinician	[*stimulus: overalls*] "What is this? Say, *overalls.*"	The next modeled trial
Child	"ovəalls."	Vowelization of medial /ɚ/
Clinician	Pulls the stimulus toward her; records the response.	No corrective feedback

Use the recording sheet with exemplars shown on the next page to establish the baserates; print it from the CD.

/ɚ/ in Word-Medial Positions

Baserate Exemplars and Recording Sheet

Use stimuli from the **Stimulus Book,** *Volume 4.*

Print this page from the CD or photocopy this page for your clinical use.

Name/Age:	Date:
Goal: To establish the baserate production of /ɚ/ in word-medial positions.	Clinician:

Scoring: Correct: ✓   Incorrect or no response: X

/ɚ/in word-medial positions	Evoked	Modeled
1. butterfly		
2. overalls		
3. nectarine		
4. tetherball		
5. underneath		
6. waterfall		
7. undersea		
8. wilderness		
9. spider web		
10. fingernail		
11. mineral		
12. bakery		
13. licorice		
14. emerald		
15. soccer ball		
16. handkerchief		
17. lumberjack		
18. somersault		
19. watermelon		
20. groceries		
Percent correct baserate		

Replace or add new exemplars as you see fit for a given child. After establishing the baserates, begin production teaching. Follow the protocols given on the next page.

/ɚ/ in Word-Medial Positions

Treatment Protocols

Use stimuli from the **Stimulus Book,** *Volume 4.*

Teach 6 to 8 exemplars using the following script.

Place a relevant stimulus in front of the child (an object, a picture, or a printed word if the child can read) and ask a question as you point to the stimulus.

Scripts for Modeled Discrete Trial Training		Note
Clinician	[*stimulus: butterfly*] "What is this? Say, *butterfly.*"	Modeling; the target vocally emphasized
Child	"buttofly."	A wrong response
Clinician	"No. That's not correct. You said *buttofly*, but it's a *butterfly*. You need to say the /ɚ/ instead of the *o* in the middle of the word."	Corrective feedback
Clinician	[*the same stimulus*] "What is this? Say, *butterfly.* Don't forget the /ɚ/ in the middle of the word. Put your tongue up and back."	The next trial
Child	"Butterfly."	A correct response
Clinician	"Way to go! You didn't miss the /ɚ/ this time!"	Verbal praise

Repeat the trials until the child gives 5 consecutively correct, imitated responses.

When the child imitates 5 correct responses in sequence, fade the modeling.

Scripts for Fading the Modeling		Note
Clinician	[*stimulus: butterfly*] "What is this? Don't forget to say the /ɚ/ instead of the *o* in the middle."	Only a prompt
Child	"buttofly."	A wrong response
Clinician	"Oh, no, you said the *o* sound instead of the /ɚ/ in the middle! It's a *butterfly*, not *buttofly*. Put the /ɚ/ in the middle."	Corrective feedback
Clinician	[*the same stimulus*] "What is this? It has the . . . sound in the middle" [*silently models the articulatory posture for the /ɚ/ sound.*]	The next trial; a partial modeling
Child	"Butterfly."	A correct response
Clinician	"That's amazing! You said *butterfly*, not *buttofly*."	Verbal praise
Clinician	[*the same stimulus*] "What is this?"	Typical question; evoked trial
Child	"Butterfly."	A correct response
Clinician	"Great job! You said it correctly! I really appreciate your hard work."	Verbal praise

If the wrong responses persist on 4 to 5 evoked trials, reinstate partial or full modeling for a few trials, again fade the modeling, and re-present the evoked trials.

When the child meets the tentative learning criterion of 10 consecutively correct, nonimitated responses for a given stimulus item, move on to the next stimulus item. With this procedure, teach 6 to 8 exemplars shown on the following recording sheet. Use different exemplars as you see fit for a given child.

/ɚ/ in Word-Medial Positions

Treatment Exemplars and Recording Sheet

Use stimuli from the **Stimulus Book,** *Volume 4.*

Print this page from CD or photocopy this page for your clinical use.

Name/Age:	Date:
Goal: Production of /ɚ/ in word-medial positions with 90% accuracy when asked an evoking question while showing a stimulus.	Clinician:

Scoring: Correct: ✓   Incorrect or no response: X

Target skills	Discrete Trials														
	1	2	3	4	5	6	7	8	9	10	11	12	13	14	15
1. butterfly															
2. overalls															
3. nectarine															
4. tetherball															
5. underneath															
6. waterfall															
7. undersea															
8. wilderness															

When the child has met the learning criterion of 10 consecutively correct evoked (nonimitated) responses for each of the 6 to 8 target exemplars, conduct a probe to see if the production has generalized to previously baserated but untrained exemplars.

If the probes do not meet the 90% correct criterion for untrained exemplars, teach additional exemplars and then probe again.

/ɚ/ in Word-Medial Positions

Probe Protocols and Recording Sheet

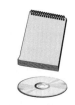

Use stimuli from the **Stimulus Book, *Volume 4.***

Print this page from the CD or photocopy this page for your clinical use.

On the probes, present only the untrained exemplars (UT). When the child fails to meet the 90% correct probe criterion, either teach 2 to 4 new exemplars or give additional training trials on already trained stimuli. If needed, select new exemplars for probes. Probe at least 10 untrained exemplars. Alternate probes and treatment until the probe criterion is met.

Scripts for Probe Trials		Note
Clinician	[*untrained stimulus: spider web*] "What is this?"	No modeling or prompts
Child	"Spider web."	A correct, generalized response
Clinician	Scores the response as correct.	No reinforcement
Clinician	[*untrained stimulus: fingernail*] "What is this?"	The second probe trial
Child	"fingonail."	A wrong probe response
Clinician	Scores the response as incorrect.	No corrective feedback

Name:	Date:	Session #:
Age:	**Clinician:**	
Diagnosis: Articulation/Phonologic Disorder	**Word medial /ɚ/ probe**	
Untrained Stimuli	**Score: + correct; – incorrect or no responses**	
1. spider web		
2. fingernail		
3. mineral		
4. bakery		
5. licorice		
6. emerald		
7. soccer ball		
8. handkerchief		
9. lumberjack		
10. somersault		
11. watermelon		
12. groceries		
Percent correct: (Criterion: 90%)		

If the child does not meet the probe criterion, give additional training on already trained exemplars or teach a few new exemplars. Subsequently, readminister the probe trials. When the child meets the 90% correct probe criterion for the exemplars, shift training to the sentence or conversational level or to another phoneme.

/ɝ/ in Word-Medial Positions

Baserate Protocols

*Use stimuli from the **Stimulus Book, Volume 4**.*

At the beginning of each trial, place a relevant stimulus (an object, a picture, or a printed word if the child can read) in front of the child. Point to the stimulus as you ask an evoking question. Do not respond in any way to the child's correct, incorrect, or lack of responses.

Scripts for Evoked Baserate Trial		Note
Clinician	[*stimulus: shirt*] "What is this?"	Evoked trial
Child	"shət."	Vowelization of medial /ɝ/
Clinician	Pulls the stimulus toward her; records the response.	No corrective feedback
Clinician	[*stimulus: bird*] "What is this?"	The next evoked trial
Child	"boəd."	Vowelization of medial /ɝ/
Clinician	Pulls the stimulus toward her; records the response.	No corrective feedback

Administer the modeled baserate trials only after completing the evoked trials on all 20 (or more) exemplars.

Scripts for Modeled Baserate Trial		Note
Clinician	[*stimulus: shirt*] "What is this? Say, *shirt.*"	Modeled trial
Child	"shət."	Vowelization of medial /ɝ/
Clinician	Pulls the stimulus toward her; records the response.	No corrective feedback
Clinician	[*stimulus: bird*] "What is this? Say, *bird.*"	The next modeled trial
Child	"boəd."	Vowelization of medial /ɝ/
Clinician	Pulls the stimulus toward her; records the response.	No corrective feedback

Use the recording sheet with exemplars shown on the next page to establish the baserates; print it from the CD.

/ɝ/ in Word-Medial Positions

Baserate Exemplars and Recording Sheet

Use stimuli from the **Stimulus Book,** *Volume 4.*

Print this page from the CD or photocopy this page for your clinical use.

Name/Age:	Date:
Goal: To establish the baserate production of /ɝ/ in word-medial positions.	Clinician:

Scoring: Correct: ✓   Incorrect or no response: X

/ɝ/ in word-medial positions	Evoked	Modeled
1. shirt		
2. bird		
3. skirt		
4. first		
5. curve		
6. circus		
7. stirrup		
8. birthday		
9. curtain		
10. birdbath		
11. fern		
12. germs		
13. herd		
14. burn		
15. curb		
16. dessert		
17. mermaid		
18. circle		
19. purple		
20. blurry		
Percent correct baserate		

Replace or add new exemplars as you see fit for a given child. After establishing the baserates, begin production teaching. Follow the protocols given on the next page.

/ɝ/ in Word-Medial Positions

Treatment Protocols

Use stimuli from the **Stimulus Book,** *Volume 4.*

Teach 6 to 8 exemplars using the following script.

Place a relevant stimulus in front of the child (an object, a picture, or a printed word if the child can read) and ask a question as you point to the stimulus.

Scripts for Modeled Discrete Trial Training		Note
Clinician	[*stimulus: shirt*] "What is this? Say, *shirt*."	Modeling; the target vocally emphasized
Child	"shət."	A wrong response
Clinician	"No. That's not correct. You said *shət*, but it's a *shirt*. You need to say the /ɝ/ in the middle of the word. Put your tongue up high and far back."	Corrective feedback
Clinician	[*the same stimulus*] "What is this? Say, *shirt*. Don't forget the /ɝ/ in the middle."	The next trial
Child	"Shirt."	A correct response
Clinician	"Way to go! You didn't miss the /ɝ/ this time!"	Verbal praise

Repeat the trials until the child gives 5 consecutively correct, imitated responses.

When the child imitates 5 correct responses in sequence, fade the modeling.

Scripts for Fading the Modeling		Note
Clinician	[*stimulus: shirt*] "What is this? Don't forget the /ɝ/ in the middle."	Only a prompt
Child	"shət."	A wrong response
Clinician	"Gee, you forgot the /ɝ/! It's a *shirt*, not *shət*. Put the /ɝ/ in the middle."	Corrective feedback
Clinician	[*the same stimulus*] "What is this? It has the . . . sound in the middle" [*silently models the articulatory posture for the /ɝ/ sound.*]	The next trial; a partial modeling
Child	"Shirt."	A correct response
Clinician	"That's great! You said *shirt*, not *shət*."	Verbal praise
Clinician	[*the same stimulus*] "What is this?"	Typical question; evoked trial
Child	"Shirt."	A correct response
Clinician	"Great job! That was perfect! You've made good progress."	Verbal praise

If the wrong responses persist on 4 to 5 evoked trials, reinstate partial or full modeling for a few trials, again fade the modeling, and re-present the evoked trials.

When the child meets the tentative learning criterion of 10 consecutively correct, nonimitated responses for a given stimulus item, move on to the next stimulus item. With this procedure, teach 6 to 8 exemplars shown on the following recording sheet. Use different exemplars as you see fit for a given child.

/ɝ/ in Word-Medial Positions

Treatment Exemplars and Recording Sheet

Use stimuli from the **Stimulus Book,** *Volume 4.*

Print this page from CD or photocopy this page for your clinical use.

Name/Age:	Date:
Goal: Production of /ɝ/ in word-medial positions with 90% accuracy when asked an evoking question while showing a stimulus.	Clinician:

Scoring: Correct: ✓   Incorrect or no response: X

Target skills	Discrete Trials														
	1	2	3	4	5	6	7	8	9	10	11	12	13	14	15
1. shirt															
2. bird															
3. skirt															
4. first															
5. curve															
6. circus															
7. stirrup															
8. birthday															

When the child has met the learning criterion of 10 consecutively correct evoked (nonimitated) responses for each of the 6 to 8 target exemplars, conduct a probe to see if the production has generalized to previously baserated but untrained exemplars.

If the probes do not meet the 90% correct criterion for untrained exemplars, teach additional exemplars and then probe again.

/ɝ/ in Word-Medial Positions

Probe Protocols and Recording Sheet

Use stimuli from the **Stimulus Book, Volume 4**.

Print this page from the CD or photocopy this page for your clinical use.

On the probes, present only the untrained exemplars (UT). When the child fails to meet the 90% correct probe criterion, either teach 2 to 4 new exemplars or give additional training trials on already trained stimuli. If needed, select new exemplars for probes. Probe at least 10 untrained exemplars. Alternate probes and treatment until the probe criterion is met.

Scripts for Probe Trials		
Clinician	[*untrained stimulus: curtain*] "What is this?"	No modeling or prompts
Child	"coətain."	A wrong probe response
Clinician	Scores the response as incorrect.	No corrective feedback
Clinician	[*untrained stimulus: birdbath*] "What is this?"	The second probe trial
Child	"bodebath."	A wrong probe response
Clinician	Scores the response as incorrect.	No corrective feedback

Name:	Date:	Session #:
Age:	**Clinician:**	
Diagnosis: Articulation/Phonologic Disorder	**Word medial /ɝ/ probe**	
Untrained Stimuli	**Score: + correct; – incorrect or no responses**	
1. curtain		
2. birdbath		
3. fern		
4. germs		
5. herd		
6. burn		
7. curb		
8. dessert		
9. mermaid		
10. circle		
11. purple		
12. blurry		
Percent correct: (Criterion: 90%)		

If the child does not meet the probe criterion, give additional training on already trained exemplars or teach a few new exemplars. Subsequently, readminister the probe trials. When the child meets the 90% correct probe criterion for the exemplars, shift training to the sentence or conversational level or to another phoneme.

/m/ in Word-Initial Positions

Baserate Protocols

Use stimuli from the **Stimulus Book,** *Volume 3.*

At the beginning of each trial, place a relevant stimulus (an object, a picture, or a printed word) in front of the child. Point to the stimulus as you ask an evoking question. Do not respond in any way to the child's correct, incorrect, or lack of responses.

Scripts for Evoked Baserate Trial		Note
Clinician	[*stimulus: man*] "This is not a woman, this is a . . . ?"	Evoked trial
Child	"æn."	Omission of initial /m/
Clinician	Pulls the stimulus toward her; records the response.	No corrective feedback
Clinician	[*stimulus: map*] "What is this called?"	The next evoked trial
Child	"æp."	Omission of initial /m/
Clinician	Pulls the stimulus toward her; records the response.	No corrective feedback

Administer the modeled baserate trials only after completing the evoked trials on all 20 (or more) exemplars.

Scripts for Modeled Baserate Trial		Note
Clinician	[*stimulus: man*] "Who is this? Say, *man.*"	Modeled trial
Child	"Man."	Correct response
Clinician	Pulls the stimulus toward her; records the response.	No reinforcement
Clinician	[*stimulus: map*] "What is this? Say, *map.*"	The next modeled trial
Child	"æp."	Omission of initial /m/
Clinician	Pulls the stimulus toward her; records the response.	No corrective feedback

Use the recording sheet with exemplars shown on the next page to establish the baserates; print it from the CD.

/m/ in Word-Initial Positions

Baserate Exemplars and Recording Sheet

Use stimuli from the **Stimulus Book,** *Volume 3.*

Print this page from the CD or photocopy this page for your clinical use.

Name/Age:	Date:
Goal: To establish the baserate production of /m/ in word-initial positions.	Clinician:

Scoring: Correct: ✓   Incorrect or no response: X

/m/ in word-initial positions	Evoked	Modeled
1. man		
2. map		
3. mat		
4. mask		
5. milk		
6. mandolin		
7. mammoth		
8. magazine		
9. medicine		
10. mailbox		
11. mice		
12. moon		
13. mop		
14. mug		
15. mitt		
16. magician		
17. mackerel		
18. magpie		
19. marigold		
20. macaroni		
Percent correct baserate		

Replace or add new exemplars as you see fit for a given child. After establishing the baserates, begin production teaching. Follow the protocols given on the next page.

/m/ in Word-Initial Positions

Treatment Protocols

*Use stimuli from the **Stimulus Book, Volume 3.***

Teach 6 to 8 exemplars using the following script.

Place a relevant stimulus in front of the child (an object, a picture, or a printed word) and ask a question as you point to the stimulus.

Scripts for Modeled Discrete Trial Training		Note
Clinician	[*stimulus: man*] "Who is this? Say, ***man***."	Modeling; the target vocally emphasized
Child	"æn."	A wrong response
Clinician	"No. That's not correct. You said æn, but it's a ***man***."	Corrective feedback
Clinician	[*the same stimulus*] "What is this? Say, ***man***. Don't forget the m sound at the beginning."	The next trial
Child	"Man."	A correct response
Clinician	"Excellent! You didn't miss the *m* sound this time!"	Verbal praise

Repeat the trials until the child gives 5 consecutively correct, imitated responses.

When the child imitates 5 correct responses in sequence, fade the modeling.

Scripts for Fading the Modeling		Note
Clinician	[*stimulus:* man] "What is this? It starts with the *m* sound."	Only a prompt
Child	"æn."	A wrong response
Clinician	"Gee, you forgot the *m* sound! It's a *man*, not æn. Put the *m* sound at the beginning."	Corrective feedback
Clinician	[*the same stimulus*] "What is this? It starts with . . . " [*silently models the lip posture for the target sound.*]	The next trial; a partial modeling
Child	"Man."	A correct response
Clinician	"That's great! You said *man* correctly, not æn."	Verbal praise
Clinician	[*the same stimulus*] "What is this?"	Typical question; evoked trial
Child	"Man."	A correct response
Clinician	"Great job! You said it correctly!"	Verbal praise

If the wrong responses persist on 4 to 5 evoked trials, reinstate partial or full modeling for a few trials, again fade the modeling, and re-present the evoked trials.

When the child meets the tentative learning criterion of 10 consecutively correct, nonimitated responses for a given stimulus item, move on to the next stimulus item. With this procedure, teach 6 to 8 exemplars shown on the following recording sheet. Use different exemplars as you see fit for a given child.

/m/ in Word-Initial Positions

Treatment Exemplars and Recording Sheet

Use stimuli from the **Stimulus Book, Volume 3**.

Print this page from CD or photocopy this page for your clinical use.

Name/Age:	Date:
Goal: Production of /m/ in word-initial positions with 90% accuracy when asked an evoking question while showing a stimulus.	Clinician:

Scoring: Correct: ✓   Incorrect or no response: X

Target skills	Discrete Trials														
	1	2	3	4	5	6	7	8	9	10	11	12	13	14	15
1. man															
2. map															
3. mat															
4. mask															
5. milk															
6. mandolin															
7. mammoth															
8. magazine															

When the child has met the learning criterion of 10 consecutively correct evoked (nonimitated) responses for each of the 6 to 8 target exemplars, conduct a probe to see if the production has generalized to previously baserated but untrained exemplars.

If the probes do not meet the 90% correct criterion for untrained exemplars, teach additional exemplars and then probe again.

/m/ in Word-Initial Positions

Probe Protocols and Recording Sheet

Use stimuli from the **Stimulus Book, *Volume 3***.

Print this page from the CD or photocopy this page for your clinical use.

On the probes, present only the untrained exemplars (UT). When the child fails to meet the 90% correct probe criterion, either teach 2 to 4 new exemplars or give additional training trials on already trained stimuli. If needed, select new exemplars for probes. Probe at least 10 untrained exemplars. Alternate probes and treatment until the probe criterion is met.

Scripts for Probe Trials		Note
Clinician	[*untrained stimulus: medicine*] "What is this?"	No modeling or prompts
Child	"Medicine."	A correct, generalized response
Clinician	Scores the response as correct.	No reinforcement
Clinician	[*untrained stimulus: mailbox*] "What is this?"	The second probe trial
Child	"ailbox."	A wrong probe response
Clinician	Scores the response as incorrect.	No corrective feedback

Name:	Date:	Session #:
Age:	**Clinician:**	
Diagnosis: Articulation/Phonologic Disorder	**Word-initial /m/ probe**	
Untrained Stimuli	**Score: + correct; – incorrect or no responses**	
1. medicine		
2. mailbox		
3. mice		
4. moon		
5. mop		
6. mug		
7. mitt		
8. magician		
9. mackerel		
10. magpie		
11. marigold		
12. macaroni		
Percent correct: (Criterion: 90%)		

If the child does not meet the probe criterion, give additional training on already trained exemplars or teach a few new exemplars. Subsequently, readminister the probe trials. When the child meets the 90% correct probe criterion for the exemplars, shift training to the sentence or conversational level or to another phoneme.

/m/ in Word-Final Positions

Baserate Protocols

Use stimuli from the **Stimulus Book, Volume 3**.

At the beginning of each trial, place a relevant stimulus (an object, a picture, or a printed word) in front of the child. Point to the stimulus as you ask an evoking question. Do not respond in any way to the child's correct, incorrect, or lack of responses.

Scripts for Evoked Baserate Trial		Note
Clinician	[*stimulus: comb*] "What is this?"	Evoked trial
Child	"co."	Omission of final /m/
Clinician	Pulls the stimulus toward her; records the response.	No corrective feedback
Clinician	[*stimulus: dime*] "What is this?"	The next evoked trial
Child	"dai."	Omission of final /m/
Clinician	Pulls the stimulus toward her; records the response.	No corrective feedback

Administer the modeled baserate trials only after completing the evoked trials on all 20 (or more) exemplars.

Scripts for Modeled Baserate Trial		Note
Clinician	[*stimulus: comb*] "What is this? Say, *comb*."	Modeled trial
Child	"Comb."	Correct response
Clinician	Pulls the stimulus toward her; records the response.	No reinforcement
Clinician	[*stimulus: dime*] "What is this? Say, *dime*."	The next modeled trial
Child	"dai."	Omission of /m/
Clinician	Pulls the stimulus toward her; records the response.	No corrective feedback

Use the recording sheet with exemplars shown on the next page to establish the baserates; print it from the CD.

/m/ in Word-Final Positions

Baserate Exemplars and Recording Sheet

Use stimuli from the **Stimulus Book,** *Volume 3.*

Print this page from the CD or photocopy this page for your clinical use.

Name/Age:	Date:
Goal: To establish the baserate production of /m/ in word-final positions.	Clinician:

Scoring: Correct: ✓   Incorrect or no response: X

/m/ in word-final positions	Evoked	Modeled
1. comb		
2. dime		
3. gum		
4. thumb		
5. plum		
6. bathroom		
7. album		
8. ice cream		
9. mushroom		
10. linoleum		
11. lime		
12. gym		
13. foam		
14. palm		
15. room		
16. chrysanthemum		
17. condominium		
18. auditorium		
19. family room		
20. lunchtime		
Percent correct baserate		

Replace or add new exemplars as you see fit for a given child. After establishing the baserates, begin production teaching. Follow the protocols given on the next page.

/m/ in Word-Final Positions

Treatment Protocols

Use stimuli from the **Stimulus Book, Volume 3**.

Teach 6 to 8 exemplars using the following script.

Place a relevant stimulus (an object, a picture, or a printed word) in front of the child and point to the stimulus as you ask an evoking question.

Scripts for Modeled Discrete Trial Training		Note
Clinician	[*stimulus: comb*] "What is this? Say, *comb*."	Modeling; the target vocally emphasized
Child	"co."	A wrong response
Clinician	"No. That's not correct. You said *co*, but it's a *comb*."	Corrective feedback
Clinician	[*the same stimulus*] "What is this? Say, *comb*. Don't forget the *m* at the end."	The next trial
Child	"Comb."	A correct response
Clinician	"Super! You didn't miss the *m* at the end of the word!"	Verbal praise

Repeat the trials until the child gives 5 consecutively correct, imitated responses.

When the child imitates 5 correct responses in sequence, fade the modeling.

Scripts for Fading the Modeling		Note
Clinician	[*stimulus: comb*] "What is this? Don't forget the *m* at the end."	Only a prompt
Child	"co."	A wrong response
Clinician	"Gee, you forgot the *m* sound! It's a *comb*, not *co*. Put the *m* at the end."	Corrective feedback
Clinician	[*the same stimulus*] "What is this? It ends with . . . " [*silently models the lip posture for the target sound.*]	The next trial; a partial modeling
Child	"Comb."	A correct response
Clinician	"You are wonderful! You said *comb*, not *co*."	Verbal praise
Clinician	[*the same stimulus*] "What is this?"	Typical question; evoked trial
Child	"Comb."	A correct response
Clinician	"I like it! You said it correctly!"	Verbal praise

If the wrong responses persist on 4 to 5 evoked trials, reinstate partial or full modeling for a few trials, again fade the modeling, and re-present the evoked trials.

When the child meets the tentative learning criterion of 10 consecutively correct, nonimitated responses for a given stimulus item, move on to the next stimulus item. With this procedure, teach 6 to 8 exemplars shown on the following recording sheet. Use different exemplars as you see fit for a given child.

/m/ in Word-Final Positions

Treatment Exemplars and Recording Sheet

Use stimuli from the **Stimulus Book, Volume 3**.

Print this page from CD or photocopy this page for your clinical use.

Name/Age:	Date:
Goal: Production of /m/ in word-final positions with 90% accuracy when asked an evoking question while showing a stimulus.	Clinician:

Scoring: Correct: ✓   Incorrect or no response: X

Target skills	Discrete Trials														
	1	2	3	4	5	6	7	8	9	10	11	12	13	14	15
1. comb															
2. dime															
3. gum															
4. thumb															
5. plum															
6. bathroom															
7. album															
8. ice cream															

When the child has met the learning criterion of 10 consecutively correct evoked (nonimitated) responses for each of the 6 to 8 target exemplars, conduct a probe to see if the production has generalized to previously baserated but untrained exemplars.

If the probes do not meet the 90% correct criterion for untrained exemplars, teach additional exemplars and then probe again.

/m/ in Word-Final Positions

Probe Protocols and Recording Sheet

Use stimuli from the **Stimulus Book,** *Volume 3.*

Print this page from the CD or photocopy this page for your clinical use.

On the probes, present only the untrained exemplars (UT). When the child fails to meet the 90% correct probe criterion, either teach 2 to 4 new exemplars or give additional training trials on already trained stimuli. If needed, select new exemplars for probes. Probe at least 10 untrained exemplars. Alternate probes and treatment until the probe criterion is met.

Scripts for Probe Trials		Note
Clinician	[*untrained stimulus: mushroom*] "What is this?"	No modeling or prompts
Child	"Mushroom."	A correct, generalized response
Clinician	Scores the response as correct.	No reinforcement
Clinician	[*untrained stimulus: linoleum*] "What is this?"	The second probe trial
Child	"linolee."	A wrong probe response
Clinician	Scores the response as incorrect.	No corrective feedback

Name:	Date:	Session #:
Age:	Clinician:	
Diagnosis: Articulation/Phonologic Disorder	**Word-final /m/probe**	
Untrained Stimuli	**Score: + correct; – incorrect or no responses**	
1. mushroom		
2. linoleum		
3. lime		
4. gym		
5. foam		
6. palm		
7. room		
8. chrysanthemum		
9. condominium		
10. auditorium		
11. family room		
12. lunchtime		
Percent correct: (Criterion: 90%)		

If the child does not meet the probe criterion, give additional training on already trained exemplars or teach a few new exemplars. Subsequently, readminister the probe trials. When the child meets the 90% correct probe criterion for the exemplars, shift training to the sentence or conversational level or to another phoneme.

/n/ in Word-Initial Positions

Baserate Protocols

Use stimuli from the **Stimulus Book, Volume 3.**

At the beginning of each trial, place a relevant stimulus (an object, a picture, or a printed word) in front of the child. Point to the stimulus as you ask an evoking question. Do not respond in any way to the child's correct, incorrect, or lack of responses.

Scripts for Evoked Baserate Trial		Note
Clinician	[*stimulus: nail*] "What is this?"	Evoked trial
Child	"ail."	Omission of initial /n/
Clinician	Pulls the stimulus toward her; records the response.	No corrective feedback
Clinician	[*stimulus: neck*] "What is this?"	The next evoked trial
Child	"ek."	Omission of initial /n/
Clinician	Pulls the stimulus toward her; records the response.	No corrective feedback

Administer the modeled baserate trials only after completing the evoked trials on all 20 (or more) exemplars.

Scripts for Modeled Baserate Trial		Note
Clinician	[*stimulus: nail*] "What is this? Say, *nail.*"	Modeled trial
Child	"Nail."	Correct response
Clinician	Pulls the stimulus toward her; records the response.	No reinforcement
Clinician	[*stimulus: neck*] "What is this? Say, *neck.*"	The next modeled trial
Child	"ek."	Omission of initial /n/
Clinician	Pulls the stimulus toward her; records the response.	No corrective feedback

Use the recording sheet with exemplars shown on the next page to establish the baserates; print it from the CD.

/n/ in Word-Initial Positions

Baserate Exemplars and Recording Sheet

*Use stimuli from the **Stimulus Book**, **Volume 3**.*

Print this page from the CD or photocopy this page for your clinical use.

Name/Age:		Date:	
Goal: To establish the baserate production of /n/ in word-initial positions.		Clinician:	

Scoring: Correct: ✓   Incorrect or no response: X

/n/ in word-initial positions	Evoked	Modeled
1. nail		
2. neck		
3. nine		
4. nurse		
5. nacho		
6. noodle		
7. necklace		
8. newspaper		
9. nightingale		
10. nutcracker		
11. nut		
12. nose		
13. needle		
14. nun		
15. night		
16. knitting		
17. newsstand		
18. neckwear		
19. needlefish		
20. nectarine		
Percent correct baserate		

Replace or add new exemplars as you see fit for a given child. After establishing the baserates, begin production teaching. Follow the protocols given on the next page.

/n/ in Word-Initial Positions

Treatment Protocols

Use stimuli from the **Stimulus Book, Volume 3**.

Teach 6 to 8 exemplars using the following script.

Place a relevant stimulus in front of the child (an object, a picture, or a printed word) and ask a question as you point to the stimulus.

Scripts for Modeled Discrete Trial Training		Note
Clinician	[*stimulus: nail*] "What is this? Say, **nail**."	Modeling; the target vocally emphasized
Child	"ail."	A wrong response
Clinician	"No. That's not correct. You said *ail*, but it's **nail**."	Corrective feedback
Clinician	[*the same stimulus*] "What is this? Say, **nail**. Don't forget the *n* sound at the beginning."	The next trial
Child	"Nail."	A correct response
Clinician	"Excellent! You didn't miss the *n* sound this time!"	Verbal praise

Repeat the trials until the child gives 5 consecutively correct, imitated responses.

When the child imitates 5 correct responses in sequence, fade the modeling.

Scripts for Fading the Modeling		Note
Clinician	[*stimulus: nail*] "What is this? Don't forget the *n* at the beginning."	Only a prompt
Child	"ail."	A wrong response
Clinician	"Oh no! I didn't hear the *n* sound! It's *nail*, not *ail*. Put the *n* at the beginning."	Corrective feedback
Clinician	[*the same stimulus*] "What is this? It starts with . . . " [*silently models the tongue posture for the target sound.*]	The next trial; a partial modeling
Child	"Nail."	A correct response
Clinician	"That's great! You said *nail*, not *ail*."	Verbal praise
Clinician	[*the same stimulus*] "What is this?"	Typical question; evoked trial
Child	"Nail."	A correct response
Clinician	"Fantastic! You work hard!"	Verbal praise

If the wrong responses persist on 4 to 5 evoked trials, reinstate partial or full modeling for a few trials, again fade the modeling, and re-present the evoked trials.

When the child meets the tentative learning criterion of 10 consecutively correct, nonimitated responses for a given stimulus item, move on to the next stimulus item. With this procedure, teach 6 to 8 exemplars shown on the following recording sheet. Use different exemplars as you see fit for a given child.

/n/ in Word-Initial Positions

Treatment Exemplars and Recording Sheet

Use stimuli from the **Stimulus Book,** *Volume 3.*

Print this page from CD or photocopy this page for your clinical use.

Name/Age:	Date:
Goal: Production of /n/ in word-initial positions with 90% accuracy when asked an evoking question while showing a stimulus.	Clinician:

Scoring: Correct: ✓   Incorrect or no response: X

Target skills	Discrete Trials														
	1	2	3	4	5	6	7	8	9	10	11	12	13	14	15
1. nail															
2. neck															
3. nine															
4. nurse															
5. nacho															
6. noodle															
7. necklace															
8. newspaper															

When the child has met the learning criterion of 10 consecutively correct evoked (nonimitated) responses for each of the 6 to 8 target exemplars, conduct a probe to see if the production has generalized to previously baserated but untrained exemplars.

If the probes do not meet the 90% correct criterion for untrained exemplars, teach additional exemplars and then probe again.

/n/ in Word-Initial Positions

Probe Protocols and Recording Sheet

Use stimuli from the **Stimulus Book, Volume 3.**

Print this page from the CD or photocopy this page for your clinical use.

On the probes, present only the untrained exemplars (UT). When the child fails to meet the 90% correct probe criterion, either teach 2 to 4 new exemplars or give additional training trials on already trained stimuli. If needed, select new exemplars for probes. Probe at least 10 untrained exemplars. Alternate probes and treatment until the probe criterion is met.

Scripts for Probe Trials		Note
Clinician	[*untrained stimulus: nightingale*] "What is this bird called?"	No modeling or prompts
Child	"Nightingale."	A correct, generalized response
Clinician	Scores the response as correct.	No reinforcement
Clinician	[*untrained stimulus: nutcracker*] "What is this?"	The second probe trial
Child	"utcracker."	A wrong probe response
Clinician	Scores the response as incorrect.	No corrective feedback

Name:	Date:	Session #:
Age:	**Clinician:**	
Diagnosis: Articulation/Phonologic Disorder	**Word-initial /n/ probe**	
Untrained Stimuli	**Score: + correct; – incorrect or no responses**	
1. nightingale		
2. nutcracker		
3. nut		
4. nose		
5. needle		
6. nun		
7. night		
8. knitting		
9. newsstand		
10. neckwear		
11. needlefish		
12. nectarine		
Percent correct: (Criterion: 90%)		

If the child does not meet the probe criterion, give additional training on already trained exemplars or teach a few new exemplars. Subsequently, readminister the probe trials. When the child meets the 90% correct probe criterion for the exemplars, shift training to the sentence or conversational level or to another phoneme.

/n/ in Word-Final Positions

Baserate Protocols

Use stimuli from the **Stimulus Book, Volume 3**.

At the beginning of each trial, place a relevant stimulus (an object, a picture, or a printed word) in front of the child. Point to the stimulus as you ask an evoking question. Do not respond in any way to the child's correct, incorrect, or lack of responses.

Scripts for Evoked Baserate Trial		Note
Clinician	[*stimulus: fan*] "What is this?"	Evoked trial
Child	"fæ."	Omission of final /n/
Clinician	Pulls the stimulus toward her; records the response.	No corrective feedback
Clinician	[*stimulus: pen*] "What is this?"	The next evoked trial
Child	"pɛ."	Omission of final /n/
Clinician	Pulls the stimulus toward her; records the response.	No corrective feedback

Administer the modeled baserate trials only after completing the evoked trials on all 20 (or more) exemplars.

Scripts for Modeled Baserate Trial		Note
Clinician	[*stimulus: fan*] "What is this? Say, *fan.*"	Modeled trial
Child	"Fan."	Correct response
Clinician	Pulls the stimulus toward her; records the response.	No reinforcement
Clinician	[*stimulus: pen*] "What is this? Say, *pen.*"	The next modeled trial
Child	"pɛ."	Omission of final /n/
Clinician	Pulls the stimulus toward her; records the response.	No corrective feedback

Use the recording sheet with exemplars shown on the next page to establish the baserates; print it from the CD.

/n/ in Word-Final Positions

Baserate Exemplars and Recording Sheet

Use stimuli from the **Stimulus Book, Volume 3**.

Print this page from the CD or photocopy this page for your clinical use.

Name/Age:	Date:
Goal: To establish the baserate production of /n/ in word-final positions.	Clinician:

Scoring: Correct: ✓   Incorrect or no response: X

/n/ in word-final positions	Evoked	Modeled
1. fan		
2. pen		
3. pin		
4. men		
5. cane		
6. accordion		
7. dandelion		
8. headphone		
9. saxophone		
10. telephone		
11. bone		
12. bean		
13. bun		
14. cone		
15. coin		
16. fisherman		
17. microphone		
18. skeleton		
19. television		
20. submarine		
Percent correct baserate		

Replace or add new exemplars as you see fit for a given child. After establishing the baserates, begin production teaching. Follow the protocols given on the next page.

/n/ in Word-Final Positions

Treatment Protocols

Use stimuli from the **Stimulus Book, Volume 3.**

Teach 6 to 8 exemplars using the following script.

Place a relevant stimulus (an object, a picture, or a printed word) in front of the child and point to the stimulus as you ask an evoking question.

Scripts for Modeled Discrete Trial Training		Note
Clinician	[*stimulus: fan*] "What is this? Say, *fan.*"	Modeling; the target vocally emphasized
Child	"fæ."	A wrong response
Clinician	"No. That's not correct. You said *fæ*, but it's *fan.*"	Corrective feedback
Clinician	[*the same stimulus*] "What is this? Say, *fan.* Don't forget the *n* sound at the end."	The next trial
Child	"Fan."	A correct response
Clinician	"Excellent! You didn't miss the *n* at the end of the word!"	Verbal praise

Repeat the trials until the child gives 5 consecutively correct, imitated responses.

When the child imitates 5 correct responses in sequence, fade the modeling.

Scripts for Fading the Modeling		Note
Clinician	[*stimulus: fan*] "What is this? Don't forget the *n* sound at the end."	Only a prompt
Child	"fæ."	A wrong response
Clinician	"Gee, I didn't hear the *n* sound! It's a *fan*, not *fæ*. Put the *n* sound at the end."	Corrective feedback
Clinician	[*the same stimulus*] "What is this? It ends with . . . " [*silently models the tongue posture for the target sound.*]	The next trial; a partial modeling
Child	"Fan."	A correct response
Clinician	"That's great! You said *fan*, not *an.*"	Verbal praise
Clinician	[*the same stimulus*] "What is this?"	Typical question; evoked trial
Child	"Fan."	A correct response
Clinician	"You are super! You got it right!"	Verbal praise

If the wrong responses persist on 4 to 5 evoked trials, reinstate partial or full modeling for a few trials, again fade the modeling, and re-present the evoked trials.

When the child meets the tentative learning criterion of 10 consecutively correct, nonimitated responses for a given stimulus item, move on to the next stimulus item. With this procedure, teach 6 to 8 exemplars shown on the following recording sheet. Use different exemplars as you see fit for a given child.

/n/ in Word-Final Positions

Treatment Exemplars and Recording Sheet

Use stimuli from the **Stimulus Book,** *Volume 3.*

Print this page from CD or photocopy this page for your clinical use.

Name/Age:	Date:
Goal: Production of /n/ in word-final positions with 90% accuracy when asked an evoking question while showing a stimulus.	Clinician:

Scoring: Correct: ✓   Incorrect or no response: X

Target skills	Discrete Trials														
	1	2	3	4	5	6	7	8	9	10	11	12	13	14	15
1. fan															
2. pen															
3. pin															
4. men															
5. cane															
6. accordion															
7. dandelion															
8. headphone															

When the child has met the learning criterion of 10 consecutively correct evoked (nonimitated) responses for each of the 6 to 8 target exemplars, conduct a probe to see if the production has generalized to previously baserated but untrained exemplars.

If the probes do not meet the 90% correct criterion for untrained exemplars, teach additional exemplars and then probe again.

/n/ in Word-Final Positions

Probe Protocols and Recording Sheet

Use stimuli from the **Stimulus Book,** *Volume 3.*

Print this page from the CD or photocopy this page for your clinical use.

On the probes, present only the untrained exemplars (UT). When the child fails to meet the 90% correct probe criterion, either teach 2 to 4 new exemplars or give additional training trials on already trained stimuli. If needed, select new exemplars for probes. Probe at least 10 untrained exemplars. Alternate probes and treatment until the probe criterion is met.

Scripts for Probe Trials		Note
Clinician	[*untrained stimulus: saxophone*] "What is this?"	No modeling or prompts
Child	"æxophone."	A wrong probe response
Clinician	Scores the response as incorrect.	No corrective feedback
Clinician	[*untrained stimulus: telephone*] "What is this?"	The second probe trial
Child	"Telephone."	A correct, generalized response
Clinician	Scores the response as correct.	No reinforcement

Name:	Date:	Session #:
Age:	**Clinician:**	
Diagnosis: Articulation/Phonologic Disorder	**Word-final /n/probe**	
Untrained Stimuli	**Score: + correct; – incorrect or no responses**	
1. saxophone		
2. telephone		
3. bone		
4. bean		
5. bun		
6. cone		
7. coin		
8. fisherman		
9. microphone		
10. skeleton		
11. television		
12. submarine		
Percent correct: (Criterion: 90%)		

If the child does not meet the probe criterion, give additional training on already trained exemplars or teach a few new exemplars. Subsequently, readminister the probe trials. When the child meets the 90% correct probe criterion for the exemplars, shift training to the sentence or conversational level or to another phoneme.

/ŋ/ in Word-Final Positions

Baserate Protocols

Use stimuli from the **Stimulus Book, Volume 3.**

English /ŋ/ does not occur in initial word positions.

At the beginning of each trial, place a relevant stimulus (an object, a picture, or a printed word) in front of the child. Point to the stimulus as you ask an evoking question. Do not respond in any way to the child's correct, incorrect, or lack of responses.

Scripts for Evoked Baserate Trial		Note
Clinician	[*stimulus: wing*] "What is this?"	Evoked trial
Child	"wi."	Omission of final /ŋ/
Clinician	Pulls the stimulus toward her; records the response.	No corrective feedback
Clinician	[*stimulus: gong*] "What is this?"	The next evoked trial
Child	"gɑ."	Omission of final /ŋ/
Clinician	Pulls the stimulus toward her; records the response.	No corrective feedback

Administer the modeled baserate trials only after completing the evoked trials on all 20 (or more) exemplars.

Scripts for Modeled Baserate Trial		Note
Clinician	[*stimulus: wing*] "What is this? Say, *wing.*"	Modeled trial
Child	"Wing."	Correct response
Clinician	Pulls the stimulus toward her; records the response.	No reinforcement
Clinician	[*stimulus: gong*] "What is this? Say, *gong.*"	The next modeled trial
Child	"gɑ."	Omission of final /ŋ/
Clinician	Pulls the stimulus toward her; records the response.	No corrective feedback

Use the recording sheet with exemplars shown on the next page to establish the baserates; print it from the CD.

/ŋ/ in Word-Final Positions

Baserate Exemplars and Recording Sheet

Use stimuli from the **Stimulus Book,** *Volume 3.*

Print this page from the CD or photocopy this page for your clinical use.

Name/Age:	Date:
Goal: To establish the baserate production of /ŋ/ in word-final positions.	Clinician:

Scoring: Correct: ✓   Incorrect or no response: X

/ŋ/ in word-final positions	Evoked	Modeled
1. wing		
2. gong		
3. long		
4. ring		
5. string		
6. smelling		
7. running		
8. camping		
9. coloring		
10. canoeing		
11. fang		
12. gang		
13. spring		
14. sling		
15. king		
16. truck driving		
17. bubble blowing		
18. butterfly catching		
19. boomerang		
20. juggling		
Percent correct baserate		

Replace or add new exemplars as you see fit for a given child. After establishing the baserates, begin production teaching. Follow the protocols given on the next page.

/ŋ/ in Word-Final Positions

Treatment Protocols

*Use stimuli from the **Stimulus Book, Volume 3**.*

Teach 6 to 8 exemplars using the following script.

Place a relevant stimulus (an object, a picture, or a printed word) in front of the child and point to the stimulus as you ask an evoking question.

Scripts for Modeled Discrete Trial Training		Note
Clinician	[*stimulus: wing*] "What is this? Say, *wing.*"	Modeling; the target vocally emphasized
Child	"wi."	A wrong response
Clinician	"No. That's not correct. You said *wi*, but it's *wing.*"	Corrective feedback
Clinician	[*the same stimulus*] "What is this? Say, *wing.* Don't forget the *ŋ* sound at the end."	The next trial
Child	"Wing."	A correct response
Clinician	"Excellent! You didn't miss the *ŋ* sound at the end of the word!"	Verbal praise

Repeat the trials until the child gives 5 consecutively correct, imitated responses.

When the child imitates 5 correct responses in sequence, fade the modeling.

Scripts for Fading the Modeling		Note
Clinician	[*stimulus: wing*] "What is this? Don't forget the *ŋ* sound at the end."	Only a prompt
Child	"wi."	A wrong response
Clinician	"Gee, you forgot the *ŋ* sound! It's *wing*, not *wi.* Put the *ŋ* sound at the end."	Corrective feedback
Clinician	[*the same stimulus*] "What is this? It ends with . . . " [*silently models the articulatory posture for the target sound.*]	The next trial; a partial modeling
Child	"Wing."	A correct response
Clinician	"That's great! You said *wing*, not *wi.*"	Verbal praise
Clinician	[*the same stimulus*] "What is this?"	Typical question; evoked trial
Child	"Wing."	A correct response
Clinician	"I like it! You said it correctly!"	Verbal praise

If the wrong responses persist on 4 to 5 evoked trials, reinstate partial or full modeling for a few trials, again fade the modeling, and re-present the evoked trials.

When the child meets the tentative learning criterion of 10 consecutively correct, nonimitated responses for a given stimulus item, move on to the next stimulus item. With this procedure, teach 6 to 8 exemplars shown on the following recording sheet. Use different exemplars as you see fit for a given child.

/ŋ/ in Word-Final Positions

Treatment Exemplars and Recording Sheet

Use stimuli from the **Stimulus Book,** *Volume 3.*

Print this page from CD or photocopy this page for your clinical use.

Name/Age:	Date:
Goal: Production of /ŋ/ in word-final positions with 90% accuracy when asked an evoking question while showing a stimulus.	Clinician:

Scoring: Correct: ✓   Incorrect or no response: X

Target skills	Discrete Trials														
	1	2	3	4	5	6	7	8	9	10	11	12	13	14	15
1. wing															
2. gong															
3. long															
4. ring															
5. string															
6. smelling															
7. running															
8. camping															

When the child has met the learning criterion of 10 consecutively correct evoked (nonimitated) responses for each of the 6 to 8 target exemplars, conduct a probe to see if the production has generalized to previously baserated but untrained exemplars.

If the probes do not meet the 90% correct criterion for untrained exemplars, teach additional exemplars and then probe again.

/ŋ/ in Word-Final Positions

Probe Protocols and Recording Sheet

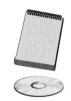

Use stimuli from the **Stimulus Book, Volume 3**.

Print this page from the CD or photocopy this page for your clinical use.

On the probes, present only the untrained exemplars (UT). When the child fails to meet the 90% correct probe criterion, either teach 2 to 4 new exemplars or give additional training trials on already trained stimuli. If needed, select new exemplars for probes. Probe at least 10 untrained exemplars. Alternate probes and treatment until the probe criterion is met.

Scripts for Probe Trials		Note
Clinician	[untrained stimulus: a child coloring] "What is she doing?"	No modeling or prompts
Child	"Coloring."	A correct, generalized response
Clinician	Scores the response as correct.	No reinforcement
Clinician	[untrained stimulus: canoeing] "What are they doing?"	The second probe trial
Child	"canoe."	A wrong probe response
Clinician	Scores the response as incorrect.	No corrective feedback

Name:	Date:	Session #:
Age:	**Clinician:**	
Diagnosis: Articulation/Phonologic Disorder	**Word-Final /ŋ/ probe**	
Untrained Stimuli	**Score: + correct; – incorrect or no responses**	
1. coloring		
2. canoeing		
3. fang		
4. gang		
5. spring		
6. sling		
7. king		
8. truck driving		
9. bubble blowing		
10. butterfly catching		
11. boomerang		
12. juggling		
Percent correct: (Criterion: 90%)		

If the child does not meet the probe criterion, give additional training on already trained exemplars or teach a few new exemplars. Subsequently, readminister the probe trials. When the child meets the 90% correct probe criterion for the exemplars, shift training to the sentence or conversational level or to another phoneme.

Part II

Teaching Phoneme Clusters

/bl/ in Word-Initial Positions

Baserate Protocols

Use stimuli from the **Stimulus Book, Volume 5**.

At the beginning of each trial, place a relevant stimulus (an object, a picture, or a printed word if the child can read) in front of the child. Point to the stimulus as you ask an evoking question. Do not respond in any way to the child's correct, incorrect, or lack of responses.

Scripts For Evoked Baserate Trial		Note
Clinician	[*stimulus: blue*] "What color is this?"	Evoked trial
Child	"bwue."	Substitution of /bw/ for /bl/
Clinician	Pulls the stimulus toward her; records the response.	No corrective feedback
Clinician	[*stimulus: block*] "What is this?"	The next evoked trial
Child	"bock."	Omission of /l/ in the /bl/ cluster
Clinician	Pulls the stimulus toward her; records the response.	No corrective feedback

Administer the modeled baserate trials only after completing the evoked trials on all 20 (or more) exemplars.

Scripts For Modeled Baserate Trial		Note
Clinician	[*stimulus: blue*] "What is this? Say, *blue*."	Modeled trial
Child	"Blue."	Correct response
Clinician	Pulls the stimulus toward her; records the response.	No reinforcement
Clinician	[*stimulus: block*] "What is this? Say, *block*."	The next modeled trial
Child	"bwock."	Substitution of /bw/ for /bl/
Clinician	Pulls the stimulus toward her; records the response.	No corrective feedback

Use the recording sheet with exemplars shown on the next page to establish the baserates; print it from the CD.

/bl/ in Word-Initial Positions

Baserate Exemplars and Recording Sheet

Use stimuli from the **Stimulus Book,** *Volume 5.*

Print this page from the CD or photocopy this page for your clinical use.

Name/Age:	Date:
Goal: To establish the baserate production of /bl/ in word-initial positions.	Clinician:

Scoring: Correct: ✓   Incorrect or no response: X

/bl/ in word-initial positions	Evoked	Modeled
1. blue		
2. block		
3. black		
4. bleach		
5. blouse		
6. blanket		
7. blender		
8. blackberry		
9. blossom		
10. bluebird		
11. blimp		
12. bluff		
13. blonde		
14. bloom		
15. blow		
16. blue whale		
17. blowtorch		
18. blister		
19. blow dryer		
20. blue jeans		
Percent correct baserate		

Replace or add new exemplars as you see fit for a given child. After establishing the baserates, begin production teaching. Follow the protocols given on the next page.

/bl/ in Word-Initial Positions

Treatment Protocols

Use stimuli from the **Stimulus Book,** *Volume 5.*

Teach 6 to 8 exemplars using the following script.

Place a relevant stimulus in front of the child (an object, a picture, or a printed word if the child can read) and ask a question as you point to the stimulus.

Scripts For Modeled Discrete Trial Training		Note
Clinician	[*stimulus: blue*] "What color is this? Say, **blue**."	Modeling; the target vocally emphasized
Child	"bwue."	A wrong response
Clinician	"No. That's not right. You said *bwue*, but it should be **blue**. The sound *l*, not *w*, comes after **b**."	Corrective feedback; the target vocally emphasized
Clinician	[*the same stimulus*] "What is this? Say, **blue**. Remember to say *l* after **b**, **bl**ue."	The next trial
Child	"Blue."	A correct response
Clinician	"Excellent! You put *b* and *l* together when you said *blue* this time! You're doing great."	Verbal praise

Repeat the trials until the child gives 5 consecutively correct, imitated responses.

When the child imitates 5 correct responses in sequence, fade the modeling.

Scripts For Fading the Modeling		Note
Clinician	[*stimulus: blue*] "What color is this? Remember to say *l* after *b*."	Only a prompt
Child	"bwue."	A wrong response
Clinician	"Oops, you said *bw* instead of *bl* at the beginning! It's *blue*, not *bwue*. Let's try it again."	Corrective feedback
Clinician	[*the same stimulus*] "What color is this? It starts with . . . " [*silently models and holds the lip and tongue posture for bl. Holds the tongue posture for l*].	The next trial; a partial modeling
Child	"Blue."	A correct response
Clinician	"That's great! You said *blue*, not *bwue*."	Verbal praise
Clinician	[*the same stimulus*] "What color is this?"	Typical question; evoked trial
Child	"Blue."	A correct response
Clinician	"Outstanding! You said it correctly! You are working very hard!"	Verbal praise

If the wrong responses persist on 4 to 5 evoked trials, reinstate partial or full modeling for a few trials, again fade the modeling, and re-present the evoked trials.

When the child meets the tentative learning criterion of 10 consecutively correct, nonimitated responses for a given stimulus item, move on to the next stimulus item. With this procedure, teach 6 to 8 exemplars shown on the following recording sheet. Use different exemplars as you see fit for a given child.

/bl/ in Word-Initial Positions

Treatment Exemplars and Recording Sheet

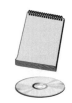

Use stimuli from the **Stimulus Book,** *Volume 5.*

Print this page from CD or photocopy this page for your clinical use.

Name/Age:	Date:
Goal: Production of /bl/ in word-initial positions with 90% accuracy when asked an evoking question while showing a stimulus.	Clinician:

Scoring: Correct: ✓   Incorrect or no response: X

Target skills	Discrete Trials														
	1	2	3	4	5	6	7	8	9	10	11	12	13	14	15
1. blue															
2. block															
3. black															
4. bleach															
5. blouse															
6. blanket															
7. blender															
8. blackberry															

When the child has met the learning criterion of 10 consecutively correct evoked (nonimitated) responses for each of the 6 to 8 target exemplars, conduct a probe to see if the production has generalized to previously baserated but untrained exemplars.

If the probes do not meet the 90% correct criterion for untrained exemplars, teach additional exemplars and then probe again.

/bl/ in Word-Initial Positions

Probe Protocols and Recording Sheet

Use stimuli from the **Stimulus Book,** *Volume 5.*

Print this page from the CD or photocopy this page for your clinical use.

On the probes, present only the untrained exemplars (UT). When the child fails to meet the 90% correct probe criterion, either teach 2 to 4 new exemplars or give additional training trials on already trained stimuli. If needed, select new exemplars for probes. Probe at least 10 untrained exemplars. Alternate probes and treatment until the probe criterion is met.

Scripts For Probe Trials		Note
Clinician	[*untrained stimulus: blossom*]. "What is this?"	No modeling or prompts
Child	No response.	Lack of generalization
Clinician	Scores it as no response.	No corrective feedback
Clinician	[*untrained stimulus: bluebird*] "What is this?"	The second probe trial
Child	"A bluebird."	A correct generalized response
Clinician	Scores the response as correct.	No reinforcement

Name:	Date:	Session #:
Age:	**Clinician:**	
Diagnosis: Articulation/Phonologic Disorder	**Word-initial /bl/ probe**	
Untrained Stimuli	**Score: + correct; – incorrect or no responses**	
1. blossom		
2. bluebird		
3. blimp		
4. bluff		
5. blonde		
6. bloom		
7. blow		
8. blue whale		
9. blowtorch		
10. blister		
11. blow dryer		
12. blue jeans		
Percent correct: (Criterion: 90%)		

If the child does not meet the probe criterion, give additional training on already trained exemplars or teach a few new exemplars. Subsequently, readminister the probe trials. When the child meets the 90% correct probe criterion for the exemplars, shift training to the sentence or conversational level or to another phoneme.

/fl/ in Word-Initial Positions

Baserate Protocols

Use stimuli from the **Stimulus Book,** *Volume 5.*

At the beginning of each trial, place a relevant stimulus (an object, a picture, or a printed word if the child can read) in front of the child. Point to the stimulus as you ask an evoking question. Do not respond in any way to the child's correct, incorrect, or lack of responses.

Scripts For Evoked Baserate Trial		**Note**
Clinician	[*stimulus: fly*] "What is this?"	Evoked trial
Child	"fwy."	Substitution of /fw/ for /fl/
Clinician	Pulls the stimulus toward her; records the response.	No corrective feedback
Clinician	[*stimulus: flag*] "What is this?"	The next evoked trial
Child	"fwag."	Substitution of /fw/ for /fl/
Clinician	Pulls the stimulus toward her; records the response.	No corrective feedback

Administer the modeled baserate trials only after completing the evoked trials on all 20 (or more) exemplars.

Scripts For Modeled Baserate Trial		**Note**
Clinician	[*stimulus: fly*] "What is this? Say, *fly.*"	Modeled trial
Child	"Fly."	Correct response
Clinician	Pulls the stimulus toward her; records the response.	No reinforcement
Clinician	[*stimulus: flag*] "What is this? Say, *flag.*"	The next modeled trial
Child	"fwag."	Substitution of /fw/ for /fl/
Clinician	Pulls the stimulus toward her; records the response.	No corrective feedback

Use the recording sheet with exemplars shown on the next page to establish the baserates; print it from the CD.

/fl/ in Word-Initial Positions

Baserate Exemplars and Recording Sheet

Use stimuli from the **Stimulus Book,** *Volume 5.*

Print this page from the CD or photocopy this page for your clinical use.

Name/Age:	Date:
Goal: To establish the baserate production of /fl/ in word-initial positions.	Clinician:

Scoring: Correct: ✓   Incorrect or no response: X

/fl/ in word-initial positions	Evoked	Modeled
1. fly		
2. flag		
3. flame		
4. flute		
5. floor		
6. flamingo		
7. flagpole		
8. flashbulb		
9. flashlight		
10. flagship		
11. flake		
12. flea		
13. float		
14. flower		
15. flat		
16. flowerpot		
17. flatfish		
18. flatware		
19. flipper		
20. flounder		
Percent correct baserate		

Replace or add new exemplars as you see fit for a given child. After establishing the baserates, begin production teaching. Follow the protocols given on the next page.

/fl/ in Word-Initial Positions

Treatment Protocols

Use stimuli from the **Stimulus Book,** *Volume 5.*

Teach 6 to 8 exemplars using the following script.

Place a relevant stimulus in front of the child (an object, a picture, or a printed word if the child can read) and ask a question as you point to the stimulus.

Scripts For Modeled Discrete Trial Training		Note
Clinician	[*stimulus: fly*] "What is this? Say, ***fly.***"	Modeling; the target vocally emphasized
Child	"fwy."	A wrong response
Clinician	"No. That's not correct. You said *fwy*, but it's a ***fly.***"	Corrective feedback
Clinician	[*the same stimulus*] "What is this? Say, ***fly***. Don't forget the ***l*** after the ***f.***"	The next trial
Child	"Fly."	A correct response
Clinician	"Excellent! You remembered to say the *l* after the *f*! That was perfect!"	Verbal praise

Repeat the trials until the child gives 5 consecutively correct, imitated responses.

When the child imitates 5 correct responses in sequence, fade the modeling.

Scripts For Fading the Modeling		Note
Clinician	[*stimulus: fly*] "What is this? Don't forget the *l* after the *f.*"	Only a prompt
Child	"fwy."	A wrong response
Clinician	"Oh no, you forgot to say the *l* after the *f*! It's a *fly*, not *fwy*. Remember to say the *f* and *l* together.	Corrective feedback
Clinician	[*the same stimulus*] "What is this? It starts with . . . " [*silently models the lip and tongue posture for the /fl/ cluster.*]	The next trial; a partial modeling
Child	"Fly."	A correct response
Clinician	"That's great! You said *fly*, not *fwy*."	Verbal praise
Clinician	[*the same stimulus*] "What is this?"	Typical question; evoked trial
Child	"Fly."	A correct response
Clinician	"That was stupendous! You said it right!"	Verbal praise

If the wrong responses persist on 4 to 5 evoked trials, reinstate partial or full modeling for a few trials, again fade the modeling, and re-present the evoked trials.

When the child meets the tentative learning criterion of 10 consecutively correct, nonimitated responses for a given stimulus item, move on to the next stimulus item. With this procedure, teach 6 to 8 exemplars shown on the following recording sheet. Use different exemplars as you see fit for a given child.

/fl/ in Word-Initial Positions

Treatment Exemplars and Recording Sheet

Use stimuli from the **Stimulus Book, Volume 5**.

Print this page from CD or photocopy this page for your clinical use.

Name/Age:	Date:
Goal: Production of /fl/ in word-initial positions with 90% accuracy when asked an evoking question while showing a stimulus.	Clinician:

Scoring: Correct: ✓ Incorrect or no response: X

Target skills	Discrete Trials														
	1	2	3	4	5	6	7	8	9	10	11	12	13	14	15
1. fly															
2. flag															
3. flame															
4. flute															
5. floor															
6. flamingo															
7. flagpole															
8. flashbulb															

When the child has met the learning criterion of 10 consecutively correct evoked (nonimitated) responses for each of the 6 to 8 target exemplars, conduct a probe to see if the production has generalized to previously baserated but untrained exemplars.

If the probes do not meet the 90% correct criterion for untrained exemplars, teach additional exemplars and then probe again.

/fl/ in Word-Initial Positions

Probe Protocols and Recording Sheet

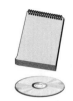

Use stimuli from the **Stimulus Book,** *Volume 5.*

Print this page from the CD or photocopy this page for your clinical use.

On the probes, present only the untrained exemplars (UT). When the child fails to meet the 90% correct probe criterion, either teach 2 to 4 new exemplars or give additional training trials on already trained stimuli. If needed, select new exemplars for probes. Probe at least 10 untrained exemplars. Alternate probes and treatment until the probe criterion is met.

Scripts For Probe Trials		Note
Clinician	[*untrained stimulus: flashlight*] "What is this?"	No modeling or prompts
Child	"Flashlight."	A correct, generalized response
Clinician	Scores the response as correct.	No reinforcement
Clinician	[*untrained stimulus: flagship*] "What is this?"	The second probe trial
Child	"fwagship."	A wrong probe response
Clinician	Scores the response as incorrect.	No corrective feedback

Name:	Date:	Session #:
Age:	**Clinician:**	
Diagnosis: Articulation/Phonologic Disorder	**Word-initial /fl/ probe**	
Untrained Stimuli	**Score: + correct; – incorrect or no responses**	
1. flashlight		
2. flagship		
3. flake		
4. flea		
5. float		
6. flower		
7. flat		
8. flowerpot		
9. flatfish		
10. flatware		
11. flipper		
12. flounder		
Percent correct: (Criterion: 90%)		

If the child does not meet the probe criterion, give additional training on already trained exemplars or teach a few new exemplars. Subsequently, readminister the probe trials. When the child meets the 90% correct probe criterion for the exemplars, shift training to the sentence or conversational level or to another phoneme.

/gl/ in Word-Initial Positions

Baserate Protocols

Use stimuli from the **Stimulus Book,** *Volume 5.*

At the beginning of each trial, place a relevant stimulus (an object, a picture, or a printed word if the child can read) in front of the child. Point to the stimulus as you ask an evoking question. Do not respond in any way to the child's correct, incorrect, or lack of responses.

Scripts For Evoked Baserate Trial		Note
Clinician	[*stimulus: drinking glass*] "What is this?"	Evoked trial
Child	"gass."	Omission of /l/ in the /gl/ cluster
Clinician	Pulls the stimulus toward her; records the response.	No corrective feedback
Clinician	[*stimulus: glove*] "What is this?"	The next evoked trial
Child	"gove."	Omission of /l/ in the /gl/ cluster
Clinician	Pulls the stimulus toward her; records the response.	No corrective feedback

Administer the modeled baserate trials only after completing the evoked trials on all 20 (or more) exemplars.

Scripts For Modeled Baserate Trial		Note
Clinician	[*stimulus: drinking glass*] "What is this? Say, *glass.*"	Modeled trial
Child	"gass."	Omission of /l/ in the /gl/ cluster
Clinician	Pulls the stimulus toward her; records the response.	No corrective feedback
Clinician	[*stimulus: glove*] "What is this? Say, *glove.*"	The next modeled trial
Child	"gove."	Omission of /l/ in the /gl/ cluster
Clinician	Pulls the stimulus toward her; records the response.	No corrective feedback

Use the recording sheet with exemplars shown on the next page to establish the baserates; print it from the CD.

/gl/ in Word-Initial Positions

Baserate Exemplars and Recording Sheet

*Use stimuli from the **Stimulus Book**, Volume 5.*

Print this page from the CD or photocopy this page for your clinical use.

Name/Age:	Date:
Goal: To establish the baserate production of /gl/ in word-initial positions.	Clinician:

Scoring: Correct: ✓   Incorrect or no response: X

/gl/ in word-initial positions	Evoked	Modeled
1. glass		
2. glove		
3. glad		
4. glue		
5. glide		
6. gladiator		
7. glow worm		
8. glacier		
9. glasses		
10. glamorous		
11. glitter		
12. glow		
13. globe		
14. glade		
15. glance		
16. glimmer		
17. gladiolus		
18. glider		
19. glossary		
20. glutton		
Percent correct baserate		

Replace or add new exemplars as you see fit for a given child. After establishing the baserates, begin production teaching. Follow the protocols given on the next page.

/gl/ in Word-Initial Positions

Treatment Protocols

Use stimuli from the **Stimulus Book,** *Volume 5.*

Teach 6 to 8 exemplars using the following script.

Place a relevant stimulus in front of the child (an object, a picture, or a printed word if the child can read) and ask a question as you point to the stimulus.

Scripts For Modeled Discrete Trial Training		Note
Clinician	[*stimulus: drinking glass*] "What is this? Say, **gl**ass.	Modeling; the target vocally emphasized
Child	"gass."	A wrong response
Clinician	"No. That's not correct. You said *gass*, but it's a **gl**ass. You need to say the *l* after the *g*."	Corrective feedback; the target vocally emphasized
Clinician	[*the same stimulus*] "What is this? Say, **gl**ass. Don't forget the *l* after the **g**."	The next trial
Child	"Glass."	A correct response
Clinician	"That is perfect! You said *g* and *l* together when you said *glass*."	Verbal praise

Repeat the trials until the child gives 5 consecutively correct, imitated responses.

When the child imitates 5 correct responses in sequence, fade the modeling.

Scripts For Fading the Modeling		Note
Clinician	[*stimulus: drinking glass*] "What is this? Don't forget to say *g* and *l* together."	Only a prompt
Child	"gass."	A wrong response
Clinician	"Oh no, you forgot the *l*! It's a *glass* not *gass*. Say the *l* after the *g*."	Corrective feedback
Clinician	[*the same stimulus*] "What is this? It starts with . . . " [*silently models the tongue posture for g and then the tongue posture for l. Holds the tongue posture for l.*]	The next trial; a partial modeling
Child	"Glass."	A correct response
Clinician	"Excellent! You said *glass*, not *gass*."	Verbal praise
Clinician	[*the same stimulus*] "What is this?"	Typical question; evoked trial
Child	"Glass."	A correct response
Clinician	"Great job! You said it correctly!"	Verbal praise

If the wrong responses persist on 4 to 5 evoked trials, reinstate partial or full modeling for a few trials, again fade the modeling, and re-present the evoked trials.

When the child meets the tentative learning criterion of 10 consecutively correct, nonimitated responses for a given stimulus item, move on to the next stimulus item. With this procedure, teach 6 to 8 exemplars shown on the following recording sheet. Use different exemplars as you see fit for a given child.

/gl/ in Word-Initial Positions

Treatment Exemplars and Recording Sheet

Use stimuli from the **Stimulus Book,** *Volume 5.*

Print this page from CD or photocopy this page for your clinical use.

Name/Age:	Date:
Goal: Production of /gl/ in word-initial positions with 90% accuracy when asked an evoking question while showing a stimulus.	Clinician:

Scoring: Correct: ✓   Incorrect or no response: X

Target skills	Discrete Trials														
	1	2	3	4	5	6	7	8	9	10	11	12	13	14	15
1. glass															
2. glove															
3. glad															
4. glue															
5. glide															
6. gladiator															
7. glow worm															
8. glacier															

When the child has met the learning criterion of 10 consecutively correct evoked (nonimitated) responses for each of the 6 to 8 target exemplars, conduct a probe to see if the production has generalized to previously baserated but untrained exemplars.

If the probes do not meet the 90% correct criterion for untrained exemplars, teach additional exemplars and then probe again.

/gl/ in Word-Initial Positions

Probe Protocols and Recording Sheet

Use stimuli from the -**Stimulus Book,** *Volume 5.*

Print this page from the CD or photocopy this page for your clinical use.

On the probes, present only the untrained exemplars (UT). When the child fails to meet the 90% correct probe criterion, either teach 2 to 4 new exemplars or give additional training trials on already trained stimuli. If needed, select new exemplars for probes. Probe at least 10 untrained exemplars. Alternate probes and treatment until the probe criterion is met.

Scripts For Probe Trials		Note
Clinician	[*untrained stimulus: (eye) glasses*] "What is this?"	No modeling or prompts
Child	"Glasses."	A correct, generalized response
Clinician	Scores the response as correct.	No reinforcement
Clinician	[*untrained stimulus:* printed word *glamorous*] "Please read this word." [*for a nonreader*] "This word is *glamorous*. What word is this?"	The second probe trial
Child	No response.	Lack of generalization
Clinician	Scores it as *no response*.	No corrective feedback

Name:	Date:	Session #:
Age:	**Clinician:**	
Diagnosis: Articulation/Phonologic Disorder	**Word-initial /gl/ probe**	
Untrained Stimuli	**Score: + correct; – incorrect or no responses**	
1. glasses		
2. glamorous		
3. glitter		
4. glow		
5. globe		
6. glade		
7. glance		
8. glimmer		
9. gladiolus		
10. glider		
11. glossary		
12. glutton		
Percent correct: (Criterion: 90%)		

If the child does not meet the probe criterion, give additional training on already trained exemplars or teach a few new exemplars. Subsequently, readminister the probe trials. When the child meets the 90% correct probe criterion for the exemplars, shift training to the sentence or conversational level or to another phoneme.

/kl/ in Word-Initial Positions

Baserate Protocols

Use stimuli from the **Stimulus Book,** *Volume 5.*

At the beginning of each trial, place a relevant stimulus (an object, a picture, or a printed word if the child can read) in front of the child. Point to the stimulus as you ask an evoking question. Do not respond in any way to the child's correct, incorrect, or lack of responses.

Scripts For Evoked Baserate Trial		Note
Clinician	[*stimulus: clown*] "What is this?"	Evoked trial
Child	"cown."	Omission of /l/ in /kl/ cluster
Clinician	Pulls the stimulus toward her; records the response.	No corrective feedback
Clinician	[*stimulus: claw*] "What is this?"	The next evoked trial
Child	"taw."	Substitution of /t/ for /kl/
Clinician	Pulls the stimulus toward her; records the response.	No corrective feedback

Administer the modeled baserate trials only after completing the evoked trials on all 20 (or more) exemplars.

Scripts For Modeled Baserate Trial		Note
Clinician	[*stimulus: clown*] "What is this? Say, *clown.*"	Modeled trial
Child	"cown."	Omission of /l/ in /kl/ cluster
Clinician	Pulls the stimulus toward her; records the response.	No corrective feedback
Clinician	[*stimulus: claw*] "What is this? Say, *claw.*"	The next modeled trial
Child	"caw."	Substitution of /k/ for /kl/
Clinician	Pulls the stimulus toward her; records the response.	No corrective feedback

Use the recording sheet with exemplars shown on the next page to establish the baserates; print it from the CD.

/kl/ in Word-Initial Positions

Baserate Exemplars and Recording Sheet

Use stimuli from the **Stimulus Book,** *Volume 5.*

Print this page from the CD or photocopy this page for your clinical use.

Name/Age:	Date:
Goal: To establish the baserate production of /kl/ in word-initial positions.	Clinician:

Scoring: Correct: ✓ Incorrect or no response: X

/kl/ in word-initial positions	Evoked	Modeled
1. clown		
2. claw		
3. clean		
4. clap		
5. clam		
6. climbing		
7. clarinet		
8. classroom		
9. clothing		
10. clipboard		
11. close		
12. club		
13. clip		
14. clock		
15. cloud		
16. clippers		
17. clothespin		
18. cluster		
19. cleaver		
20. closet		
Percent correct baserate		

Replace or add new exemplars as you see fit for a given child. After establishing the baserates, begin production teaching. Follow the protocols given on the next page.

/kl/ in Word-Initial Positions
Treatment Protocols

Use stimuli from the **Stimulus Book, Volume 5**.

Teach 6 to 8 exemplars using the following script.

Place a relevant stimulus in front of the child (an object, a picture, or a printed word if the child can read) and ask a question as you point to the stimulus.

Scripts For Modeled Discrete Trial Training		Note
Clinician	[*stimulus: clown*] "What is this? Say, **clown.**"	Modeling; the target vocally emphasized
Child	"cown."	A wrong response
Clinician	"No. That's not correct. You said *cown*, but it's a **clown.** The *l* sound comes after the **k** sound, **clown.**"	Corrective feedback
Clinician	[*the same stimulus*] "What is this? Say, **clown.** Remember that the *l* sound comes after the **k** sound."	The next trial
Child	"cown."	A wrong response
Clinician	"Oh no! You forgot to say the *l* after the *k*. Remember to do it next time."	Corrective feedback

Repeat the trials until the child gives 5 consecutively correct, imitated responses.

When the child imitates 5 correct responses in sequence, fade the modeling.

Scripts For Fading the Modeling		Note
Clinician	[*stimulus: clown*] "What is this? Don't forget to say the *l* after the *k*."	Only a prompt
Child	"cown."	A wrong response
Clinician	"Oh, oh, you forgot to say the *l* after the *k*! It's a *clown*, not cown. Remember to say the *l* in *clown*.	Corrective feedback
Clinician	[*the same stimulus*] "What is this? It starts with . . . " [*silently models the tongue posture for the /kl/ cluster. Holds the tongue posture for l.*]	The next trial; a partial modeling
Child	"Clown."	A correct response
Clinician	"That's great! You said *clown*, not *cown*."	Verbal praise
Clinician	[*the same stimulus*] "What is this?"	Typical question; evoked trial
Child	"Clown."	A correct response
Clinician	"Great job! You said it correctly!"	Verbal praise

If the wrong responses persist on 4 to 5 evoked trials, reinstate partial or full modeling for a few trials, again fade the modeling, and re-present the evoked trials.

When the child meets the tentative learning criterion of 10 consecutively correct, nonimitated responses for a given stimulus item, move on to the next stimulus item. With this procedure, teach 6 to 8 exemplars shown on the following recording sheet. Use different exemplars as you see fit for a given child.

/kl/ in Word-Initial Positions

Treatment Exemplars and Recording Sheet

Use stimuli from the **Stimulus Book,** *Volume 5.*

Print this page from CD or photocopy this page for your clinical use.

Name/Age:	Date:
Goal: Production of /kl/ in word-initial positions with 90% accuracy when asked an evoking question while showing a stimulus.	Clinician:

Scoring: Correct: ✓   Incorrect or no response: X

Target skills	Discrete Trials														
	1	2	3	4	5	6	7	8	9	10	11	12	13	14	15
1. clown															
2. claw															
3. clean															
4. clap															
5. clam															
6. climbing															
7. clarinet															
8. classroom															

When the child has met the learning criterion of 10 consecutively correct evoked (nonimitated) responses for each of the 6 to 8 target exemplars, conduct a probe to see if the production has generalized to previously baserated but untrained exemplars.

If the probes do not meet the 90% correct criterion for untrained exemplars, teach additional exemplars and then probe again.

/kl/ in Word-Initial Positions

Probe Protocols and Recording Sheet

Use stimuli from the **Stimulus Book, Volume 5**.

Print this page from the CD or photocopy this page for your clinical use.

On the probes, present only the untrained exemplars (UT). When the child fails to meet the 90% correct probe criterion, either teach 2 to 4 new exemplars or give additional training trials on already trained stimuli. If needed, select new exemplars for probes. Probe at least 10 untrained exemplars. Alternate probes and treatment until the probe criterion is met.

Scripts For Probe Trials		Note
Clinician	[*untrained stimulus: clothing*] "What is this?"	No modeling or prompts
Child	"toething."	A wrong probe response
Clinician	Scores the response as incorrect.	No corrective feedback
Clinician	[*untrained stimulus: clipboard*] "What is this?"	The second probe trial
Child	"cipboard."	A wrong probe response
Clinician	Scores the response as incorrect.	No corrective feedback

Name:	Date:	Session #:
Age:	**Clinician:**	
Diagnosis: Articulation/Phonologic Disorder	**Word-initial /kl/ probe**	
Untrained Stimuli	**Score: + correct; – incorrect or no responses**	
1. clothing		
2. clipboard		
3. close		
4. climb		
5. clip		
6. clock		
7. cloud		
8. clippers		
9. clothespin		
10. cluster		
11. cleaver		
12. classmate		
Percent correct: (Criterion: 90%)		

If the child does not meet the probe criterion, give additional training on already trained exemplars or teach a few new exemplars. Subsequently, readminister the probe trials. When the child meets the 90% correct probe criterion for the exemplars, shift training to the sentence or conversational level or to another phoneme.

/pl/ in Word-Initial Positions

Baserate Protocols

Use stimuli from the **Stimulus Book,** *Volume 5.*

At the beginning of each trial, place a relevant stimulus (an object, a picture, or a printed word if the child can read) in front of the child. Point to the stimulus as you ask an evoking question. Do not respond in any way to the child's correct, incorrect, or lack of responses.

Scripts For Evoked Baserate Trial		Note
Clinician	[*stimulus: plane*] "What is this?"	Evoked trial
Child	"pane."	Omission of /l/ in /pl/ cluster
Clinician	Pulls the stimulus toward her; records the response.	No corrective feedback
Clinician	[*stimulus: plate*] "What is this?"	The next evoked trial
Child	"pwate."	Substitution of /pw/ for /pl/
Clinician	Pulls the stimulus toward her; records the response.	No corrective feedback

Administer the modeled baserate trials only after completing the evoked trials on all 20 (or more) exemplars.

Scripts For Modeled Baserate Trial		Note
Clinician	[*stimulus: plane*] "What is this? Say, *plane*."	Modeled trial
Child	"pwane."	Substitution of /pw/ for /pl/
Clinician	Pulls the stimulus toward her; records the response.	No corrective feedback
Clinician	[*stimulus: plate*] "What is this? Say, *plate*."	The next modeled trial
Child	"pwate."	Substitution of /pw/ for /pl/
Clinician	Pulls the stimulus toward her; records the response.	No corrective feedback

Use the recording sheet with exemplars shown on the next page to establish the baserates; print it from the CD.

/pl/ in Word-Initial Positions

Baserate Exemplars and Recording Sheet

Use stimuli from the **Stimulus Book,** *Volume 5.*

Print this page from the CD or photocopy this page for your clinical use.

Name/Age:	Date:
Goal: To establish the baserate production of /pl/ in word-initial positions.	Clinician:

Scoring: Correct: ✓   Incorrect or no response: X

/pl/ in word-initial positions	Evoked	Modeled
1. plane		
2. plate		
3. play		
4. plus		
5. plant		
6. place mat		
7. plantation		
8. platform		
9. platypus		
10. playground		
11. planet		
12. plow		
13. pliers		
14. plug		
15. plum		
16. playpen		
17. plumber		
18. playmate		
19. playhouse		
20. plunger		
Percent correct baserate		

Replace or add new exemplars as you see fit for a given child. After establishing the baserates, begin production teaching. Follow the protocols given on the next page.

/pl/ in Word-Initial Positions

Treatment Protocols

Use stimuli from the **Stimulus Book, Volume 5**.

Teach 6 to 8 exemplars using the following script.

Place a relevant stimulus in front of the child (an object, a picture, or a printed word if the child can read) and ask a question as you point to the stimulus.

Scripts For Modeled Discrete Trial Training		Note
Clinician	[*stimulus: plane*] "What is this? Say, **plane**."	Modeling; the target vocally emphasized
Child	"pwane."	A wrong response
Clinician	"No. That's not correct. You said *pwane*, but it's a **plane**. The **l**, not *w*, comes after the **p**."	Corrective feedback
Clinician	[*the same stimulus*] "What is this? Say, **plane**."	The next trial
Child	"Plane."	A correct response
Clinician	"Way to go! You didn't forget to say the *l* after the *p*!"	Verbal praise

Repeat the trials until the child gives 5 consecutively correct, imitated responses.

When the child imitates 5 correct responses in sequence, fade the modeling.

Scripts For Fading the Modeling		Note
Clinician	[*stimulus: plane*] "What is this? Don't forget to say the *l* after the *p*."	Only a prompt
Child	"pwane."	A wrong response
Clinician	"Oops, you forgot to say the *l* after the *p*! You said *pwane*, but it should be *plane*."	Corrective feedback
Clinician	[*the same stimulus*] "What is this? It starts with . . . " [*silently models the lip and tongue posture for the /pl/ cluster.*]	The next trial; a partial modeling
Child	"Plane."	A correct response
Clinician	"That's great! You said *plane*, not *pwane*."	Verbal praise
Clinician	[*the same stimulus*] "What is this?"	Typical question; evoked trial
Child	"Plane."	A correct response
Clinician	"That was magnificent. You remembered to say the *l* after the *p*!"	Verbal praise

If the wrong responses persist on 4 to 5 evoked trials, reinstate partial or full modeling for a few trials, again fade the modeling, and re-present the evoked trials.

When the child meets the tentative learning criterion of 10 consecutively correct, nonimitated responses for a given stimulus item, move on to the next stimulus item. With this procedure, teach 6 to 8 exemplars shown on the following recording sheet. Use different exemplars as you see fit for a given child.

/pl/ in Word-Initial Positions

Treatment Exemplars and Recording Sheet

Use stimuli from the **Stimulus Book, Volume 5**.

Print this page from CD or photocopy this page for your clinical use.

Name/Age:	Date:
Goal: Production of /pl/ in word-initial positions with 90% accuracy when asked an evoking question while showing a stimulus.	Clinician:

Scoring: Correct: ✓   Incorrect or no response: X

Target skills	Discrete Trials														
	1	2	3	4	5	6	7	8	9	10	11	12	13	14	15
1. plane															
2. plate															
3. play															
4. plus															
5. plant															
6. place mat															
7. plantation															
8. platform															

When the child has met the learning criterion of 10 consecutively correct evoked (nonimitated) responses for each of the 6 to 8 target exemplars, conduct a probe to see if the production has generalized to previously baserated but untrained exemplars.

If the probes do not meet the 90% correct criterion for untrained exemplars, teach additional exemplars and then probe again.

/pl/ in Word-Initial Positions

Probe Protocols and Recording Sheet

Use stimuli from the **Stimulus Book,** *Volume 5.*

Print this page from the CD or photocopy this page for your clinical use.

On the probes, present only the untrained exemplars (UT). When the child fails to meet the 90% correct probe criterion, either teach 2 to 4 new exemplars or give additional training trials on already trained stimuli. If needed, select new exemplars for probes. Probe at least 10 untrained exemplars. Alternate probes and treatment until the probe criterion is met.

Scripts For Probe Trials		Note
Clinician	[*untrained stimulus: platypus*] "What is this?"	No modeling or prompts
Child	No response.	Lack of generalization
Clinician	Scores it as *no response*.	No corrective feedback
Clinician	[*untrained stimulus: playground*] "What is this?"	The second probe trial
Child	"A playground."	A correct response
Clinician	Scores the response as correct.	No reinforcement

Name:	Date:	Session #:
Age:	**Clinician:**	
Diagnosis: Articulation/Phonologic Disorder	**Word-initial /pl/ probe**	
Untrained Stimuli	**Score: + correct; – incorrect or no responses**	
1. platypus		
2. playground		
3. planet		
4. plow		
5. pliers		
6. plug		
7. plum		
8. playpen		
9. plumber		
10. playmate		
11. playhouse		
12. plunger		
Percent correct: (Criterion: 90%)		

If the child does not meet the probe criterion, give additional training on already trained exemplars or teach a few new exemplars. Subsequently, readminister the probe trials. When the child meets the 90% correct probe criterion for the exemplars, shift training to the sentence or conversational level or to another phoneme.

/sl/ in Word-Initial Positions

Baserate Protocols

Use stimuli from the **Stimulus Book,** *Volume 5.*

At the beginning of each trial, place a relevant stimulus (an object, a picture, or a printed word if the child can read) in front of the child. Point to the stimulus as you ask an evoking question. Do not respond in any way to the child's correct, incorrect, or lack of responses.

Scripts For Evoked Baserate Trial		Note
Clinician	[*stimulus: slide*] "What is this?"	Evoked trial
Child	"ide."	Omission of initial /sl/ cluster
Clinician	Pulls the stimulus toward her; records the response.	No corrective feedback
Clinician	[*stimulus: sled*] "What is this?"	The next evoked trial
Child	"wed."	Substitution of /w/ for /sl/ cluster
Clinician	Pulls the stimulus toward her; records the response.	No corrective feedback

Administer the modeled baserate trials only after completing the evoked trials on all 20 (or more) exemplars.

Scripts For Modeled Baserate Trial		Note
Clinician	[*stimulus: slide*] "What is this? Say, *slide*."	Modeled trial
Child	"lide."	Omission of /s/ in /sl/ cluster
Clinician	Pulls the stimulus toward her; records the response.	No corrective feedback
Clinician	[*stimulus: sled*] "What is this? Say, *sled*."	The next modeled trial
Child	"Sled."	Correct response
Clinician	Pulls the stimulus toward her; records the response.	No reinforcement

Use the recording sheet with exemplars shown on the next page to establish the baserates; print it from the CD.

/sl/ in Word-Initial Positions

Baserate Exemplars and Recording Sheet

Use stimuli from the **Stimulus Book,** *Volume 5*.

Print this page from the CD or photocopy this page for your clinical use.

Name/Age:	Date:
Goal: To establish the baserate production of /sl/ in word-initial positions.	Clinician:

Scoring: Correct: ✓   Incorrect or no response: X

/sl/ in word-initial positions	Evoked	Modeled
1. slide		
2. sled		
3. slate		
4. slope		
5. sleep		
6. slender		
7. sleeping bag		
8. sled dog		
9. slingshot		
10. slippers		
11. sling		
12. slipped		
13. sloppy		
14. sleeve		
15. slice		
16. slippery		
17. sleepwear		
18. sleeveless		
19. slipcover		
20. slumber		
Percent correct baserate		

Replace or add new exemplars as you see fit for a given child. After establishing the baserates, begin production teaching. Follow the protocols given on the next page.

/sl/ in Word-Initial Positions

Treatment Protocols

Use stimuli from the **Stimulus Book,** *Volume 5.*

Teach 6 to 8 exemplars using the following script.

Place a relevant stimulus in front of the child (an object, a picture, or a printed word if the child can read) and ask a question as you point to the stimulus.

Scripts For Modeled Discrete Trial Training		Note
Clinician	[*stimulus: slide*] "What is this? Say, **sl**ide."	Modeling; the target vocally emphasized
Child	"lide."	A wrong response
Clinician	"No. That's not correct. You said *lide*, but it's a **sl**ide. You need to say the **s** sound at the beginning, **sl**ide."	Corrective feedback
Clinician	[*the same stimulus*] "What is this? Say **sl**ide. Don't forget the **s** at the beginning."	The next trial
Child	"Slide."	A correct response
Clinician	"Amazing! You didn't forget the *s* this time!"	Verbal praise

Repeat the trials until the child gives 5 consecutively correct, imitated responses.

When the child imitates 5 correct responses in sequence, fade the modeling.

Scripts For Fading the Modeling		Note
Clinician	[*stimulus: slide*] "What is this? Don't forget the *s* at the beginning."	Only a prompt
Child	"lide."	A wrong response
Clinician	"Oh no, you forgot the *s*! It's a *sl*ide, not *lide*. Put the *s* at the beginning."	Corrective feedback
Clinician	[*the same stimulus*] "What is this? It starts with . . . " [*silently stretches lips and points to teeth to model visible posture for /s/.*]	The next trial; a partial modeling
Child	"Slide."	A correct response
Clinician	"That's great! You said *slide*, not *lide*."	Verbal praise
Clinician	[*the same stimulus*] "What is this?"	Typical question; evoked trial
Child	"Slide."	A correct response
Clinician	"Outstanding! You said it correctly!"	Verbal praise

If the wrong responses persist on 4 to 5 evoked trials, reinstate partial or full modeling for a few trials, again fade the modeling, and re-present the evoked trials.

When the child meets the tentative learning criterion of 10 consecutively correct, nonimitated responses for a given stimulus item, move on to the next stimulus item. With this procedure, teach 6 to 8 exemplars shown on the following recording sheet. Use different exemplars as you see fit for a given child.

/sl/ in Word-Initial Positions

Treatment Exemplars and Recording Sheet

*Use stimuli from the **Stimulus Book, Volume 5**.*

Print this page from CD or photocopy this page for your clinical use.

Name/Age:	Date:
Goal: Production of /sl/ in word-initial positions with 90% accuracy when asked an evoking question while showing a stimulus.	Clinician:

Scoring: Correct: ✓   Incorrect or no response: X

Target skills	Discrete Trials														
	1	2	3	4	5	6	7	8	9	10	11	12	13	14	15
1. slide															
2. sled															
3. slate															
4. slope															
5. sleep															
6. slender															
7. sleeping bag															
8. sled dog															

When the child has met the learning criterion of 10 consecutively correct evoked (nonimitated) responses for each of the 6 to 8 target exemplars, conduct a probe to see if the production has generalized to previously baserated but untrained exemplars.

If the probes do not meet the 90% correct criterion for untrained exemplars, teach additional exemplars and then probe again.

/sl/ in Word-Initial Positions

Probe Protocols and Recording Sheet

Use stimuli from the **Stimulus Book,** *Volume 5.*

Print this page from the CD or photocopy this page for your clinical use.

On the probes, present only the untrained exemplars (UT). When the child fails to meet the 90% correct probe criterion, either teach 2 to 4 new exemplars or give additional training trials on already trained stimuli. If needed, select new exemplars for probes. Probe at least 10 untrained exemplars. Alternate probes and treatment until the probe criterion is met.

Scripts For Probe Trials		Note
Clinician	[*untrained stimulus: slingshot*] "What is this?"	No modeling or prompts
Child	"Slingshot."	A correct, generalized response
Clinician	Scores the response as correct.	No reinforcement
Clinician	[*untrained stimulus: slippers*] "What are these?"	The second probe trial
Child	"Slippers."	A correct, generalized response
Clinician	Scores the response as correct.	No reinforcement

Name:	Date:	Session #:
Age:	**Clinician:**	
Diagnosis: Articulation/Phonologic Disorder	**Word-initial /sl/ probe**	
Untrained Stimuli	**Score: + correct; – incorrect or no responses**	
1. slingshot		
2. slippers		
3. sled		
4. slipped		
5. sloppy		
6. sleeve		
7. slice		
8. slippery		
9. sleepwear		
10. sleeveless		
11. slipcover		
12. slumber		
Percent correct: (Criterion: 90%)		

If the child does not meet the probe criterion, give additional training on already trained exemplars or teach a few new exemplars. Subsequently, readminister the probe trials. When the child meets the 90% correct probe criterion for the exemplars, shift training to the sentence or conversational level or to another phoneme.

/br/ in Word-Initial Positions

Baserate Protocols

Use stimuli from the **Stimulus Book,** *Volume 5.*

At the beginning of each trial, place a relevant stimulus (an object, a picture, or a printed word if the child can read) in front of the child. Point to the stimulus as you ask an evoking question. Do not respond in any way to the child's correct, incorrect, or lack of responses.

Scripts For Evoked Baserate Trial		Note
Clinician	[*stimulus: broom*] "What is this?"	Evoked trial
Child	"boom."	Omission of /r/ in /br/ cluster
Clinician	Pulls the stimulus toward her; records the response.	No corrective feedback
Clinician	[*stimulus: brown*] "What color is this?"	The next evoked trial
Child	"bwown."	Substitution of /bw/ for /br/
Clinician	Pulls the stimulus toward her; records the response.	No corrective feedback

Administer the modeled baserate trials only after completing the evoked trials on all 20 (or more) exemplars.

Scripts For Modeled Baserate Trial		Note
Clinician	[*stimulus: broom*] "What is this? Say, *broom.*"	Modeled trial
Child	"bwoom."	Substitution of /bw/ for /br/
Clinician	Pulls the stimulus toward her; records the response.	No corrective feedback
Clinician	[*stimulus: brown*] "What color is this? Say, *brown.*"	The next modeled trial
Child	"Brown."	Correct response
Clinician	Pulls the stimulus toward her; records the response.	No reinforcement

Use the recording sheet with exemplars shown on the next page to establish the baserates; print it from the CD.

/br/ in Word-Initial Positions

Baserate Exemplars and Recording Sheet

*Use stimuli from the **Stimulus Book, Volume 5**.*

Print this page from the CD or photocopy this page for your clinical use.

Name/Age:	Date:
Goal: To establish the baserate production of /br/ in word-initial positions.	Clinician:

Scoring: Correct: ✓   Incorrect or no response: X

/br/ in word-initial positions	Evoked	Modeled
1. broom		
2. brown		
3. brush		
4. braces		
5. braid		
6. breakfast		
7. bracelet		
8. bronco		
9. broccoli		
10. broken		
11. brain		
12. branch		
13. brick		
14. bridge		
15. brook		
16. briefcase		
17. bracket		
18. broomstick		
19. brunette		
20. brontosaur		
Percent correct baserate		

Replace or add new exemplars as you see fit for a given child. After establishing the baserates, begin production teaching. Follow the protocols given on the next page.

/br/ in Word-Initial Positions

Treatment Protocols

Use stimuli from the **Stimulus Book,** *Volume 5.*

Teach 6 to 8 exemplars using the following script.

Place a relevant stimulus in front of the child (an object, a picture, or a printed word if the child can read) and ask a question as you point to the stimulus.

Scripts For Modeled Discrete Trial Training		Note
Clinician	[*stimulus: broom*] "What is this? Say, **broom**."	Modeling; the target vocally emphasized
Child	"bwoom."	A wrong response
Clinician	"No. That's not correct. You said *bwoom*, but it's a **broom**. The **r** sound comes after the **b**."	Corrective feedback
Clinician	[*the same stimulus*] "What is this? Say, **broom**. Don't forget the **r** after the **b** when you say **br**oom."	The next trial
Child	"Broom."	A correct response
Clinician	"Excellent! You didn't miss the *r* this time!"	Verbal praise

Repeat the trials until the child gives 5 consecutively correct, imitated responses.

When the child imitates 5 correct responses in sequence, fade the modeling.

Scripts For Fading the Modeling		Note
Clinician	[*stimulus: broom*] "What is this? Remember to say the *r* sound after the *b*."	Only a prompt
Child	"bwoom."	A wrong response
Clinician	"Gee, you forgot to say the *b* and the *r* together! It's not a *bwoom*. It's a *broom*. The *r* sound, not *w*, comes after *b*."	Corrective feedback
Clinician	[*the same stimulus*] "What is this? It starts with . . . " [*silently models the visible lip and tongue posture for the /br/ cluster.*]	The next trial; a partial modeling
Child	"Broom."	A correct response
Clinician	"That's great! You said *broom*, not *bwoom*."	Verbal praise
Clinician	[*the same stimulus*] "What is this?"	Typical question; evoked trial
Child	"Broom."	A correct response
Clinician	"Great job! You said it correctly!"	Verbal praise

If the wrong responses persist on 4 to 5 evoked trials, reinstate partial or full modeling for a few trials, again fade the modeling, and re-present the evoked trials.

When the child meets the tentative learning criterion of 10 consecutively correct, nonimitated responses for a given stimulus item, move on to the next stimulus item. With this procedure, teach 6 to 8 exemplars shown on the following recording sheet. Use different exemplars as you see fit for a given child.

/br/ in Word-Initial Positions

Treatment Exemplars and Recording Sheet

Use stimuli from the **Stimulus Book, *Volume 5***.

Print this page from CD or photocopy this page for your clinical use.

Name/Age:	Date:
Goal: Production of /br/ in word-initial positions with 90% accuracy when asked an evoking question while showing a stimulus.	Clinician:

Scoring: Correct: ✓   Incorrect or no response: X

Target skills	Discrete Trials														
	1	2	3	4	5	6	7	8	9	10	11	12	13	14	15
1. broom															
2. brown															
3. brush															
4. braces															
5. braid															
6. breakfast															
7. bracelet															
8. bronco															

When the child has met the learning criterion of 10 consecutively correct evoked (nonimitated) responses for each of the 6 to 8 target exemplars, conduct a probe to see if the production has generalized to previously baserated but untrained exemplars.

If the probes do not meet the 90% correct criterion for untrained exemplars, teach additional exemplars and then probe again.

/br/ in Word-Initial Positions

Probe Protocols and Recording Sheet

Use stimuli from the **Stimulus Book,** *Volume 5.*

Print this page from the CD or photocopy this page for your clinical use.

On the probes, present only the untrained exemplars (UT). When the child fails to meet the 90% correct probe criterion, either teach 2 to 4 new exemplars or give additional training trials on already trained stimuli. If needed, select new exemplars for probes. Probe at least 10 untrained exemplars. Alternate probes and treatment until the probe criterion is met.

Scripts For Probe Trials		Note
Clinician	[*untrained stimulus: broccoli*] "What is this?"	No modeling or prompts
Child	"Broccoli."	A correct, generalized response
Clinician	Scores the response as correct.	No reinforcement
Clinician	[*untrained stimulus: broken*] "The boy dropped the glass. The glass is _____."	The second probe trial
Child	"boken."	A wrong probe response
Clinician	Scores the response as incorrect.	No corrective feedback

Name:	Date:	Session #:
Age:	**Clinician:**	
Diagnosis: Articulation/Phonologic Disorder	**Word-initial /br/ probe**	
Untrained Stimuli	**Score: + correct; – incorrect or no responses**	
1. broccoli		
2. broken		
3. brain		
4. branch		
5. brick		
6. bridge		
7. brook		
8. briefcase		
9. bracket		
10. broomstick		
11. brunette		
12. brontosaur		
Percent correct: (Criterion: 90%)		

If the child does not meet the probe criterion, give additional training on already trained exemplars or teach a few new exemplars. Subsequently, readminister the probe trials. When the child meets the 90% correct probe criterion for the exemplars, shift training to the sentence or conversational level or to another phoneme.

/dr/ in Word-Initial Positions

Baserate Protocols

Use stimuli from the **Stimulus Book,** *Volume 5.*

At the beginning of each trial, place a relevant stimulus (an object, a picture, or a printed word if the child can read) in front of the child. Point to the stimulus as you ask an evoking question. Do not respond in any way to the child's correct, incorrect, or lack of responses.

Scripts For Evoked Baserate Trial		Note
Clinician	[*stimulus: dress*] "What is this?"	Evoked trial
Child	"A dwess."	Substitution of /dw/ for /dr/
Clinician	Pulls the stimulus toward her; records the response.	No corrective feedback
Clinician	[*stimulus: drinking*] "What is the boy doing?"	The next evoked trial
Child	"dwinking."	Substitution of /dw/ for /dr/
Clinician	Pulls the stimulus toward her; records the response.	No corrective feedback

Administer the modeled baserate trials only after completing the evoked trials on all 20 (or more) exemplars.

Scripts For Modeled Baserate Trial		Note
Clinician	[*stimulus: dress*] "What is this? Say, *dress.*"	Modeled trial
Child	"Dress."	Correct response
Clinician	Pulls the stimulus toward her; records the response.	No reinforcement
Clinician	[*stimulus: drinking*] "What is the *boy* doing? Say, *drinking.*"	The next modeled trial
Child	"dwinking."	Substitution of /dw/ for /dr/
Clinician	Pulls the stimulus toward her; records the response.	No corrective feedback

Use the recording sheet with exemplars shown on the next page to establish the baserates; print it from the CD.

/dr/ in Word-Initial Positions

Baserate Exemplars and Recording Sheet

Use stimuli from the **Stimulus Book,** *Volume 5.*

Print this page from the CD or photocopy this page for your clinical use.

Name/Age:	Date:
Goal: To establish the baserate production of /dr/ in word-initial positions.	Clinician:

Scoring: Correct: ✓   Incorrect or no response: X

/dr/ in word-initial positions	Evoked	Modeled
1. dress		
2. drinking		
3. drape		
4. drawing		
5. drawer		
6. dragons		
7. dragonfly		
8. drainpipe		
9. drawbridge		
10. drumstick		
11. dreaming		
12. dresser		
13. dragging		
14. dryer		
15. drip		
16. driveway		
17. drawstring		
18. drugstore		
19. dromedary		
20. drummer boy		
Percent correct baserate		

Replace or add new exemplars as you see fit for a given child. After establishing the baserates, begin production teaching. Follow the protocols given on the next page.

/dr/ in Word-Initial Positions

Treatment Protocols

Use stimuli from the **Stimulus Book,** *Volume 5.*

Teach 6 to 8 exemplars using the following script.

Place a relevant stimulus in front of the child (an object, a picture, or a printed word if the child can read) and ask a question as you point to the stimulus.

Scripts For Modeled Discrete Trial Training		Note
Clinician	[*stimulus: dress*] "What is this? Say, ***dress***."	Modeling; the target vocally emphasized
Child	"dwess."	A wrong response
Clinician	"No. That's not correct. You said *dwess*, but it's a ***dress***."	Corrective feedback
Clinician	[*the same stimulus*] "What is this? Say, ***dress***. You need to say the ***r*** sound after the ***d***."	The next trial
Child	"Dress."	A correct response
Clinician	"Excellent! You didn't miss the ***r*** this time!"	Verbal praise

Repeat the trials until the child gives 5 consecutively correct, imitated responses.

When the child imitates 5 correct responses in sequence, fade the modeling.

Scripts For Fading the Modeling		Note
Clinician	[*stimulus: dress*] "What is this? Don't forget to say the *r* after the *d*."	Only a prompt
Child	"dwess."	A wrong response
Clinician	"Oops, you forgot the *r* sound after the *d*. It's a *dress*, not *dwess*. Say the *d* and the *r* together."	Corrective feedback
Clinician	[*the same stimulus*] "What is this? It starts with . . . " [*silently models the tongue posture for the /dr/ cluster.*]	The next trial; a partial modeling
Child	"Dress."	A correct response
Clinician	"That's excellent! You said *dress*, not *dwess*."	Verbal praise
Clinician	[*the same stimulus*] "What is this?"	Typical question; evoked trial
Child	"Dress."	A correct response
Clinician	"That was perfect! You said it correctly!"	Verbal praise

If the wrong responses persist on 4 to 5 evoked trials, reinstate partial or full modeling for a few trials, again fade the modeling, and re-present the evoked trials.

When the child meets the tentative learning criterion of 10 consecutively correct, nonimitated responses for a given stimulus item, move on to the next stimulus item. With this procedure, teach 6 to 8 exemplars shown on the following recording sheet. Use different exemplars as you see fit for a given child.

/dr/ in Word-Initial Positions

Treatment Exemplars and Recording Sheet

Use stimuli from the **Stimulus Book**, **Volume 5**.

Print this page from CD or photocopy this page for your clinical use.

Name/Age:	Date:
Goal: Production of /dr/ in word-initial positions with 90% accuracy when asked an evoking question while showing a stimulus.	Clinician:

Scoring: Correct: ✓   Incorrect or no response: X

Target skills	Discrete Trials														
	1	2	3	4	5	6	7	8	9	10	11	12	13	14	15
1. dress															
2. drinking															
3. drape															
4. drawing															
5. drawer															
6. dragons															
7. dragonfly															
8. drainpipe															

When the child has met the learning criterion of 10 consecutively correct evoked (nonimitated) responses for each of the 6 to 8 target exemplars, conduct a probe to see if the production has generalized to previously baserated but untrained exemplars.

If the probes do not meet the 90% correct criterion for untrained exemplars, teach additional exemplars and then probe again.

/dr/ in Word-Initial Positions

Probe Protocols and Recording Sheet

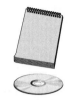

Use stimuli from the **Stimulus Book,** *Volume 5.*

Print this page from the CD or photocopy this page for your clinical use.

On the probes, present only the untrained exemplars (UT). When the child fails to meet the 90% correct probe criterion, either teach 2 to 4 new exemplars or give additional training trials on already trained stimuli. If needed, select new exemplars for probes. Probe at least 10 untrained exemplars. Alternate probes and treatment until the probe criterion is met.

Scripts For Probe Trials		Note
Clinician	[*untrained stimulus: drawbridge*] "What is this?"	No modeling or prompts
Child	"No response."	Lack of generalization
Clinician	Scores it as *no response.*	No corrective feedback
Clinician	[*untrained stimulus: drumstick*] "What is this?"	The second probe trial
Child	"dwumstick."	A wrong probe response
Clinician	Scores the response as incorrect.	No corrective feedback

Name:	Date:	Session #:
Age:	**Clinician:**	
Diagnosis: Articulation/Phonologic Disorder	**Word-initial /dr/ probe**	
Untrained Stimuli	**Score: + correct; – incorrect or no responses**	
1. drawbridge		
2. drumstick		
3. dreaming		
4. dresser		
5. dragging		
6. dryer		
7. drip		
8. driveway		
9. drawstring		
10. drugstore		
11. dromedary		
12. drummer boy		
Percent correct: (Criterion: 90%)		

If the child does not meet the probe criterion, give additional training on already trained exemplars or teach a few new exemplars. Subsequently, readminister the probe trials. When the child meets the 90% correct probe criterion for the exemplars, shift training to the sentence or conversational level or to another phoneme.

/fr/ in Word-Initial Positions

Baserate Protocols

Use stimuli from the **Stimulus Book,** *Volume 6.*

At the beginning of each trial, place a relevant stimulus (an object, a picture, or a printed word if the child can read) in front of the child. Point to the stimulus as you ask an evoking question. Do not respond in any way to the child's correct, incorrect, or lack of responses.

Scripts For Evoked Baserate Trial		Note
Clinician	[*stimulus: frog*] "What is this?"	Evoked trial
Child	"fog."	Omission of /r/ in /fr/ cluster
Clinician	Pulls the stimulus toward her; records the response.	No corrective feedback
Clinician	[*stimulus: freckles*] "What do you see on the girl's face?"	The next evoked trial
Child	"fweckles."	Substitution of /fw/ for /fr/
Clinician	Pulls the stimulus toward her; records the response.	No corrective feedback

Administer the modeled baserate trials only after completing the evoked trials on all 20 (or more) exemplars.

Scripts For Modeled Baserate Trial		Note
Clinician	[*stimulus: frog*] "What is this? Say, *frog.*"	Modeled trial
Child	"fog."	Omission of /r/ in /fr/ cluster
Clinician	Pulls the stimulus toward her; records the response.	No corrective feedback
Clinician	[*stimulus: freckles*] "What do you see on the girl's face? Say, *freckles.*"	The next modeled trial
Child	"fweckles."	Omission of /r/ in /fr/ cluster
Clinician	Pulls the stimulus toward her; records the response.	No corrective feedback

Use the recording sheet with exemplars shown on the next page to establish the baserates; print it from the CD.

/fr/ in Word-Initial Positions

Baserate Exemplars and Recording Sheet

Use stimuli from the **Stimulus Book,** *Volume 6.*

Print this page from the CD or photocopy this page for your clinical use.

Name/Age:	Date:
Goal: To establish the baserate production of /fr/ in word-initial positions.	Clinician:

Scoring: Correct: ✓   Incorrect or no response: X

/fr/ in word-initial positions	Evoked	Modeled
1. frog		
2. freckles		
3. freight		
4. fry		
5. friend		
6. fraction		
7. Friday		
8. fragment		
9. frosting		
10. fruitcake		
11. frame		
12. fruit		
13. front		
14. frost		
15. frowning		
16. freezer		
17. frying		
18. fruit salad		
19. frogman		
20. fracture		
Percent correct baserate		

Replace or add new exemplars as you see fit for a given child. After establishing the baserates, begin production teaching. Follow the protocols given on the next page.

/fr/ in Word-Initial Positions

Treatment Protocols

Use stimuli from the **Stimulus Book, Volume 6.**

Teach 6 to 8 exemplars using the following script.

Place a relevant stimulus in front of the child (an object, a picture, or a printed word if the child can read) and ask a question as you point to the stimulus.

Scripts For Modeled Discrete Trial Training		Note
Clinician	[*stimulus: frog*] "What is this? Say, **frog**."	Modeling; the target vocally emphasized
Child	"fog."	A wrong response
Clinician	"No. That's not correct. You said *fog*, but it's a **frog**. You need to say an **r** after the **f**."	Corrective feedback
Clinician	[*the same stimulus*] "What is this? Say, **frog**. Don't forget to say the **r** sound after the **f**, **frog**."	The next trial
Child	"Frog."	A correct response
Clinician	"Excellent! You didn't miss the **r** this time!"	Verbal praise

Repeat the trials until the child gives 5 consecutively correct, imitated responses.

When the child imitates 5 correct responses in sequence, fade the modeling.

Scripts For Fading the Modeling		Note
Clinician	[*stimulus: frog*] "What is this? Don't forget the *r* after the *f*."	Only a prompt
Child	"fog."	A wrong response
Clinician	"Gee, you forgot the *r*! It's a *frog*, not *fog*. Say the *r* after the *f*."	Corrective feedback
Clinician	[*the same stimulus*] "What is this? It starts with . . . " [*silently models the lip and tongue posture for the /fr/ cluster.*]	The next trial; a partial modeling
Child	"Frog."	A correct response
Clinician	"That's great! You said *frog*, not *fog*."	Verbal praise
Clinician	[*the same stimulus*] "What is this?"	Typical question; evoked trial
Child	"Frog."	A correct response
Clinician	"Great job! You said it perfectly! You are working very hard."	Verbal praise

If the wrong responses persist on 4 to 5 evoked trials, reinstate partial or full modeling for a few trials, again fade the modeling, and re-present the evoked trials.

When the child meets the tentative learning criterion of 10 consecutively correct, nonimitated responses for a given stimulus item, move on to the next stimulus item. With this procedure, teach 6 to 8 exemplars shown on the following recording sheet. Use different exemplars as you see fit for a given child.

/fr/ in Word-Initial Positions

Treatment Exemplars and Recording Sheet

Use stimuli from the **Stimulus Book,** *Volume 6.*

Print this page from CD or photocopy this page for your clinical use.

Name/Age:	Date:
Goal: Production of /fr/ in word-initial positions with 90% accuracy when asked an evoking question while showing a stimulus.	Clinician:

Scoring: Correct: ✓   Incorrect or no response: X

Target skills	Discrete Trials														
	1	2	3	4	5	6	7	8	9	10	11	12	13	14	15
1. frog															
2. freckles															
3. freight															
4. fry															
5. friend															
6. fraction															
7. Friday															
8. fragment															

When the child has met the learning criterion of 10 consecutively correct evoked (nonimitated) responses for each of the 6 to 8 target exemplars, conduct a probe to see if the production has generalized to previously baserated but untrained exemplars.

If the probes do not meet the 90% correct criterion for untrained exemplars, teach additional exemplars and then probe again.

/fr/ in Word-Initial Positions

Probe Protocols and Recording Sheet

Use stimuli from the **Stimulus Book, Volume 6.**

Print this page from the CD or photocopy this page for your clinical use.

On the probes, present only the untrained exemplars (UT). When the child fails to meet the 90% correct probe criterion, either teach 2 to 4 new exemplars or give additional training trials on already trained stimuli. If needed, select new exemplars for probes. Probe at least 10 untrained exemplars. Alternate probes and treatment until the probe criterion is met.

Scripts for Probe Trials		Note
Clinician	[*untrained stimulus: frosting*] "What is covering the cake?"	No modeling or prompts
Child	"Frosting."	A correct, generalized response
Clinician	Scores the response as correct.	No reinforcement
Clinician	[*untrained stimulus: fruitcake*] "What is this?"	The second probe trial
Child	"fuitcake."	A wrong probe response
Clinician	Scores the response as incorrect.	No corrective feedback

Name:	Date:	Session #:
Age:	**Clinician:**	
Diagnosis: Articulation/Phonologic Disorder	**Word-initial /fr/ probe**	
Untrained Stimuli	**Score: + correct; – incorrect or no responses**	
1. frosting		
2. fruitcake		
3. frame		
4. fruit		
5. front		
6. frost		
7. frowning		
8. freezer		
9. frying		
10. fruit salad		
11. frogman		
12. fracture		
Percent correct: (Criterion: 90%)		

If the child does not meet the probe criterion, give additional training on already trained exemplars or teach a few new exemplars. Subsequently, readminister the probe trials. When the child meets the 90% correct probe criterion for the exemplars, shift training to the sentence or conversational level or to another phoneme.

/gr/ in Word-Initial Positions

Baserate Protocols

Use stimuli from the **Stimulus Book,** *Volume 6.*

At the beginning of each trial, place a relevant stimulus (an object, a picture, or a printed word if the child can read) in front of the child. Point to the stimulus as you ask an evoking question. Do not respond in any way to the child's correct, incorrect, or lack of responses.

Scripts For Evoked Baserate Trial		Note
Clinician	[*stimulus: grapes*] "What are these?"	Evoked trial
Child	"apes."	Omission of /gr/ cluster
Clinician	Pulls the stimulus toward her; records the response.	No corrective feedback
Clinician	[*stimulus: gray*] "What color is this?"	The next evoked trial
Child	"day."	Substitution of /d/ for /gr/
Clinician	Pulls the stimulus toward her; records the response.	No corrective feedback

Administer the modeled baserate trials only after completing the evoked trials on all 20 (or more) exemplars.

Scripts For Modeled Baserate Trial		Note
Clinician	[*stimulus: grapes*] "What are these? Say, *grapes.*"	Modeled trial
Child	"gapes."	Omission of /r/ in /gr/ cluster
Clinician	Pulls the stimulus toward her; records the response.	No corrective feedback
Clinician	[*stimulus: gray*] "What is this? Say, *gray.*"	The next modeled trial
Child	"gay."	Substitution of /g/ for /gr/
Clinician	Pulls the stimulus toward her; records the response.	No corrective feedback

Use the recording sheet with exemplars shown on the next page to establish the baserates; print it from the CD.

/gr/ in Word-Initial Positions

Baserate Exemplars and Recording Sheet

Use stimuli from the **Stimulus Book,** *Volume 6.*

Print this page from the CD or photocopy this page for your clinical use.

Name/Age:	Date:
Goal: To establish the baserate production of /gr/ in word-initial positions.	Clinician:

Scoring: Correct: ✓   Incorrect or no response: X

/gr/ in word-initial positions	Evoked	Modeled
1. grapes		
2. gray		
3. grade		
4. grin		
5. grill		
6. grizzly bear		
7. grandma		
8. grapefruit		
9. grapevine		
10. grasshopper		
11. grass		
12. green		
13. group		
14. groom		
15. ground		
16. Great Dane		
17. grand piano		
18. greyhound		
19. groceries		
20. groundhog		
Percent correct baserate		

Replace or add new exemplars as you see fit for a given child. After establishing the baserates, begin production teaching. Follow the protocols given on the next page.

/gr/ in Word-Initial Positions

Treatment Protocols

Use stimuli from the **Stimulus Book,** *Volume 6.*

Teach 6 to 8 exemplars using the following script.

Place a relevant stimulus in front of the child (an object, a picture, or a printed word if the child can read) and ask a question as you point to the stimulus.

Scripts For Modeled Discrete Trial Training		Note
Clinician	[*stimulus: grapes*] "What are these? Say, **gr***apes.*"	Modeling; the target vocally emphasized
Child	"gapes."	A wrong response
Clinician	"No. That's not correct. You said *gapes*, but it's **gr***apes.* The word starts with **g** and **r** together. You left out the **r**."	Corrective feedback
Clinician	[*the same stimulus*] "What are these? Say, **gr***apes.* Don't forget the **r** after the **g** this time."	The next trial
Child	"gapes."	A wrong response
Clinician	"Oh no! You forgot to say the **r** after the *g* again. Remember that the sound **r** comes after the **g**, **gr***apes.*"	Corrective feedback

Repeat the trials until the child gives 5 consecutively correct, imitated responses.

When the child imitates 5 correct responses in sequence, fade the modeling.

Scripts For Fading the Modeling		Note
Clinician	[*stimulus: grapes*] "What are these? Don't forget to say the *r* sound after the *g* sound this time."	Only a prompt
Child	"gapes."	A wrong response
Clinician	"Oh no, you forgot the *r*! It's *grapes*, not *gapes*. Say the *g* and the *r* together."	Corrective feedback
Clinician	[*the same stimulus*] "What are these? It starts with . . . " [*silently models the tongue posture for the* /gr/ *cluster.*]	The next trial; a partial modeling
Child	"Grapes."	A correct response
Clinician	"Alright! You said *grapes*, not *gapes*."	Verbal praise
Clinician	[*the same stimulus*] "What are these?"	Typical question; evoked trial
Child	"Grapes."	A correct response
Clinician	"That was excellent! You said it perfectly!"	Verbal praise

If the wrong responses persist on 4 to 5 evoked trials, reinstate partial or full modeling for a few trials, again fade the modeling, and re-present the evoked trials.

When the child meets the tentative learning criterion of 10 consecutively correct, nonimitated responses for a given stimulus item, move on to the next stimulus item. With this procedure, teach 6 to 8 exemplars shown on the following recording sheet. Use different exemplars as you see fit for a given child.

/gr/ in Word-Initial Positions

Treatment Exemplars and Recording Sheet

Use stimuli from the **Stimulus Book,** *Volume 6.*

Print this page from CD or photocopy this page for your clinical use.

Name/Age:	Date:
Goal: Production of /gr/ in word-initial positions with 90% accuracy when asked an evoking question while showing a stimulus.	Clinician:

Scoring: Correct: ✓   Incorrect or no response: X

Target skills	Discrete Trials														
	1	2	3	4	5	6	7	8	9	10	11	12	13	14	15
1. grapes															
2. gray															
3. grade															
4. grin															
5. grill															
6. grizzly bear															
7. grandma															
8. grapefruit															

When the child has met the learning criterion of 10 consecutively correct evoked (nonimitated) responses for each of the 6 to 8 target exemplars, conduct a probe to see if the production has generalized to previously baserated but untrained exemplars.

If the probes do not meet the 90% correct criterion for untrained exemplars, teach additional exemplars and then probe again.

/gr/ in Word-Initial Positions

Probe Protocols and Recording Sheet

Use stimuli from the **Stimulus Book,** *Volume 6.*

Print this page from the CD or photocopy this page for your clinical use.

On the probes, present only the untrained exemplars (UT). When the child fails to meet the 90% correct probe criterion, either teach 2 to 4 new exemplars or give additional training trials on already trained stimuli. If needed, select new exemplars for probes. Probe at least 10 untrained exemplars. Alternate probes and treatment until the probe criterion is met.

Scripts for Probe Trials		Note
Clinician	[*untrained stimulus: grapevine*] "What is this?"	No modeling or prompts
Child	"Grapevine."	A correct, generalized response
Clinician	Scores the response as correct.	No reinforcement
Clinician	[*untrained stimulus: grasshopper*] "What is this?"	The second probe trial
Child	"Grasshopper."	A correct, generalized response
Clinician	Scores the response as correct .	No reinforcement

Name:	Date:	Session #:
Age:	Clinician:	
Diagnosis: Articulation/Phonologic Disorder	Word-initial /gr/ probe	
Untrained Stimuli	**Score: + correct; – incorrect or no responses**	
1. grapevine		
2. grasshopper		
3. grass		
4. green		
5. group		
6. groom		
7. gravy		
8. Great Dane		
9. greenhouse		
10. greyhound		
11. groceries		
12. groundhog		
Percent correct: (Criterion: 90%)		

If the child does not meet the probe criterion, give additional training on already trained exemplars or teach a few new exemplars. Subsequently, readminister the probe trials. When the child meets the 90% correct probe criterion for the exemplars, shift training to the sentence or conversational level or to another phoneme.

/kr/ in Word-Initial Positions

Baserate Protocols

Use stimuli from the **Stimulus Book, Volume 6**.

At the beginning of each trial, place a relevant stimulus (an object, a picture, or a printed word if the child can read) in front of the child. Point to the stimulus as you ask an evoking question. Do not respond in any way to the child's correct, incorrect, or lack of responses.

Scripts For Evoked Baserate Trial		Note
Clinician	[*stimulus: crab*] "What is this?"	Evoked trial
Child	"cab."	Omission of /r/ in /kr/ cluster
Clinician	Pulls the stimulus toward her; records the response.	No corrective feedback
Clinician	[*stimulus: crown*] "What is this?"	The next evoked trial
Child	"clown."	Substitution of /kl/ for /kr/
Clinician	Pulls the stimulus toward her; records the response.	No corrective feedback

Administer the modeled baserate trials only after completing the evoked trials on all 20 (or more) exemplars.

Scripts For Modeled Baserate Trial		Note
Clinician	[*stimulus: crab*] "What is this? Say, *crab.*"	Modeled trial
Child	"cab."	Omission of /r/ in /kr/ cluster
Clinician	Pulls the stimulus toward her; records the response.	No corrective feedback
Clinician	[*stimulus: crown*] "What is this? Say, *crown.*"	The next modeled trial
Child	"Crown."	Correct response
Clinician	Pulls the stimulus toward her; records the response.	No reinforcement

Use the recording sheet with exemplars shown on the next page to establish the baserates; print it from the CD.

/kr/ in Word-Initial Positions

Baserate Exemplars and Recording Sheet

Use stimuli from the **Stimulus Book,** *Volume 6.*

Print this page from the CD or photocopy this page for your clinical use.

Name/Age:	Date:
Goal: To establish the baserate production of /kr/ in word-initial positions.	Clinician:

Scoring: Correct: ✓   Incorrect or no response: X

/kr/ in word-initial positions	Evoked	Modeled
1. crab		
2. crown		
3. creek		
4. cradle		
5. crane		
6. crowd		
7. crayfish		
8. crock pot		
9. cranberry		
10. crayon		
11. crawling		
12. crust		
13. crib		
14. cry		
15. crow		
16. crutches		
17. cricket		
18. crimson		
19. crocodile		
20. crescent		
Percent correct baserate		

Replace or add new exemplars as you see fit for a given child. After establishing the baserates, begin production teaching. Follow the protocols given on the next page.

/kr/ in Word-Initial Positions

Treatment Protocols

Use stimuli from the **Stimulus Book, Volume 6.**

Teach 6 to 8 exemplars using the following script.

Place a relevant stimulus in front of the child (an object, a picture, or a printed word if the child can read) and ask a question as you point to the stimulus.

Scripts For Modeled Discrete Trial Training		Note
Clinician	[*stimulus: crab*] "What is this? Say, **crab**."	Modeling; the target vocally emphasized
Child	"cwab."	A wrong response
Clinician	"No. That's not correct. You said *cwab*, but it's a **crab**. The **r** sound, not *w*, comes after /k/."	Corrective feedback
Clinician	[*the same stimulus*] "What is this? Say **crab** Remember that the **r** sound comes after the /k/, **crab**."	The next trial
Child	"Crab."	A correct response
Clinician	"Excellent! You said the **r** sound after the /k/ when you said *crab*! Way to go!"	Verbal praise

Repeat the trials until the child gives 5 consecutively correct, imitated responses.

When the child imitates 5 correct responses in sequence, fade the modeling.

Scripts For Fading the Modeling		Note
Clinician	[*stimulus: crab*] "What is this? Don't forget to say the *r* after the /k/."	Only a prompt
Child	"cwab."	A wrong response
Clinician	"Gee, you said the *w* sound instead of the *r* sound after the /k/! It's a *crab*, not *cwab*. Remember that the *r* sound comes after the /k/."	Corrective feedback
Clinician	[*the same stimulus*] "What is this? It starts with . . . " [*silently models the tongue posture for the /kr/ cluster.*]	The next trial; a partial modeling
Child	"Crab."	A correct response
Clinician	"That's great! You said *crab*, not *cwab*."	Verbal praise
Clinician	[*the same stimulus*] "What is this?"	Typical question; evoked trial
Child	"Crab."	A correct response
Clinician	"Outstanding! You said it correctly!"	Verbal praise

If the wrong responses persist on 4 to 5 evoked trials, reinstate partial or full modeling for a few trials, again fade the modeling, and re-present the evoked trials.

When the child meets the tentative learning criterion of 10 consecutively correct, nonimitated responses for a given stimulus item, move on to the next stimulus item. With this procedure, teach 6 to 8 exemplars shown on the following recording sheet. Use different exemplars as you see fit for a given child.

/kr/ in Word-Initial Positions

Treatment Exemplars and Recording Sheet

Use stimuli from the **Stimulus Book,** *Volume 6.*

Print this page from CD or photocopy this page for your clinical use.

Name/Age:	Date:
Goal: Production of /kr/ in word-initial positions with 90% accuracy when asked an evoking question while showing a stimulus.	Clinician:

Scoring: Correct: ✓   Incorrect or no response: X

Target skills	Discrete Trials														
	1	2	3	4	5	6	7	8	9	10	11	12	13	14	15
1. crab															
2. crown															
3. creek															
4. cradle															
5. crane															
6. crowd															
7. crayfish															
8. crock pot															

When the child has met the learning criterion of 10 consecutively correct evoked (nonimitated) responses for each of the 6 to 8 target exemplars, conduct a probe to see if the production has generalized to previously baserated but untrained exemplars.

If the probes do not meet the 90% correct criterion for untrained exemplars, teach additional exemplars and then probe again.

/kr/ in Word-Initial Positions

Probe Protocols and Recording Sheet

Use stimuli from the **Stimulus Book,** *Volume 6.*

Print this page from the CD or photocopy this page for your clinical use.

On the probes, present only the untrained exemplars (UT). When the child fails to meet the 90% correct probe criterion, either teach 2 to 4 new exemplars or give additional training trials on already trained stimuli. If needed, select new exemplars for probes. Probe at least 10 untrained exemplars. Alternate probes and treatment until the probe criterion is met.

Scripts for Probe Trials		Note
Clinician	[*untrained stimulus: cranberry*] "What is this?"	No modeling or prompts
Child	"Cranberry."	A correct, generalized response
Clinician	Scores the response as correct.	No reinforcement
Clinician	[*untrained stimulus: crayon*] "What is this?"	The second probe trial
Child	"Crayon."	A correct, generalized response
Clinician	Scores the response as correct.	No reinforcement

Name:	Date:	Session #:
Age:	**Clinician:**	
Diagnosis: Articulation/Phonologic Disorder	**Word-initial /kr/ probe**	
Untrained Stimuli	**Score: + correct; – incorrect or no responses**	
1. cranberry		
2. crayon		
3. crawling		
4. crust		
5. crib		
6. cry		
7. crown		
8. crutches		
9. cricket		
10. crimson		
11. crocodile		
12. crescent		
Percent correct: (Criterion: 90%)		

If the child does not meet the probe criterion, give additional training on already trained exemplars or teach a few new exemplars. Subsequently, readminister the probe trials. When the child meets the 90% correct probe criterion for the exemplars, shift training to the sentence or conversational level or to another phoneme.

/pr/ in Word-Initial Positions

Baserate Protocols

Use stimuli from the **Stimulus Book,** *Volume 5.*

At the beginning of each trial, place a relevant stimulus (an object, a picture, or a printed word if the child can read) in front of the child. Point to the stimulus as you ask an evoking question. Do not respond in any way to the child's correct, incorrect, or lack of responses.

Scripts For Evoked Baserate Trial		Note
Clinician	[*stimulus: prawn*] "What is this?"	Evoked trial
Child	"I don't know."	Does not know word
Clinician	Pulls the stimulus toward her; records the response. Makes note that child does not know word.	No corrective feedback
Clinician	[*stimulus: proud*] "The boy won first place. He feels very _____?"	The next evoked trial
Child	"pwoud."	Substitution of /pw/ for /pr/
Clinician	Pulls the stimulus toward her; records the response.	No corrective feedback

Administer the modeled baserate trials only after completing the evoked trials on all 20 (or more) exemplars.

Scripts For Modeled Baserate Trial		Note
Clinician	[*stimulus: prawn*] "What is this? Say, *prawn*."	Modeled trial
Child	"pawn."	Omission of /r/ in /pr/ cluster
Clinician	Pulls the stimulus toward her; records the response.	No corrective feedback
Clinician	[*stimulus: proud*] "The boy won first place. He feels very proud. Say, *proud*."	The next modeled trial
Child	"Proud."	Correct response
Clinician	Pulls the stimulus toward her; records the response.	No reinforcement

Use the recording sheet with exemplars shown on the next page to establish the baserates; print it from the CD.

/pr/ in Word-Initial Positions

Baserate Exemplars and Recording Sheet

Use stimuli from the **Stimulus Book,** *Volume 5.*

Print this page from the CD or photocopy this page for your clinical use.

Name/Age:	Date:
Goal: To establish the baserate production of /pr/ in word-initial positions.	Clinician:

Scoring: Correct: ✓   Incorrect or no response: X

/pr/ in word-initial positions	Evoked	Modeled
1. prawn		
2. proud		
3. prince		
4. print		
5. pretty		
6. prairie dog		
7. precipitate		
8. present		
9. propeller		
10. pretzel		
11. pressing		
12. prong		
13. prize		
14. prune		
15. pry		
16. professor		
17. president		
18. protractor		
19. primrose		
20. profile		
Percent correct baserate		

Replace or add new exemplars as you see fit for a given child. After establishing the baserates, begin production teaching. Follow the protocols given on the next page.

/pr/ in Word-Initial Positions

Treatment Protocols

Use stimuli from the **Stimulus Book, Volume 5**.

Teach 6 to 8 exemplars using the following script.

Place a relevant stimulus in front of the child (an object, a picture, or a printed word if the child can read) and ask a question as you point to the stimulus.

Scripts For Modeled Discrete Trial Training		Note
Clinician	[*stimulus: prawn*] "What is this? This is a **pr**awn. Say, **pr**awn."	Modeling; the target vocally emphasized
Child	"pwawn."	A wrong response
Clinician	"No. That's not correct. You said *pwawn*, but it's a **pr**awn. The **r** sound comes after the **p**."	Corrective feedback
Clinician	[*the same stimulus*] "What is this? Say, **pr**awn. Don't forget to say the **r** after the **p**."	The next trial
Child	"Prawn."	A correct response
Clinician	"Excellent! You didn't miss the **r** this time!"	Verbal praise

Repeat the trials until the child gives 5 consecutively correct, imitated responses.

When the child imitates 5 correct responses in sequence, fade the modeling.

Scripts For Fading the Modeling		Note
Clinician	[*stimulus: prawn*] "What is this? Don't forget to the say the *r* after the *p*."	Only a prompt
Child	"pwawn."	A wrong response
Clinician	"Uh oh, you forgot to say the *r* after the *p*! It's a *prawn*, not *pwawn*. The *r* sound, not *w*, comes after the *p*."	Corrective feedback
Clinician	[*the same stimulus*] "What is this? It starts with . . . " [*silently models the lip and tongue posture for the /pr/ cluster.*]	The next trial; a partial modeling
Child	"Prawn."	A correct response
Clinician	"That's great! You said *prawn*, not *pwawn*."	Verbal praise
Clinician	[*the same stimulus*] "What is this?"	Typical question; evoked trial
Child	"Prawn."	A correct response
Clinician	"That was magnificent! You are such a hard worker."	Verbal praise

If the wrong responses persist on 4 to 5 evoked trials, reinstate partial or full modeling for a few trials, again fade the modeling, and re-present the evoked trials.

When the child meets the tentative learning criterion of 10 consecutively correct, nonimitated responses for a given stimulus item, move on to the next stimulus item. With this procedure, teach 6 to 8 exemplars shown on the following recording sheet. Use different exemplars as you see fit for a given child.

/pr/ in Word-Initial Positions

Treatment Exemplars and Recording Sheet

Use stimuli from the **Stimulus Book, Volume 5**.

Print this page from CD or photocopy this page for your clinical use.

Name/Age:	Date:
Goal: Production of /pr/ in word-initial positions with 90% accuracy when asked an evoking question while showing a stimulus.	Clinician:

Scoring: Correct: ✓   Incorrect or no response: X

Target skills	Discrete Trials														
	1	2	3	4	5	6	7	8	9	10	11	12	13	14	15
1. prawn															
2. proud															
3. prince															
4. print															
5. pretty															
6. prairie dog															
7. precipitate															
8. present															

When the child has met the learning criterion of 10 consecutively correct evoked (nonimitated) responses for each of the 6 to 8 target exemplars, conduct a probe to see if the production has generalized to previously baserated but untrained exemplars.

If the probes do not meet the 90% correct criterion for untrained exemplars, teach additional exemplars and then probe again.

/pr/ in Word-Initial Positions

Probe Protocols and Recording Sheet

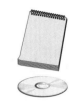

Use stimuli from the **Stimulus Book, Volume 5**.

Print this page from the CD or photocopy this page for your clinical use.

On the probes, present only the untrained exemplars (UT). When the child fails to meet the 90% correct probe criterion, either teach 2 to 4 new exemplars or give additional training trials on already trained stimuli. If needed, select new exemplars for probes. Probe at least 10 untrained exemplars. Alternate probes and treatment until the probe criterion is met.

Scripts for Probe Trials		Note
Clinician	[*untrained stimulus: propeller*] "What is this?"	No modeling or prompts
Child	"Propeller."	A correct, generalized response
Clinician	Scores the response as correct.	No reinforcement
Clinician	[*untrained stimulus: pretzel*] "What is this?"	The second probe trial
Child	"Pretzel."	A correct, generalized response
Clinician	Scores the response as correct.	No reinforcement

Name:	Date:	Session #:
Age:	**Clinician:**	
Diagnosis: Articulation/Phonologic Disorder	**Word-initial /pr/ probe**	
Untrained Stimuli	**Score: + correct; – incorrect or no responses**	
1. propeller		
2. pretzel		
3. pressing		
4. prong		
5. prize		
6. prune		
7. pry		
8. professor		
9. president		
10. protractor		
11. primrose		
12. profile		
Percent correct: (Criterion: 90%)		

If the child does not meet the probe criterion, give additional training on already trained exemplars or teach a few new exemplars. Subsequently, readminister the probe trials. When the child meets the 90% correct probe criterion for the exemplars, shift training to the sentence or conversational level or to another phoneme.

/tr/ in Word-Initial Positions

Baserate Protocols

Use stimuli from the **Stimulus Book, *Volume 5***.

At the beginning of each trial, place a relevant stimulus (an object, a picture, or a printed word if the child can read) in front of the child. Point to the stimulus as you ask an evoking question. Do not respond in any way to the child's correct, incorrect, or lack of responses.

Scripts For Evoked Baserate Trial		Note
Clinician	[*stimulus: tree*] "What is this?"	Evoked trial
Child	"Tee."	Omission of /r/ in the /tr/ cluster
Clinician	Pulls the stimulus toward her; records the response.	No corrective feedback
Clinician	[*stimulus: train*] "What is this?"	The next evoked trial
Child	"tane."	Omission of /r/ in the /tr/ cluster
Clinician	Pulls the stimulus toward her; records the response.	No corrective feedback

Administer the modeled baserate trials only after completing the evoked trials on all 20 (or more) exemplars.

Scripts For Modeled Baserate Trial		Note
Clinician	[*stimulus: tree*] "What is this? Say, *tree*."	Modeled trial
Child	"Tree."	Correct response
Clinician	Pulls the stimulus toward her; records the response.	No reinforcement
Clinician	[*stimulus: train*] "What is this? Say, *train*."	The next modeled trial
Child	"tane."	Omission of /r/ in /tr/ cluster
Clinician	Pulls the stimulus toward her; records the response.	No corrective feedback

Use the recording sheet with exemplars shown on the next page to establish the baserates; print it from the CD.

/tr/ in Word-Initial Positions

Baserate Exemplars and Recording Sheet

*Use stimuli from the **Stimulus Book**, **Volume 5**.*

Print this page from the CD or photocopy this page for your clinical use.

Name/Age:	Date:
Goal: To establish the baserate production of /tr/ in word-initial positions.	Clinician:

Scoring: Correct: ✓ Incorrect or no response: X

/tr/ in word-initial positions	Evoked	Modeled
1. tree		
2. train		
3. track		
4. trunk		
5. trail		
6. trumpet		
7. traffic light		
8. trophies		
9. trampoline		
10. triangle		
11. trap		
12. trout		
13. treat		
14. trash		
15. truck		
16. tricycle		
17. tripod		
18. trellis		
19. trapeze		
20. treadmill		
Percent correct baserate		

Replace or add new exemplars as you see fit for a given child. After establishing the baserates, begin production teaching. Follow the protocols given on the next page.

/tr/ in Word-Initial Positions

Treatment Protocols

Use stimuli from the **Stimulus Book,** *Volume 5.*

Teach 6 to 8 exemplars using the following script.

Place a relevant stimulus in front of the child (an object, a picture, or a printed word if the child can read) and ask a question as you point to the stimulus.

Scripts For Modeled Discrete Trial Training		Note
Clinician	[*stimulus: tree*] "What is this? Say, ***tree.***"	Modeling; the target vocally emphasized
Child	"tee."	A wrong response
Clinician	"No. That's not correct. You said *tee*, but it's a ***tree.***"	Corrective feedback
Clinician	[*the same stimulus*] "What is this? Say, ***tree***. You need to say an ***r*** after the ***t***."	The next trial
Child	"Tree."	A correct response
Clinician	"Excellent! You didn't forget the ***r*** this time!"	Verbal praise

Repeat the trials until the child gives 5 consecutively correct, imitated responses.

When the child imitates 5 correct responses in sequence, fade the modeling.

Scripts For Fading the Modeling		Note
Clinician	[*stimulus: tree*] "What is this? Don't forget to say the *r* after the *t*."	Only a prompt
Child	"tee."	A wrong response
Clinician	"Oops, you forgot the *r*! It's a *tree*, not *tee*. Remember that the *r* sound comes after the *t*."	Corrective feedback
Clinician	[*the same stimulus*] "What is this? It starts with . . . " [*silently models the tongue posture for the /tr/ cluster.*]	The next trial; a partial modeling
Child	"Tree."	A correct response
Clinician	"That's excellent! You said *tree*, not *tee*."	Verbal praise
Clinician	[*the same stimulus*] "What is this?"	Typical question; evoked trial
Child	"Tree."	A correct response
Clinician	"Great job! That was perfect!"	Verbal praise

If the wrong responses persist on 4 to 5 evoked trials, reinstate partial or full modeling for a few trials, again fade the modeling, and re-present the evoked trials.

When the child meets the tentative learning criterion of 10 consecutively correct, nonimitated responses for a given stimulus item, move on to the next stimulus item. With this procedure, teach 6 to 8 exemplars shown on the following recording sheet. Use different exemplars as you see fit for a given child.

/tr/ in Word-Initial Positions

Treatment Exemplars and Recording Sheet

Use stimuli from the **Stimulus Book, Volume 5**.

Print this page from CD or photocopy this page for your clinical use.

Name/Age:	Date:
Goal: Production of /tr/ in word-initial positions with 90% accuracy when asked an evoking question while showing a stimulus.	Clinician:

Scoring: Correct: ✓   Incorrect or no response: X

Target skills	Discrete Trials														
	1	2	3	4	5	6	7	8	9	10	11	12	13	14	15
1. tree															
2. train															
3. track															
4. trunk															
5. trail															
6. trumpet															
7. traffic light															
8. trophies															

When the child has met the learning criterion of 10 consecutively correct evoked (nonimitated) responses for each of the 6 to 8 target exemplars, conduct a probe to see if the production has generalized to previously baserated but untrained exemplars.

If the probes do not meet the 90% correct criterion for untrained exemplars, teach additional exemplars and then probe again.

/tr/ in Word-Initial Positions

Probe Protocols and Recording Sheet

Use stimuli from the **Stimulus Book,** *Volume 5.*

Print this page from the CD or photocopy this page for your clinical use.

On the probes, present only the untrained exemplars (UT). When the child fails to meet the 90% correct probe criterion, either teach 2 to 4 new exemplars or give additional training trials on already trained stimuli. If needed, select new exemplars for probes. Probe at least 10 untrained exemplars. Alternate probes and treatment until the probe criterion is met.

Scripts for Probe Trials		Note
Clinician	[*untrained stimulus: trampoline*] "What is this?"	No modeling or prompts
Child	"A tampoline."	A wrong probe response
Clinician	Scores the response as incorrect.	No corrective feedback
Clinician	[*untrained stimulus: triangle*] "What is this?"	The second probe trial
Child	"Triangle."	A correct, generalized response
Clinician	Scores the response as correct	No reinforcement

Name:	Date:	Session #:
Age:	**Clinician:**	
Diagnosis: Articulation/Phonologic Disorder	**Word-initial /tr/ probe**	
Untrained Stimuli	**Score: + correct; – incorrect or no responses**	
1. trampoline		
2. triangle		
3. trap		
4. trout		
5. treat		
6. trash		
7. truck		
8. tricycle		
9. tripod		
10. trellis		
11. trapeze		
12. treadmill		
Percent correct: (Criterion: 90%)		

If the child does not meet the probe criterion, give additional training on already trained exemplars or teach a few new exemplars. Subsequently, readminister the probe trials. When the child meets the 90% correct probe criterion for the exemplars, shift training to the sentence or conversational level or to another phoneme.

/sk/ in Word-Initial Positions
Baserate Protocols

Use stimuli from the **Stimulus Book,** *Volume 6.*

At the beginning of each trial, place a relevant stimulus (an object, a picture, or a printed word if the child can read) in front of the child. Point to the stimulus as you ask an evoking question. Do not respond in any way to the child's correct, incorrect, or lack of responses.

Scripts For Evoked Baserate Trial		Note
Clinician	[*stimulus: skunk*] "What is this?"	Evoked trial
Child	"A kunk."	Omission of /s/ in /sk/ cluster
Clinician	Pulls the stimulus toward her; records the response.	No corrective feedback
Clinician	[*stimulus: school*] "Where do children go to learn?"	The next evoked trial
Child	"To kool."	Omission of /s/ in /sk/ cluster
Clinician	Pulls the stimulus toward her; records the response.	No corrective feedback

Administer the modeled baserate trials only after completing the evoked trials on all 20 (or more) exemplars.

Scripts For Modeled Baserate Trial		Note
Clinician	[*stimulus: skunk*] "What is this? Say, *skunk.*"	Modeled trial
Child	"kunk."	Omission of /s/ in /sk/ cluster
Clinician	Pulls the stimulus toward her; records the response.	No corrective feedback
Clinician	[*stimulus: school*] "Where do children go to learn? Say, *school.*"	The next modeled trial
Child	"School."	Correct response
Clinician	Pulls the stimulus toward her; records the response.	No reinforcement

Use the recording sheet with exemplars shown on the next page to establish the baserates; print it from the CD.

/sk/ in Word-Initial Positions

Baserate Exemplars and Recording Sheet

Use stimuli from the **Stimulus Book**, *Volume 6*.

Print this page from the CD or photocopy this page for your clinical use.

Name/Age:	Date:
Goal: To establish the baserate production of /sk/ in word-initial positions.	Clinician:

Scoring: Correct: ✓   Incorrect or no response: X

/sk/ in word-initial positions	Evoked	Modeled
1. skunk		
2. school		
3. scoop		
4. sky		
5. scowl		
6. scorpion		
7. skillet		
8. skeleton		
9. scarecrow		
10. scooter		
11. skate		
12. skull		
13. skin		
14. skis		
15. scar		
16. school bus		
17. ski lift		
18. skateboard		
19. schooner		
20. skipper		
Percent correct baserate		

Replace or add new exemplars as you see fit for a given child. After establishing the baserates, begin production teaching. Follow the protocols given on the next page.

/sk/ in Word-Initial Positions

Treatment Protocols

Use stimuli from the **Stimulus Book, Volume 6.**

Teach 6 to 8 exemplars using the following script.

Place a relevant stimulus in front of the child (an object, a picture, or a printed word if the child can read) and ask a question as you point to the stimulus.

Scripts For Modeled Discrete Trial Training		Note
Clinician	[*stimulus: skunk*] "What is this? Say, **sk**unk."	Modeling; the target vocally emphasized
Child	"kunk."	A wrong response
Clinician	"No. That's not correct. You said *kunk*, but it's a **sk**unk. You need to say the **s** sound at the beginning."	Corrective feedback
Clinician	[*the same stimulus*] "What is this? Say, **sk**unk. Don't forget the **s** at the beginning."	The next trial
Child	"kunk."	A wrong response
Clinician	"Oops! You said *kunk* again. Remember to say the **s** sound at the beginning, **sk**unk."	Corrective feedback

Repeat the trials until the child gives 5 consecutively correct, imitated responses.

When the child imitates 5 correct responses in sequence, fade the modeling.

Scripts For Fading the Modeling		Note
Clinician	[*stimulus: skunk*] "What is this? Don't forget the *s* at the beginning. You need to say the *s* and the *k* together."	Only a prompt
Child	"kunk."	A wrong response
Clinician	"Uh, oh, you forgot the *s*! It's a *skunk*, not *kunk*. Put the *s* at the beginning."	Corrective feedback
Clinician	[*the same stimulus*] "What is this? It starts with . . ." [*silently models the articulatory posture for the /sk/ cluster.*]	The next trial; a partial modeling
Child	"Skunk."	A correct response
Clinician	"That's outstanding! You said *skunk*, not *kunk*."	Verbal praise
Clinician	[*the same stimulus*] "What is this?"	Typical question; evoked trial
Child	"Skunk."	A correct response
Clinician	"Great job! You said it correctly!"	Verbal praise

If the wrong responses persist on 4 to 5 evoked trials, reinstate partial or full modeling for a few trials, again fade the modeling, and re-present the evoked trials.

When the child meets the tentative learning criterion of 10 consecutively correct, nonimitated responses for a given stimulus item, move on to the next stimulus item. With this procedure, teach 6 to 8 exemplars shown on the following recording sheet. Use different exemplars as you see fit for a given child.

/sk/ in Word-Initial Positions

Treatment Exemplars and Recording Sheet

Use stimuli from the **Stimulus Book,** *Volume 6.*

Print this page from CD or photocopy this page for your clinical use.

Name/Age:	Date:
Goal: Production of /sk/ in word-initial positions with 90% accuracy when asked an evoking question while showing a stimulus.	Clinician:

Scoring: Correct: ✓   Incorrect or no response: X

Target skills	Discrete Trials														
	1	2	3	4	5	6	7	8	9	10	11	12	13	14	15
1. skunk															
2. school															
3. scoop															
4. sky															
5. scowl															
6. scorpion															
7. skillet															
8. skeleton															

When the child has met the learning criterion of 10 consecutively correct evoked (nonimitated) responses for each of the 6 to 8 target exemplars, conduct a probe to see if the production has generalized to previously baserated but untrained exemplars.

If the probes do not meet the 90% correct criterion for untrained exemplars, teach additional exemplars and then probe again.

/sk/ in Word-Initial Positions

Probe Protocols and Recording Sheet

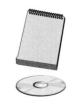

Use stimuli from the **Stimulus Book,** *Volume 6.*

Print this page from the CD or photocopy this page for your clinical use.

On the probes, present only the untrained exemplars (UT). When the child fails to meet the 90% correct probe criterion, either teach 2 to 4 new exemplars or give additional training trials on already trained stimuli. If needed, select new exemplars for probes. Probe at least 10 untrained exemplars. Alternate probes and treatment until the probe criterion is met.

Scripts for Probe Trials		Note
Clinician	[*untrained stimulus: scarecrow*] "What is this?"	No modeling or prompts
Child	"I don't know."	Lack of generalization
Clinician	Scores it as *no response.*	No corrective feedback
Clinician	[*untrained stimulus: scooter*] "What is this?"	The second probe trial
Child	"Scooter."	A correct, generalized response
Clinician	Scores the response as correct.	No reinforcement

Name:	Date:	Session #:
Age:	**Clinician:**	
Diagnosis: Articulation/Phonologic Disorder	**Word-initial /sk/ probe**	
Untrained Stimuli	**Score: + correct; – incorrect or no responses**	
1. scarecrow		
2. scooter		
3. skate		
4. skull		
5. skin		
6. skis		
7. scar		
8. school bus		
9. ski lift		
10. skateboard		
11. schooner		
12. skipper		
Percent correct: (Criterion: 90%)		

If the child does not meet the probe criterion, give additional training on already trained exemplars or teach a few new exemplars. Subsequently, readminister the probe trials. When the child meets the 90% correct probe criterion for the exemplars, shift training to the sentence or conversational level or to another phoneme.

/sn/ in Word-Initial Positions

Baserate Protocols

Use stimuli from the **Stimulus Book,** *Volume 6.*

At the beginning of each trial, place a relevant stimulus (an object, a picture, or a printed word if the child can read) in front of the child. Point to the stimulus as you ask an evoking question. Do not respond in any way to the child's correct, incorrect, or lack of responses.

Scripts For Evoked Baserate Trial		Note
Clinician	[*stimulus: snake*] "What is this?"	Evoked trial
Child	"nake."	Omission of /s/ in /sn/ cluster
Clinician	Pulls the stimulus toward her; records the response.	No corrective feedback
Clinician	[*stimulus: sneezing*] "What is the boy doing?"	The next evoked trial
Child	"neezing."	Omission of /s/ in /sn/ cluster
Clinician	Pulls the stimulus toward her; records the response.	No corrective feedback

Administer the modeled baserate trials only after completing the evoked trials on all 20 (or more) exemplars.

Scripts For Modeled Baserate Trial		Note
Clinician	[*stimulus: snake*] "What is this? Say, *snake.*"	Modeled trial
Child	"Snake."	Correct response
Clinician	Pulls the stimulus toward her; records the response.	No reinforcement
Clinician	[*stimulus: sneezing*] "What is the boy doing? Say, *sneezing.*"	The next modeled trial
Child	"neezing."	Omission of /s/ in /sn/ cluster
Clinician	Pulls the stimulus toward her; records the response.	No corrective feedback

Use the recording sheet with exemplars shown on the next page to establish the baserates; print it from the CD.

/sn/ in Word-Initial Positions

Baserate Exemplars and Recording Sheet

Use stimuli from the **Stimulus Book,** *Volume 6.*

Print this page from the CD or photocopy this page for your clinical use.

Name/Age:	Date:
Goal: To establish the baserate production of /sn/ in word-initial positions.	Clinician:

Scoring: Correct: ✓   Incorrect or no response: X

/sn/ in word-initial positions	Evoked	Modeled
1. snake		
2. sneezing		
3. snail		
4. snap		
5. snoozing		
6. sneakers		
7. snowball		
8. snowflake		
9. snapshot		
10. snap pea (bean)		
11. snow		
12. snack		
13. sniffing		
14. snout		
15. snipping		
16. snowshoe		
17. snowmobile		
18. snakebite		
19. snorkeling		
20. snowplow		
Percent correct baserate		

Replace or add new exemplars as you see fit for a given child. After establishing the baserates, begin production teaching. Follow the protocols given on the next page.

/sn/ in Word-Initial Positions

Treatment Protocols

Use stimuli from the **Stimulus Book,** *Volume 6.*

Teach 6 to 8 exemplars using the following script.

Place a relevant stimulus in front of the child (an object, a picture, or a printed word if the child can read) and ask a question as you point to the stimulus.

Scripts For Modeled Discrete Trial Training		Note
Clinician	[*stimulus: snake*] "What is this? Say, **sn**ake."	Modeling; the target vocally emphasized
Child	"nake."	A wrong response
Clinician	"Sorry. That's not correct. You said *nake*, but it's a **sn**ake. You left out the **s** at the beginning."	Corrective feedback
Clinician	[*the same stimulus*] "What is this? Say, **sn**ake. Don't forget the **s** at the beginning."	The next trial
Child	"Snake."	A correct response
Clinician	"Marvelous! You remembered to say the **s** at the beginning of the word!"	Verbal praise

Repeat the trials until the child gives 5 consecutively correct, imitated responses.

When the child imitates 5 correct responses in sequence, fade the modeling.

Scripts For Fading the Modeling		Note
Clinician	[*stimulus: snake*] "What is this? Don't forget the *s* at the beginning."	Only a prompt
Child	"nake."	A wrong response
Clinician	"Gee, you forgot the *s*! It's not a *nake*. It's a *snake*. Put the *s* at the beginning."	Corrective feedback
Clinician	[*the same stimulus*] "What is this? It starts with . . . " [*silently models the articulatory posture for the /sn/ cluster.*]	The next trial; a partial modeling
Child	"Snake."	A correct response
Clinician	"Wow! You said *snake*, not *nake*. Way to go!"	Verbal praise
Clinician	[*the same stimulus*] "What is this?"	Typical question; evoked trial
Child	"Snake."	A correct response
Clinician	"Great job! You said it perfectly that time!"	Verbal praise

If the wrong responses persist on 4 to 5 evoked trials, reinstate partial or full modeling for a few trials, again fade the modeling, and re-present the evoked trials.

When the child meets the tentative learning criterion of 10 consecutively correct, nonimitated responses for a given stimulus item, move on to the next stimulus item. With this procedure, teach 6 to 8 exemplars shown on the following recording sheet. Use different exemplars as you see fit for a given child.

/sn/ in Word-Initial Positions

Treatment Exemplars and Recording Sheet

Use stimuli from the **Stimulus Book,** *Volume 6.*

Print this page from CD or photocopy this page for your clinical use.

Name/Age:	Date:
Goal: Production of /sn/ in word-initial positions with 90% accuracy when asked an evoking question while showing a stimulus.	Clinician:

Scoring: Correct: ✓ Incorrect or no response: X

Target skills	Discrete Trials														
	1	2	3	4	5	6	7	8	9	10	11	12	13	14	15
1. snake															
2. sneezing															
3. snail															
4. snap															
5. snoozing															
6. sneakers															
7. snowball															
8. snowflake															

When the child has met the learning criterion of 10 consecutively correct evoked (nonimitated) responses for each of the 6 to 8 target exemplars, conduct a probe to see if the production has generalized to previously baserated but untrained exemplars.

If the probes do not meet the 90% correct criterion for untrained exemplars, teach additional exemplars and then probe again.

/sn/ in Word-Initial Positions

Probe Protocols and Recording Sheet

Use stimuli from the **Stimulus Book,** *Volume 6.*

Print this page from the CD or photocopy this page for your clinical use.

On the probes, present only the untrained exemplars (UT). When the child fails to meet the 90% correct probe criterion, either teach 2 to 4 new exemplars or give additional training trials on already trained stimuli. If needed, select new exemplars for probes. Probe at least 10 untrained exemplars. Alternate probes and treatment until the probe criterion is met.

Scripts for Probe Trials		Note
Clinician	[*untrained stimulus: snapshot*] "What is this?"	No modeling or prompts
Child	"I don't know."	Lack of generalization
Clinician	Scores the response as incorrect.	No corrective feedback
Clinician	[*untrained stimulus: snap pea*] "What is this?"	The second probe trial
Child	"Snap pea."	A correct response
Clinician	Scores the response as correct.	No reinforcement

Name:	Date:	Session #:
Age:	**Clinician:**	
Diagnosis: Articulation/Phonologic Disorder	**Word-initial /sn/ probe**	
Untrained Stimuli	**Score: + correct; – incorrect or no responses**	
1. snapshot		
2. snap pea (bean)		
3. snow		
4. snack		
5. sniffing		
6. snout		
7. snipping		
8. snowshoe		
9. snowmobile		
10. snakebite		
11. snorkeling		
12. snowplow		
Percent correct: (Criterion: 90%)		

If the child does not meet the probe criterion, give additional training on already trained exemplars or teach a few new exemplars. Subsequently, readminister the probe trials. When the child meets the 90% correct probe criterion for the exemplars, shift training to the sentence or conversational level or to another phoneme.

/sp/ in Word-Initial Positions

Baserate Protocols

Use stimuli from the **Stimulus Book,** *Volume 6.*

At the beginning of each trial, place a relevant stimulus (an object, a picture, or a printed word if the child can read) in front of the child. Point to the stimulus as you ask an evoking question. Do not respond in any way to the child's correct, incorrect, or lack of responses.

Scripts For Evoked Baserate Trial		Note
Clinician	[*stimulus: spider*] "What is this?"	Evoked trial
Child	"pider."	Omission of /s/ in /sp/ cluster
Clinician	Pulls the stimulus toward her; records the response.	No corrective feedback
Clinician	[*stimulus: spots*] "What are these?"	The next evoked trial
Child	"pots."	Omission of /s/ in /sp/ cluster
Clinician	Pulls the stimulus toward her; records the response.	No corrective feedback

Administer the modeled baserate trials only after completing the evoked trials on all 20 (or more) exemplars.

Scripts For Modeled Baserate Trial		Note
Clinician	[*stimulus: spider*] "What is this? Say, *spider.*"	Modeled trial
Child	"Spider."	Correct response
Clinician	Pulls the stimulus toward her; records the response.	No reinforcement
Clinician	[*stimulus: spots*] "What are these? Say, *spots.*"	The next modeled trial
Child	"pots."	Omission of /s/ in /sp/ cluster
Clinician	Pulls the stimulus toward her; records the response.	No corrective feedback

Use the recording sheet with exemplars shown on the next page to establish the baserates; print it from the CD.

/sp/ in Word-Initial Positions

Baserate Exemplars and Recording Sheet

Use stimuli from the **Stimulus Book,** *Volume 6.*

Print this page from the CD or photocopy this page for your clinical use.

Name/Age:	Date:
Goal: To establish the baserate production of /sp/ in word-initial positions.	Clinician:

Scoring: Correct: ✓   Incorrect or no response: X

/sp/ in word-initial positions	Evoked	Modeled
1. spider		
2. spots		
3. spokes		
4. spout		
5. spilled		
6. spaghetti		
7. spaceship		
8. spareribs		
9. spider web		
10. sparrow		
11. spoon		
12. spike		
13. spear		
14. spinning		
15. sponge		
16. spatula		
17. speedboat		
18. spoonful		
19. space suit		
20. spinach		
Percent correct baserate		

Replace or add new exemplars as you see fit for a given child. After establishing the baserates, begin production teaching. Follow the protocols given on the next page.

/sp/ in Word-Initial Positions
Treatment Protocols

Use stimuli from the **Stimulus Book,** *Volume 6.*

Teach 6 to 8 exemplars using the following script.

Place a relevant stimulus in front of the child (an object, a picture, or a printed word if the child can read) and ask a question as you point to the stimulus.

Scripts For Modeled Discrete Trial Training		Note
Clinician	[*stimulus: spider*] "What is this? Say, **sp***ider.*"	Modeling; the target vocally emphasized
Child	"pider."	A wrong response
Clinician	"No. That's not correct. You said *pider*, but it's a **sp***ider.* You need to say the **s** sound at the beginning."	Corrective feedback
Clinician	[*the same stimulus*] "What is this? Say, *spider.* Don't forget the **s** at the beginning."	The next trial
Child	"Spider."	A correct response
Clinician	"Excellent! You didn't miss the *s* this time!"	Verbal praise

Repeat the trials until the child gives 5 consecutively correct, imitated responses.

When the child imitates 5 correct responses in sequence, fade the modeling.

Scripts For Fading the Modeling		Note
Clinician	[*stimulus: spider*] "What is this? Don't forget the *s* at the beginning."	Only a prompt
Child	"pider."	A wrong response
Clinician	"Gee, you forgot the *s*! It's a *spider*, not *pider*. Put the *s* at the beginning."	Corrective feedback
Clinician	[*the same stimulus*] "What is this? It starts with . . . " [*silently models the lip posture for the /sp/ cluster.*]	The next trial; a partial modeling
Child	"Spider."	A correct response
Clinician	"That's great! You said *spider*, not *pider*."	Verbal praise
Clinician	[*the same stimulus*] "What is this?"	Typical question; evoked trial
Child	"Spider."	A correct response
Clinician	"Great job! You said it correctly!"	Verbal praise

If the wrong responses persist on 4 to 5 evoked trials, reinstate partial or full modeling for a few trials, again fade the modeling, and re-present the evoked trials.

When the child meets the tentative learning criterion of 10 consecutively correct, nonimitated responses for a given stimulus item, move on to the next stimulus item. With this procedure, teach 6 to 8 exemplars shown on the following recording sheet. Use different exemplars as you see fit for a given child.

/sp/ in Word-Initial Positions

Treatment Exemplars and Recording Sheet

Use stimuli from the **Stimulus Book,** *Volume 6.*

Print this page from CD or photocopy this page for your clinical use.

Name/Age:	Date:
Goal: Production of /sp/ in word-initial positions with 90% accuracy when asked an evoking question while showing a stimulus.	Clinician:

Scoring: Correct: ✓   Incorrect or no response: X

Target skills	Discrete Trials														
	1	2	3	4	5	6	7	8	9	10	11	12	13	14	15
1. spider															
2. spots															
3. spokes															
4. spout															
5. spilled															
6. spaghetti															
7. spaceship															
8. spareribs															

When the child has met the learning criterion of 10 consecutively correct evoked (nonimitated) responses for each of the 6 to 8 target exemplars, conduct a probe to see if the production has generalized to previously baserated but untrained exemplars.

If the probes do not meet the 90% correct criterion for untrained exemplars, teach additional exemplars and then probe again.

/sp/ in Word-Initial Positions

Probe Protocols and Recording Sheet

*Use stimuli from the **Stimulus Book, Volume 6**.*

Print this page from the CD or photocopy this page for your clinical use.

On the probes, present only the untrained exemplars (UT). When the child fails to meet the 90% correct probe criterion, either teach 2 to 4 new exemplars or give additional training trials on already trained stimuli. If needed, select new exemplars for probes. Probe at least 10 untrained exemplars. Alternate probes and treatment until the probe criterion is met.

Scripts for Probe Trials		Note
Clinician	[*untrained stimulus: spider web*] "What is this?"	No modeling or prompts
Child	"Spider web."	A correct, generalized response
Clinician	Scores the response as correct.	No reinforcement
Clinician	[*untrained stimulus: sparrow*] "What is this?"	The second probe trial
Child	"Sparrow."	A correct, generalized response
Clinician	Scores the response as correct.	No reinforcement

Name:	Date:	Session #:
Age:	**Clinician:**	
Diagnosis: Articulation/Phonologic Disorder	**Word-initial /sp/ probe**	
Untrained Stimuli	**Score: + correct; – incorrect or no responses**	
1. spider web		
2. sparrow		
3. spoon		
4. spike		
5. spear		
6. spinning		
7. sponge		
8. spatula		
9. speedboat		
10. spoonful		
11. space suit		
12. spinach		
Percent correct: (Criterion: 90%)		

If the child does not meet the probe criterion, give additional training on already trained exemplars or teach a few new exemplars. Subsequently, readminister the probe trials. When the child meets the 90% correct probe criterion for the exemplars, shift training to the sentence or conversational level or to another phoneme.

/st/ in Word-Initial Positions

Baserate Protocols

Use stimuli from the **Stimulus Book, Volume 6**.

At the beginning of each trial, place a relevant stimulus (an object, a picture, or a printed word if the child can read) in front of the child. Point to the stimulus as you ask an evoking question. Do not respond in any way to the child's correct, incorrect, or lack of responses.

Scripts For Evoked Baserate Trial		Note
Clinician	[*stimulus: star*] "What is this?"	Evoked trial
Child	"tar."	Omission of /s/ in /st/ cluster
Clinician	Pulls the stimulus toward her; records the response.	No corrective feedback
Clinician	[*stimulus: stick*] "What is this?"	The next evoked trial
Child	"tick."	Omission of /s/ in /st/ cluster
Clinician	Pulls the stimulus toward her; records the response.	No corrective feedback

Administer the modeled baserate trials only after completing the evoked trials on all 20 (or more) exemplars.

Scripts For Modeled Baserate Trial		Note
Clinician	[*stimulus: star*] "What is this? Say, *star.*"	Modeled trial
Child	"tar."	Omission of /s/ in /st/ cluster
Clinician	Pulls the stimulus toward her; records the response.	No corrective feedback
Clinician	[*stimulus: stick*] "What is this? Say, *stick.*"	The next modeled trial
Child	"tick."	Omission of /s/ in /st/ cluster
Clinician	Pulls the stimulus toward her; records the response.	No corrective feedback

Use the recording sheet with exemplars shown on the next page to establish the baserates; print it from the CD.

/st/ in Word-Initial Positions

Baserate Exemplars and Recording Sheet

*Use stimuli from the **Stimulus Book, Volume 6**.*

Print this page from the CD or photocopy this page for your clinical use.

Name/Age:	Date:
Goal: To establish the baserate production of /st/ in word-initial positions.	Clinician:

Scoring: Correct: ✓   Incorrect or no response: X

/st/ in word-initial positions	Evoked	Modeled
1. star		
2. stick		
3. stop		
4. steak		
5. stairs		
6. stadium		
7. starfish		
8. stomach		
9. staircase		
10. stapler		
11. stem		
12. stone		
13. stork		
14. stool		
15. stamp		
16. stagecoach		
17. stoplight		
18. statue		
19. steamboat		
20. stethoscope		
Percent correct baserate		

Replace or add new exemplars as you see fit for a given child. After establishing the baserates, begin production teaching. Follow the protocols given on the next page.

/st/ in Word-Initial Positions

Treatment Protocols

Use stimuli from the **Stimulus Book,** *Volume 6.*

Teach 6 to 8 exemplars using the following script.

Place a relevant stimulus in front of the child (an object, a picture, or a printed word if the child can read) and ask a question as you point to the stimulus.

Scripts For Modeled Discrete Trial Training		Note
Clinician	[*stimulus: star*] "What is this? Say, **st**ar."	Modeling; the target vocally emphasized
Child	"tar."	A wrong response
Clinician	"No. That's not correct. You said *tar*, but it's a **st**ar. You need to say the **s** sound at the beginning of the word, **st**ar."	Corrective feedback
Clinician	[*the same stimulus*] "What is this? Say, **st**ar. Remember that you need to say the **s** sound at the beginning."	The next trial
Child	"Star."	A correct response
Clinician	"Magnificent! You remembered the **s** sound at the beginning of the word **st**ar!"	Verbal praise

Repeat the trials until the child gives 5 consecutively correct, imitated responses.

When the child imitates 5 correct responses in sequence, fade the modeling.

Scripts For Fading the Modeling		Note
Clinician	[*stimulus: star*] "What is this? Don't forget the *s* at the beginning."	Only a prompt
Child	"tar."	A wrong response
Clinician	"Oops, you forgot the *s* at the beginning! It's a s*tar*, not *tar*. Remember to say the *s* at the beginning."	Corrective feedback
Clinician	[*the same stimulus*] "What is this? It starts with . . . " [*silently models the lip and tongue posture for the /st/ cluster.*]	The next trial; a partial modeling
Child	"Star."	A correct response
Clinician	"That's perfect! You said *star*, not *tar*."	Verbal praise
Clinician	[*the same stimulus*] "What is this?"	Typical question; evoked trial
Child	"Star."	A correct response
Clinician	"You said it correctly. You are doing fantastic!"	Verbal praise

If the wrong responses persist on 4 to 5 evoked trials, reinstate partial or full modeling for a few trials, again fade the modeling, and re-present the evoked trials.

When the child meets the tentative learning criterion of 10 consecutively correct, nonimitated responses for a given stimulus item, move on to the next stimulus item. With this procedure, teach 6 to 8 exemplars shown on the following recording sheet. Use different exemplars as you see fit for a given child.

/st/ in Word-Initial Positions

Treatment Exemplars and Recording Sheet

Use stimuli from the **Stimulus Book,** *Volume 6.*

Print this page from CD or photocopy this page for your clinical use.

Name/Age:	Date:
Goal: Production of /st/ in word-initial positions with 90% accuracy when asked an evoking question while showing a stimulus.	Clinician:

Scoring: Correct: ✓   Incorrect or no response: X

Target skills	Discrete Trials														
	1	2	3	4	5	6	7	8	9	10	11	12	13	14	15
1. star															
2. stick															
3. stop															
4. steak															
5. stairs															
6. stadium															
7. starfish															
8. stomach															

When the child has met the learning criterion of 10 consecutively correct evoked (nonimitated) responses for each of the 6 to 8 target exemplars, conduct a probe to see if the production has generalized to previously baserated but untrained exemplars.

If the probes do not meet the 90% correct criterion for untrained exemplars, teach additional exemplars and then probe again.

/st/ in Word-Initial Positions

Probe Protocols and Recording Sheet

Use stimuli from the **Stimulus Book**, *Volume 6*.

Print this page from the CD or photocopy this page for your clinical use.

On the probes, present only the untrained exemplars (UT). When the child fails to meet the 90% correct probe criterion, either teach 2 to 4 new exemplars or give additional training trials on already trained stimuli. If needed, select new exemplars for probes. Probe at least 10 untrained exemplars. Alternate probes and treatment until the probe criterion is met.

Scripts for Probe Trials		Note
Clinician	[*untrained stimulus: staircase*] "What is this?"	No modeling or prompts
Child	"Staircase."	A correct, generalized response
Clinician	Scores the response as correct.	No reinforcement
Clinician	[*untrained stimulus: stapler*] "What is this?"	The second probe trial
Child	"Stapler."	A correct, generalized response
Clinician	Scores the response as correct.	No reinforcement

Name:	Date:	Session #:
Age:	**Clinician:**	
Diagnosis: Articulation/Phonologic Disorder	**Word-initial /st/ probe**	
Untrained Stimuli	**Score: + correct; – incorrect or no responses**	
1. staircase		
2. stapler		
3. stem		
4. stone		
5. stork		
6. stool		
7. stamp		
8. stagecoach		
9. stoplight		
10. statue		
11. steamboat		
12. stethoscope		
Percent correct: (Criterion: 90%)		

If the child does not meet the probe criterion, give additional training on already trained exemplars or teach a few new exemplars. Subsequently, readminister the probe trials. When the child meets the 90% correct probe criterion for the exemplars, shift training to the sentence or conversational level or to another phoneme.

/sw/ in Word-Initial Positions

Baserate Protocols

Use stimuli from the **Stimulus Book**, *Volume 6.*

At the beginning of each trial, place a relevant stimulus (an object, a picture, or a printed word if the child can read) in front of the child. Point to the stimulus as you ask an evoking question. Do not respond in any way to the child's correct, incorrect, or lack of responses.

Scripts For Evoked Baserate Trial		Note
Clinician	[*stimulus: swing*] "What is this?"	Evoked trial
Child	"A wing."	Omission of /s/ in /sw/ cluster
Clinician	Pulls the stimulus toward her; records the response.	No corrective feedback
Clinician	[*stimulus: swan*] "What is this?"	The next evoked trial
Child	"wan."	Omission of /s/ in /sw/ cluster
Clinician	Pulls the stimulus toward her; records the response.	No corrective feedback

Administer the modeled baserate trials only after completing the evoked trials on all 20 (or more) exemplars.

Scripts For Modeled Baserate Trial		Note
Clinician	[*stimulus: swing*] "What is this? Say, *swing.*"	Modeled trial
Child	"wing."	Omission of /s/ in /sw/ cluster
Clinician	Pulls the stimulus toward her; records the response.	No corrective feedback
Clinician	[*stimulus: swan*] "What is this? Say, *swan.*"	The next modeled trial
Child	"wan."	Omission of /s/ in /sw/ cluster
Clinician	Pulls the stimulus toward her; records the response.	No corrective feedback

Use the recording sheet with exemplars shown on the next page to establish the baserates; print it from the CD.

/sw/ in Word-Initial Positions

Baserate Exemplars and Recording Sheet

Use stimuli from the **Stimulus Book,** *Volume 6.*

Print this page from the CD or photocopy this page for your clinical use.

Name/Age:	Date:
Goal: To establish the baserate production of /sw/ in word-initial positions.	Clinician:

Scoring: Correct: ✓ Incorrect or no response: X

/sw/ in word-initial positions	Evoked	Modeled
1. swing		
2. swan		
3. swim		
4. swab		
5. sweeping		
6. swallow		
7. sweater		
8. sweet pea		
9. sweating		
10. sweet potato		
11. swollen		
12. swatting		
13. swine		
14. swamp		
15. swarm		
16. swimsuit		
17. sweat shirt		
18. swim mask		
19. swaddle		
20. Swiss cheese		
Percent correct baserate		

Replace or add new exemplars as you see fit for a given child. After establishing the baserates, begin production teaching. Follow the protocols given on the next page.

/sw/ in Word-Initial Positions

Treatment Protocols

Use stimuli from the **Stimulus Book,** *Volume 6.*

Teach 6 to 8 exemplars using the following script.

Place a relevant stimulus in front of the child (an object, a picture, or a printed word if the child can read) and ask a question as you point to the stimulus.

Scripts For Modeled Discrete Trial Training		Note
Clinician	[*stimulus: swing*] "What is this? Say, **sw***ing.*"	Modeling; the target vocally emphasized
Child	"wing."	A wrong response
Clinician	"No. That's not right. You said *wing*, but it's a **sw***ing.* You need to say an **s** sound in front of the *w* sound."	Corrective feedback
Clinician	[*the same stimulus*] "What is this? Say, **sw***ing.* Don't forget to say an **s** sound before the **w**."	The next trial
Child	"Swing."	A correct response
Clinician	"Fantastic! You said the **s** sound at the very beginning!"	Verbal praise

Repeat the trials until the child gives 5 consecutively correct, imitated responses.

When the child imitates 5 correct responses in sequence, fade the modeling.

Scripts For Fading the Modeling		Note
Clinician	[*stimulus: swing*] "What is this? Don't forget the *s* at the very beginning."	Only a prompt
Child	"wing."	A wrong response
Clinician	"Oh no, you forgot the *s*! It's a *swing*, not *wing*. Say the *s* sound before the *w* sound."	Corrective feedback
Clinician	[*the same stimulus*] "What is this? It starts with . . . " [*silently models the articulatory posture for the /sw/ cluster.*]	The next trial; a partial modeling
Child	"Swing."	A correct response
Clinician	"That's great! You said *swing*, not *wing*."	Verbal praise
Clinician	[*the same stimulus*] "What is this?"	Typical question; evoked trial
Child	"Swing."	A correct response
Clinician	"Great job! You said it correctly!"	Verbal praise

If the wrong responses persist on 4 to 5 evoked trials, reinstate partial or full modeling for a few trials, again fade the modeling, and re-present the evoked trials.

When the child meets the tentative learning criterion of 10 consecutively correct, nonimitated responses for a given stimulus item, move on to the next stimulus item. With this procedure, teach 6 to 8 exemplars shown on the following recording sheet. Use different exemplars as you see fit for a given child.

/sw/ in Word-Initial Positions

Treatment Exemplars and Recording Sheet

Use stimuli from the **Stimulus Book,** *Volume 6.*

Print this page from CD or photocopy this page for your clinical use.

Name/Age:	Date:
Goal: Production of /sw/ in word-initial positions with 90% accuracy when asked an evoking question while showing a stimulus.	Clinician:

Scoring: Correct: ✓   Incorrect or no response: X

Target skills	Discrete Trials														
	1	2	3	4	5	6	7	8	9	10	11	12	13	14	15
1. swing															
2. swan															
3. swim															
4. swab															
5. sweeping															
6. swallow															
7. sweater															
8. sweet pea															

When the child has met the learning criterion of 10 consecutively correct evoked (nonimitated) responses for each of the 6 to 8 target exemplars, conduct a probe to see if the production has generalized to previously baserated but untrained exemplars.

If the probes do not meet the 90% correct criterion for untrained exemplars, teach additional exemplars and then probe again.

/sw/ in Word-Initial Positions

Probe Protocols and Recording Sheet

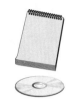

Use stimuli from the **Stimulus Book,** ***Volume 6.***

Print this page from the CD or photocopy this page for your clinical use.

On the probes, present only the untrained exemplars (UT). When the child fails to meet the 90% correct probe criterion, either teach 2 to 4 new exemplars or give additional training trials on already trained stimuli. If needed, select new exemplars for probes. Probe at least 10 untrained exemplars. Alternate probes and treatment until the probe criterion is met.

Scripts for Probe Trials		**Note**
Clinician	[*untrained stimulus: sweating*] "The man is very hot. He is _____?"	No modeling or prompts
Child	"Sweating."	A correct, generalized response
Clinician	Scores the response as correct.	No reinforcement
Clinician	[*untrained stimulus: sweet potato*] "What is this?"	The second probe trial
Child	"No response."	Lack of generalization
Clinician	Scores it as *no response.*	No corrective feedback

Name:	**Date:**	**Session #:**
Age:	**Clinician:**	
Diagnosis: Articulation/Phonologic Disorder	**Word-initial /sw/ probe**	
Untrained Stimuli	**Score: + correct; – incorrect or no responses**	
1. sweating		
2. sweet potato		
3. swollen		
4. swatting		
5. swine		
6. swamp		
7. swarm		
8. swimsuit		
9. sweat shirt		
10. swim mask		
11. swaddle		
12. Swiss cheese		
Percent correct: (Criterion: 90%)		

If the child does not meet the probe criterion, give additional training on already trained exemplars or teach a few new exemplars. Subsequently, readminister the probe trials. When the child meets the 90% correct probe criterion for the exemplars, shift training to the sentence or conversational level or to another phoneme.

/spr/ in Word-Initial Positions

Baserate Protocols

Use stimuli from the **Stimulus Book,** *Volume 6.*

At the beginning of each trial, place a relevant stimulus (an object, a picture, or a printed word if the child can read) in front of the child. Point to the stimulus as you ask an evoking question. Do not respond in any way to the child's correct, incorrect, or lack of responses.

Scripts For Evoked Baserate Trial		Note
Clinician	[*stimulus: spring*] "What season comes after winter?"	Evoked trial
Child	"sping."	Omission of /r/ in /spr/ cluster
Clinician	Pulls the stimulus toward her; records the response.	No corrective feedback
Clinician	[*stimulus: sprig*] "What is this?"	The next evoked trial
Child	"I don't know."	Does not know word
Clinician	Pulls the stimulus toward her; records the response. Notes that child does not know word.	No corrective feedback

Administer the modeled baserate trials only after completing the evoked trials on all 20 (or more) exemplars.

Scripts For Modeled Baserate Trial		Note
Clinician	[*stimulus: spring*] "What season comes after winter? Say, *spring.*"	Modeled trial
Child	"sping."	Omission of /r/ in /spr/ cluster
Clinician	Pulls the stimulus toward her; records the response.	No corrective feedback
Clinician	[*stimulus: sprig*] "What is this? Say, *sprig.*"	The next modeled trial
Child	"spig."	Omission of initial /r/ in /spr/ cluster
Clinician	Pulls the stimulus toward her; records the response.	No corrective feedback

Use the recording sheet with exemplars shown on the next page to establish the baserates; print it from the CD.

/spr/ in Word-Initial Positions

Baserate Exemplars and Recording Sheet

Use stimuli from the **Stimulus Book,** *Volume 6.*

Print this page from the CD or photocopy this page for your clinical use.

Name/Age:	Date:
Goal: To establish the baserate production of /spr/ in word-initial positions.	Clinician:

Scoring: Correct: ✓   Incorrect or no response: X

/spr/ in word-initial positions	Evoked	Modeled
1. spring		
2. sprig		
3. spraying		
4. sprain		
5. sprouting		
6. Springfield		
7. springboard		
8. springtime		
9. sprinkling		
10. spray gun		
11. sprawl		
12. spreading		
13. sprinkle		
14. spree		
15. sprint		
16. spring fever		
17. sprinkler		
18. sprocket		
19. spreadsheet		
20. spreader		
Percent correct baserate		

Replace or add new exemplars as you see fit for a given child. After establishing the baserates, begin production teaching. Follow the protocols given on the next page.

/spr/ in Word-Initial Positions

Treatment Protocols

Use stimuli from the **Stimulus Book,** *Volume 6.*

Teach 6 to 8 exemplars using the following script.

Place a relevant stimulus in front of the child (an object, a picture, or a printed word if the child can read) and ask a question as you point to the stimulus.

Scripts For Modeled Discrete Trial Training		Note
Clinician	[*stimulus: spring*] "What season comes after winter? Say, **spring.**"	Modeling; the target vocally emphasized
Child	"sping."	A wrong response
Clinician	"No. That's not correct. You said *sping*, but it's **spring.** You need to say the *r* sound after the *s* and the *p* sounds. You need to say all three sounds together. "	Corrective feedback
Clinician	[*the same stimulus*] "What season comes after winter? Say, **spring.** Don't forget the *r* sound after the *s* and the *p* sounds."	The next trial
Child	"Spring."	A correct response
Clinician	"Excellent! You didn't miss the *r* this time!"	Verbal praise

Repeat the trials until the child gives 5 consecutively correct, imitated responses.

When the child imitates 5 correct responses in sequence, fade the modeling.

Scripts For Fading the Modeling		Note
Clinician	[*stimulus: spring*] "What season comes after winter? Don't forget the *r* sound after the *s* and the *p* sounds."	Only a prompt
Child	"sping."	A wrong response
Clinician	"Uh, oh, you forgot the *r* in *spring*! It's *spring*, not *sping*. Remember to say the *r*.	Corrective feedback
Clinician	[*the same stimulus*] "What is this? It starts with . . . " [*silently models the articulatory posture for the /spr/ cluster.*]	The next trial; a partial modeling
Child	"Spring."	A correct response
Clinician	"That's great! You said *spring*, not *sping*."	Verbal praise
Clinician	[*the same stimulus*] "What is this?"	Typical question; evoked trial
Child	"Spring."	A correct response
Clinician	"That was fantastic! You said it correctly!"	Verbal praise

If the wrong responses persist on 4 to 5 evoked trials, reinstate partial or full modeling for a few trials, again fade the modeling, and re-present the evoked trials.

When the child meets the tentative learning criterion of 10 consecutively correct, nonimitated responses for a given stimulus item, move on to the next stimulus item. With this procedure, teach 6 to 8 exemplars shown on the following recording sheet. Use different exemplars as you see fit for a given child.

/spr/ in Word-Initial Positions

Treatment Exemplars and Recording Sheet

Use stimuli from the **Stimulus Book,** *Volume 6.*

Print this page from CD or photocopy this page for your clinical use.

Name/Age:	Date:
Goal: Production of /spr/ in word-initial positions with 90% accuracy when asked an evoking question while showing a stimulus.	Clinician:

Scoring: Correct: ✓   Incorrect or no response: X

Target skills	Discrete Trials														
	1	2	3	4	5	6	7	8	9	10	11	12	13	14	15
1. spring															
2. sprig															
3. spraying															
4. sprain															
5. sprouting															
6. Springfield															
7. springboard															
8. springtime															

When the child has met the learning criterion of 10 consecutively correct evoked (nonimitated) responses for each of the 6 to 8 target exemplars, conduct a probe to see if the production has generalized to previously baserated but untrained exemplars.

If the probes do not meet the 90% correct criterion for untrained exemplars, teach additional exemplars and then probe again.

/spr/ in Word-Initial Positions

Probe Protocols and Recording Sheet

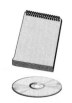

*Use stimuli from the **Stimulus Book, Volume 6.***

Print this page from the CD or photocopy this page for your clinical use.

On the probes, present only the untrained exemplars (UT). When the child fails to meet the 90% correct probe criterion, either teach 2 to 4 new exemplars or give additional training trials on already trained stimuli. If needed, select new exemplars for probes. Probe at least 10 untrained exemplars. Alternate probes and treatment until the probe criterion is met.

Scripts for Probe Trials		Note
Clinician	[*untrained stimulus: sprinkler*] "What is this?"	No modeling or prompts
Child	"Sprinkler."	A correct, generalized response
Clinician	Scores the response as correct.	No reinforcement
Clinician	[*untrained stimulus: spray gun*] "What is this?"	The second probe trial
Child	"spay gun."	A wrong probe response
Clinician	Scores the response as incorrect.	No corrective feedback

Name:	Date:	Session #:
Age:	**Clinician:**	
Diagnosis: Articulation/Phonologic Disorder	**Word-initial /spr/ probe**	
Untrained Stimuli	**Score: + correct; – incorrect or no responses**	
1. sprinkling		
2. spray gun		
3. sprawl		
4. spreading		
5. sprinkle		
6. spree		
7. sprint		
8. spring fever		
9. sprinkler		
10. sprocket		
11. spreadsheet		
12. spreader		
Percent correct: (Criterion: 90%)		

If the child does not meet the probe criterion, give additional training on already trained exemplars or teach a few new exemplars. Subsequently, readminister the probe trials. When the child meets the 90% correct probe criterion for the exemplars, shift training to the sentence or conversational level or to another phoneme.

/str/ in Word-Initial Positions

Baserate Protocols

Use stimuli from the **Stimulus Book,** *Volume 6*.

At the beginning of each trial, place a relevant stimulus (an object, a picture, or a printed word if the child can read) in front of the child. Point to the stimulus as you ask an evoking question. Do not respond in any way to the child's correct, incorrect, or lack of responses.

Scripts For Evoked Baserate Trial		Note
Clinician	[*stimulus: straw*] "What is this?"	Evoked trial
Child	"A traw."	Omission of /s/ in /str/ cluster
Clinician	Pulls the stimulus toward her; records the response.	No corrective feedback
Clinician	[*stimulus: stream*] "What is this?"	The next evoked trial
Child	No response.	
Clinician	Pulls the stimulus toward her; records the response.	No corrective feedback

Administer the modeled baserate trials only after completing the evoked trials on all 20 (or more) exemplars.

Scripts For Modeled Baserate Trial		Note
Clinician	[*stimulus: straw*] "What is this? Say, *straw*."	Modeled trial
Child	"Straw."	Correct response
Clinician	Pulls the stimulus toward her; records the response.	No reinforcement
Clinician	[*stimulus: stream*] "What is this? Say, *stream*."	The next modeled trial
Child	"tream."	Omission of /s/ in /str/ cluster
Clinician	Pulls the stimulus toward her; records	No corrective feedback

Use the recording sheet with exemplars shown on the next page to establish the baserates; print it from the CD.

/str/ in Word-Initial Positions

Baserate Exemplars and Recording Sheet

Use stimuli from the **Stimulus Book,** *Volume 6.*

Print this page from the CD or photocopy this page for your clinical use.

Name/Age:	Date:
Goal: To establish the baserate production of /str/ in word-initial positions.	Clinician:

Scoring: Correct: ✓   Incorrect or no response: X

/str/ in word-initial positions	Evoked	Modeled
1. straw		
2. stream		
3. straight		
4. string		
5. strip	˙	
6. strawberry		
7. stretching		
8. straggler		
9. stroller		
10. straightedge		
11. strong		
12. stripes		
13. striking		
14. street		
15. strap		
16. stranger		
17. strapless		
18. streamer		
19. streetcar		
20. string beans		
Percent correct baserate		

Replace or add new exemplars as you see fit for a given child. After establishing the baserates, begin production teaching. Follow the protocols given on the next page.

/str/ in Word-Initial Positions

Treatment Protocols

Use stimuli from the **Stimulus Book,** *Volume 6.*

Teach 6 to 8 exemplars using the following script.

Place a relevant stimulus in front of the child (an object, a picture, or a printed word if the child can read) and ask a question as you point to the stimulus.

Scripts For Modeled Discrete Trial Training		Note
Clinician	[*stimulus: straw*] "What is this? Say, **straw**."	Modeling; the target vocally emphasized
Child	"traw."	A wrong response
Clinician	"No. That's not correct. You said *traw*, but it's a **straw**."	Corrective feedback
Clinician	[*the same stimulus*] "What is this? Say, **straw**. You need to say the **s** sound at the very beginning, **straw**."	The next trial
Child	"Straw."	A correct response
Clinician	"Stupendous! You didn't leave out the **s** at the beginning of the word *straw*."	Verbal praise

Repeat the trials until the child gives 5 consecutively correct, imitated responses.

When the child imitates 5 correct responses in sequence, fade the modeling.

Scripts For Fading the Modeling		Note
Clinician	[*stimulus: straw*] "What is this? Don't forget the *s* at the beginning."	Only a prompt
Child	"traw."	A wrong response
Clinician	"Oh, no, you forgot the *s* at the beginning of the word! It's a *straw*, not *traw*. Remember to say the *s* sound at the beginning."	Corrective feedback
Clinician	[*the same stimulus*] "What is this? It starts with . . . " [*silently models the articulatory posture for the /str/ cluster.*]	The next trial; a partial modeling
Child	"Straw."	A correct response
Clinician	"That's fantastic! You said *straw*, not *traw*."	Verbal praise
Clinician	[*the same stimulus*] "What is this?"	Typical question; evoked trial
Child	"Straw."	A correct response
Clinician	"Wow! You said it correctly! You are working very hard. Keep up the good work."	Verbal praise

If the wrong responses persist on 4 to 5 evoked trials, reinstate partial or full modeling for a few trials, again fade the modeling, and re-present the evoked trials.

When the child meets the tentative learning criterion of 10 consecutively correct, nonimitated responses for a given stimulus item, move on to the next stimulus item. With this procedure, teach 6 to 8 exemplars shown on the following recording sheet. Use different exemplars as you see fit for a given child.

/str/ in Word-Initial Positions

Treatment Exemplars and Recording Sheet

Use stimuli from the **Stimulus Book, Volume 6.**

Print this page from CD or photocopy this page for your clinical use.

Name/Age:	Date:
Goal: Production of /str/ in word-initial positions with 90% accuracy when asked an evoking question while showing a stimulus.	Clinician:

Scoring: Correct: ✓   Incorrect or no response: X

Target skills	Discrete Trials														
	1	2	3	4	5	6	7	8	9	10	11	12	13	14	15
1. straw															
2. stream															
3. straight															
4. string															
5. strip															
6. strawberry															
7. stretching															
8. straggler															

When the child has met the learning criterion of 10 consecutively correct evoked (nonimitated) responses for each of the 6 to 8 target exemplars, conduct a probe to see if the production has generalized to previously baserated but untrained exemplars.

If the probes do not meet the 90% correct criterion for untrained exemplars, teach additional exemplars and then probe again.

/str/ in Word-Initial Positions

Probe Protocols and Recording Sheet

Use stimuli from the **Stimulus Book,** *Volume 6.*

Print this page from the CD or photocopy this page for your clinical use.

On the probes, present only the untrained exemplars (UT). When the child fails to meet the 90% correct probe criterion, either teach 2 to 4 new exemplars or give additional training trials on already trained stimuli. If needed, select new exemplars for probes. Probe at least 10 untrained exemplars. Alternate probes and treatment until the probe criterion is met.

Scripts for Probe Trials		Note
Clinician	[*untrained stimulus: stroller*] "What is this?"	No modeling or prompts
Child	"troller."	A wrong probe response
Clinician	Scores the response as incorrect.	No corrective feedback
Clinician	[*untrained stimulus: straightedge*] "What is this?"	The second probe trial
Child	"I don't know."	Lack of generalization
Clinician	Scores the response as incorrect. Notes that child does not know word.	No corrective feedback

Name:	Date:	Session #:
Age:	**Clinician:**	
Diagnosis: Articulation/Phonologic Disorder	**Word-initial /str/ probe**	
Untrained Stimuli	**Score: + correct; – incorrect or no responses**	
1. stroller		
2. straightedge		
3. strong		
4. stripes		
5. striking		
6. street		
7. strap		
8. stranger		
9. strapless		
10. streamer		
11. streetcar		
12. string beans		
Percent correct: (Criterion: 90%)		

If the child does not meet the probe criterion, give additional training on already trained exemplars or teach a few new exemplars. Subsequently, readminister the probe trials. When the child meets the 90% correct probe criterion for the exemplars, shift training to the sentence or conversational level or to another phoneme.

/ld/ in Word-Final Positions

Baserate Protocols

Use stimuli from the **Stimulus Book,** *Volume 7.*

At the beginning of each trial, place a relevant stimulus (an object, a picture, or a printed word if the child can read) in front of the child. Point to the stimulus as you ask an evoking question. Do not respond in any way to the child's correct, incorrect, or lack of responses.

Scripts For Evoked Baserate Trial		Note
Clinician	[*stimulus: child*] "This person is not an adult. She is a _____?"	Evoked trial
Child	"tʃaiod."	Vowelization of /l/ in /ld/ cluster
Clinician	Pulls the stimulus toward her; records the response.	No corrective feedback
Clinician	[*stimulus: bald*] "The baby doesn't have any hair. The baby is _____?"	The next evoked trial
Child	"bad."	Vowelization of /l/ in /ld/ cluster
Clinician	Pulls the stimulus toward her; records the response.	No corrective feedback

Administer the modeled baserate trials only after completing the evoked trials on all 20 (or more) exemplars.

Scripts For Modeled Baserate Trial		Note
Clinician	[*stimulus: child*] "This person is not an adult. She is a child? Say, *child.*"	Modeled trial
Child	"tʃaiod."	Vowelization of /l/ in /ld/ cluster
Clinician	Pulls the stimulus toward her; records the response.	No corrective feedback
Clinician	[*stimulus: bald*] "The baby doesn't have any hair. The baby is bald. Say, *bald.*"	The next modeled trial
Child	"bad."	Vowelization of /l/ in /ld/ cluster
Clinician	Pulls the stimulus toward her; records the response.	No corrective feedback

Use the recording sheet with exemplars shown on the next page to establish the baserates; print it from the CD.

/ld/ in Word-Final Positions

Baserate Exemplars and Recording Sheet

Use stimuli from the **Stimulus Book,** *Volume 7.*

Print this page from the CD or photocopy this page for your clinical use.

Name/Age:	Date:
Goal: To establish the baserate production of /ld/ in word-final positions.	Clinician:

Scoring: Correct: ✓   Incorrect or no response: X

/ld/ in word-final positions	Evoked	Modeled
1. child		
2. bald		
3. old		
4. gold		
5. spilled		
6. cornfield		
7. threshold		
8. outfield		
9. emerald		
10. marigold		
11. shield		
12. build		
13. sold		
14. field		
15. cold		
16. billfold		
17. unfold		
18. windshield		
19. household		
20. airfield		
Percent correct baserate		

Replace or add new exemplars as you see fit for a given child. After establishing the baserates, begin production teaching. Follow the protocols given on the next page.

/ld/ in Word-Final Positions

Treatment Protocols

Use stimuli from the **Stimulus Book, Volume 7.**

Teach 6 to 8 exemplars using the following script.

Place a relevant stimulus (an object, a picture, or a printed word if the child can read) in front of the child and point to the stimulus as you ask an evoking question.

Scripts For Modeled Discrete Trial Training		Note
Clinician	[*stimulus: child*] "This person is not an adult. She is a child?" Say, *child.*"	Modeling; the target vocally emphasized
Child	"tʃaiod."	A wrong response
Clinician	"No. That's not correct. You said tʃaiod, but she is a *child*. You need to say the *l* sound before the *d* sound at the end."	Corrective feedback
Clinician	[*the same stimulus*] "What is this? Say, *child.* Don't forget to say the *l* sound before the *d* at the end."	The next trial
Child	"Child."	A correct response
Clinician	"Excellent! You remembered to say the *l* sound this time.	Verbal praise

Repeat the trials until the child gives 5 consecutively correct, imitated responses.

When the child imitates 5 correct responses in sequence, fade the modeling.

Scripts For Fading the Modeling		Note
Clinician	[*stimulus: child*] "What is this? Don't forget the *l* sound before you say the *d* sound at the end."	Only a prompt
Child	"tʃaiod."	A wrong response
Clinician	"Gee, you forgot the *l*! It's a *child*, not *tʃaiod*. Remember to say the *l* sound before you say the *d* sound at the end."	Corrective feedback
Clinician	[*the same stimulus*] "What is this? It ends with . . . " [*silently models the articulatory posture for the /ld/ cluster.*]	The next trial; a partial modeling
Child	"Child."	A correct response
Clinician	"That's great! You said *child*, not *tʃaiod*."	Verbal praise
Clinician	[*the same stimulus*] "What is this?"	Typical question; evoked trial
Child	"Child."	A correct response
Clinician	"Amazing! That was perfect!"	Verbal praise

If the wrong responses persist on 4 to 5 evoked trials, reinstate partial or full modeling for a few trials, again fade the modeling, and re-present the evoked trials.

When the child meets the tentative learning criterion of 10 consecutively correct, nonimitated responses for a given stimulus item, move on to the next stimulus item. With this procedure, teach 6 to 8 exemplars shown on the following recording sheet. Use different exemplars as you see fit for a given child.

/ld/ in Word-Final Positions

Treatment Exemplars and Recording Sheet

Use stimuli from the **Stimulus Book,** *Volume 7*.

Print this page from CD or photocopy this page for your clinical use.

Name/Age:	Date:
Goal: Production of /ld/ in word-final positions with 90% accuracy when asked an evoking question while showing a stimulus.	Clinician:

Scoring: Correct: ✓   Incorrect or no response: X

Target skills	Discrete Trials														
	1	2	3	4	5	6	7	8	9	10	11	12	13	14	15
1. child															
2. bald															
3. old															
4. gold															
5. spilled															
6. cornfield															
7. threshold															
8. outfield															

When the child has met the learning criterion of 10 consecutively correct evoked (nonimitated) responses for each of the 6 to 8 target exemplars, conduct a probe to see if the production has generalized to previously baserated but untrained exemplars.

If the probes do not meet the 90% correct criterion for untrained exemplars, teach additional exemplars and then probe again.

/ld/ in Word-Final Positions

Probe Protocols and Recording Sheet

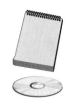

Use stimuli from the **Stimulus Book, Volume 7**.

Print this page from the CD or photocopy this page for your clinical use.

On the probes, present only the untrained exemplars (UT). When the child fails to meet the 90% correct probe criterion, either teach 2 to 4 new exemplars or give additional training trials on already trained stimuli. If needed, select new exemplars for probes. Probe at least 10 untrained exemplars. Alternate probes and treatment until the probe criterion is met.

Scripts for Probe Trials		Note
Clinician	[untrained stimulus: emerald] "What is this?"	No modeling or prompts
Child	"Emerald."	A correct, generalized response
Clinician	Scores the response as correct.	No reinforcement
Clinician	[untrained stimulus: marigold] "What is this?"	The second probe trial
Child	"Marigold."	A correct, generalized response
Clinician	Scores the response as correct.	No reinforcement

Name:	Date:	Session #:
Age:	**Clinician:**	
Diagnosis: Articulation/Phonologic Disorder	**Word-final /ld/ probe**	
Untrained Stimuli	**Score: + correct; – incorrect or no responses**	
1. emerald		
2. marigold		
3. shield		
4. build		
5. sold		
6. field		
7. cold		
8. billfold		
9. unfold		
10. windshield		
11. household		
12. airfield		
Percent correct: (Criterion: 90%)		

If the child does not meet the probe criterion, give additional training on already trained exemplars or teach a few new exemplars. Subsequently, readminister the probe trials. When the child meets the 90% correct probe criterion for the exemplars, shift training to the sentence or conversational level or to another phoneme.

/lɚ/ in Word-Final Positions

Baserate Protocols

*Use stimuli from the **Stimulus Book, Volume 7.***

At the beginning of each trial, place a relevant stimulus (an object, a picture, or a printed word if the child can read) in front of the child. Point to the stimulus as you ask an evoking question. Do not respond in any way to the child's correct, incorrect, or lack of responses.

Scripts For Evoked Baserate Trial		Note
Clinician	[*stimulus: dollar*] "What is this?"	Evoked trial
Child	"A dolla."	Omission of /ɚ/ in /lɚ/ cluster
Clinician	Pulls the stimulus toward her; records the response.	No corrective feedback
Clinician	[*stimulus: collar*] "What is this?"	The next evoked trial
Child	"A colla."	Omission of /ɚ/ in /lɚ/ cluster
Clinician	Pulls the stimulus toward her; records the response.	No corrective feedback

Administer the modeled baserate trials only after completing the evoked trials on all 20 (or more) exemplars.

Scripts For Modeled Baserate Trial		Note
Clinician	[*stimulus: dollar*] "What is this? Say, *dollar.*"	Modeled trial
Child	"dolla."	Omission of /ɚ/ in /lɚ/ cluster
Clinician	Pulls the stimulus toward her; records the response.	No corrective feedback
Clinician	[*stimulus: collar*] "What is this? Say, *collar.*"	The next modeled trial
Child	"colla."	Omission of /ɚ/ in /lɚ/ cluster
Clinician	Pulls the stimulus toward her; records the response.	No corrective feedback

Use the recording sheet with exemplars shown on the next page to establish the baserates; print it from the CD.

/lɚ/ in Word-Final Positions

Baserate Exemplars and Recording Sheet

Use stimuli from the **Stimulus Book, Volume 7**.

Print this page from the CD or photocopy this page for your clinical use.

Name/Age:	Date:
Goal: To establish the baserate production of /lɚ/ in word-final positions.	Clinician:

Scoring: Correct: ✓ Incorrect or no response: X

/lɚ/ in word-final positions	Evoked	Modeled
1. dollar		
2. collar		
3. cooler		
4. dealer		
5. pillar		
6. watercolor		
7. multicolor		
8. semitrailer		
9. caterpillar		
10. muscular		
11. molar		
12. sailor		
13. trailer		
14. smaller		
15. tailor		
16. patroller		
17. sand dollar		
18. two-wheeler		
19. regular		
20. tubular		
Percent correct baserate		

Replace or add new exemplars as you see fit for a given child. After establishing the baserates, begin production teaching. Follow the protocols given on the next page.

/lɚ/ in Word-Final Positions

Treatment Protocols

Use stimuli from the **Stimulus Book,** *Volume 7.*

Teach 6 to 8 exemplars using the following script.

Place a relevant stimulus (an object, a picture, or a printed word if the child can read) in front of the child and point to the stimulus as you ask an evoking question.

Scripts For Modeled Discrete Trial Training		Note
Clinician	[*stimulus: dollar*] "What is this? Say, *do**llar**."*	Modeling; the target vocally emphasized
Child	"dolla."	A wrong response
Clinician	"No. That's not correct. You said dolla, but it's a *dollar*. You need to say the /ɚ/ sound after the *l* at the end of the word."	Corrective feedback
Clinician	[*the same stimulus*] "What is this? Say, *dollar*. Don't forget the /ɚ/ sound at the end. You need to say the *l* and the /ɚ/ together, /lɚ/."	The next trial
Child	"Dollar."	A correct response
Clinician	"Magnificent! You didn't miss the /ɚ/ at the end of the word!"	Verbal praise

Repeat the trials until the child gives 5 consecutively correct, imitated responses.

When the child imitates 5 correct responses in sequence, fade the modeling.

Scripts For Fading the Modeling		Note
Clinician	[*stimulus: dollar*] "What is this? Don't forget the /ɚ/ at the end."	Only a prompt
Child	"dolla."	A wrong response
Clinician	"Oops, you forgot the /ɚ/! It's a *dollar*, not *dolla*. Put the /ɚ/ sound after the *l* sound at the end of the word."	Corrective feedback
Clinician	[*the same stimulus*] "What is this? It ends with . . . " [*silently models the articulatory posture for the /lɚ/ cluster.*]	The next trial; a partial modeling
Child	"Dollar."	A correct response
Clinician	"That's great! You said *dollar*, not *dolla*."	Verbal praise
Clinician	[*the same stimulus*] "What is this?"	Typical question; evoked trial
Child	"Dollar."	A correct response
Clinician	"Beautiful! You said it perfectly!"	Verbal praise

If the wrong responses persist on 4 to 5 evoked trials, reinstate partial or full modeling for a few trials, again fade the modeling, and re-present the evoked trials.

When the child meets the tentative learning criterion of 10 consecutively correct, nonimitated responses for a given stimulus item, move on to the next stimulus item. With this procedure, teach 6 to 8 exemplars shown on the following recording sheet. Use different exemplars as you see fit for a given child.

/lɚ/ in Word-Final Positions

Treatment Exemplars and Recording Sheet

Use stimuli from the **Stimulus Book,** *Volume 7.*

Print this page from CD or photocopy this page for your clinical use.

Name/Age:	Date:
Goal: Production of /lɚ/ in word-final positions with 90% accuracy when asked an evoking question while showing a stimulus.	Clinician:

Scoring: Correct: ✓   Incorrect or no response: X

Target skills	Discrete Trials														
	1	2	3	4	5	6	7	8	9	10	11	12	13	14	15
1. dollar															
2. collar															
3. cooler															
4. dealer															
5. pillar															
6. watercolor															
7. multicolor															
8. semitrailer															

When the child has met the learning criterion of 10 consecutively correct evoked (nonimitated) responses for each of the 6 to 8 target exemplars, conduct a probe to see if the production has generalized to previously baserated but untrained exemplars.

If the probes do not meet the 90% correct criterion for untrained exemplars, teach additional exemplars and then probe again.

/lɚ/ in Word-Final Positions

Probe Protocols and Recording Sheet

Use stimuli from the **Stimulus Book, Volume 7**.

Print this page from the CD or photocopy this page for your clinical use.

On the probes, present only the untrained exemplars (UT). When the child fails to meet the 90% correct probe criterion, either teach 2 to 4 new exemplars or give additional training trials on already trained stimuli. If needed, select new exemplars for probes. Probe at least 10 untrained exemplars. Alternate probes and treatment until the probe criterion is met.

Scripts for Probe Trials		Note
Clinician	[untrained stimulus: caterpillar] "What is this?"	No modeling or prompts
Child	"A caterpillar."	A correct, generalized response
Clinician	Scores the response as correct.	No reinforcement
Clinician	[untrained stimulus: muscular] "The man exercises a lot. He is very _____?"	The second probe trial
Child	"Muscula."	A wrong probe response
Clinician	Scores the response as incorrect.	No corrective feedback

Name:	Date:	Session #:
Age:	**Clinician:**	
Diagnosis: Articulation/Phonologic Disorder	**Word-final /lɚ/probe**	
Untrained Stimuli	**Score: + correct; – incorrect or no responses**	
1. caterpillar		
2. muscular		
3. molar		
4. sailor		
5. trailer		
6. smaller		
7. polar		
8. patroller		
9. sand dollar		
10. two-wheeler		
11. regular		
12. tubular		
Percent correct: (Criterion: 90%)		

If the child does not meet the probe criterion, give additional training on already trained exemplars or teach a few new exemplars. Subsequently, readminister the probe trials. When the child meets the 90% correct probe criterion for the exemplars, shift training to the sentence or conversational level or to another phoneme.

/lt/ in Word-Final Positions

Baserate Protocols

Use stimuli from the **Stimulus Book,** *Volume 7.*

At the beginning of each trial, place a relevant stimulus (an object, a picture, or a printed word if the child can read) in front of the child. Point to the stimulus as you ask an evoking question. Do not respond in any way to the child's correct, incorrect, or lack of responses.

Scripts For Evoked Baserate Trial		Note
Clinician	[*stimulus: belt*] "What is this?"	Evoked trial
Child	"bɛot."	Vowelization of /l/ in /lt/ cluster
Clinician	Pulls the stimulus toward her; records the response.	No corrective feedback
Clinician	[*stimulus: colt*] "A young male (boy) horse is called a _____?"	The next evoked trial
Child	"I don't know."	Does not know word
Clinician	Pulls the stimulus toward her; records the response. Notes that child does not know word.	No corrective feedback

Administer the modeled baserate trials only after completing the evoked trials on all 20 (or more) exemplars.

Scripts For Modeled Baserate Trial		Note
Clinician	[*stimulus: belt*] "What is this? Say, *belt.*"	Modeled trial
Child	"bɛot."	Vowelization of /l/ in /lt/ cluster
Clinician	Pulls the stimulus toward her; records the response.	No corrective feedback
Clinician	[*stimulus: colt*] "A young male (boy) horse is called a colt? Say, *colt.*"	The next modeled trial
Child	"cət."	Vowelization of /l/ in /lt/ cluster
Clinician	Pulls the stimulus toward her; records the response.	No corrective feedback

Use the recording sheet with exemplars shown on the next page to establish the baserates; print it from the CD.

/lt/ in Word-Final Positions

Baserate Exemplars and Recording Sheet

Use stimuli from the **Stimulus Book,** *Volume 7.*

Print this page from the CD or photocopy this page for your clinical use.

Name/Age:	Date:
Goal: To establish the baserate production of /lt/ in word-final positions.	Clinician:

Scoring: Correct: ✓   Incorrect or no response: X

/lt/ in word-final positions	Evoked	Modeled
1. belt		
2. colt		
3. salt		
4. quilt		
5. melt		
6. cobalt		
7. adult		
8. pole vault		
9. seat belt		
10. asphalt		
11. guilt		
12. bolt		
13. felt		
14. malt		
15. tilt		
16. fan belt		
17. result		
18. bank vault		
19. somersault		
20. insult		
Percent correct baserate		

Replace or add new exemplars as you see fit for a given child. After establishing the baserates, begin production teaching. Follow the protocols given on the next page.

/lt/ in Word-Final Positions

Treatment Protocols

Use stimuli from the **Stimulus Book, *Volume 7.***

Teach 6 to 8 exemplars using the following script.

Place a relevant stimulus (an object, a picture, or a printed word if the child can read) in front of the child and point to the stimulus as you ask an evoking question.

Scripts For Modeled Discrete Trial Training		Note
Clinician	[*stimulus: belt*] "What is this? Say, ***belt***."	Modeling; the target vocally emphasized
Child	"bɛot."	A wrong response
Clinician	"No. That's not correct. You said *bɛot*, but it's a ***belt***. You need to say the ***l*** sound before the ***t*** sound at the end."	Corrective feedback
Clinician	[*the same stimulus*] "What is this? Say, ***belt***. Remember to say the ***l*** sound before the ***t*** at the end of the word. You need to say the ***l*** and ***t*** together, ***lt***."	The next trial
Child	"Belt."	A correct response
Clinician	"Way to go! You put the ***l*** and ***t*** together in the word ***belt***.	Verbal praise

Repeat the trials until the child gives 5 consecutively correct, imitated responses.

When the child imitates 5 correct responses in sequence, fade the modeling.

Scripts For Fading the Modeling		Note
Clinician	[*stimulus: belt*] "What is this? Don't forget the ***l*** sound before the ***t*** sound at the end."	Only a prompt
Child	"bɛot."	A wrong response
Clinician	"Oops, you forgot the ***l***! It's a ***belt***, not *bɛot*. Say the ***l*** before the ***t*** at the end."	Corrective feedback
Clinician	[*the same stimulus*] "What is this? It ends with . . . " [*silently models the articulatory posture for the /lt/ cluster.*]	The next trial; a partial modeling
Child	"Belt."	A correct response
Clinician	"That's great! You said *belt*, not *bɛot*."	Verbal praise
Clinician	[*the same stimulus*] "What is this?"	Typical question; evoked trial
Child	"Belt."	A correct response
Clinician	"That was fantastic! You said it correctly!"	Verbal praise

If the wrong responses persist on 4 to 5 evoked trials, reinstate partial or full modeling for a few trials, again fade the modeling, and re-present the evoked trials.

When the child meets the tentative learning criterion of 10 consecutively correct, nonimitated responses for a given stimulus item, move on to the next stimulus item. With this procedure, teach 6 to 8 exemplars shown on the following recording sheet. Use different exemplars as you see fit for a given child.

/lt/ in Word-Final Positions

Treatment Exemplars and Recording Sheet

Use stimuli from the **Stimulus Book, Volume 7**.

Print this page from CD or photocopy this page for your clinical use.

Name/Age:	Date:
Goal: Production of /lt/ in word-final positions with 90% accuracy when asked an evoking question while showing a stimulus.	Clinician:

Scoring: Correct: ✓   Incorrect or no response: X

Target skills	Discrete Trials														
	1	2	3	4	5	6	7	8	9	10	11	12	13	14	15
1. belt															
2. colt															
3. salt															
4. quilt															
5. melt															
6. cobalt															
7. adult															
8. pole vault															

When the child has met the learning criterion of 10 consecutively correct evoked (nonimitated) responses for each of the 6 to 8 target exemplars, conduct a probe to see if the production has generalized to previously baserated but untrained exemplars.

If the probes do not meet the 90% correct criterion for untrained exemplars, teach additional exemplars and then probe again.

/lt/ in Word-Final Positions

Probe Protocols and Recording Sheet

Use stimuli from the **Stimulus Book,** *Volume 7.*

Print this page from the CD or photocopy this page for your clinical use.

On the probes, present only the untrained exemplars (UT). When the child fails to meet the 90% correct probe criterion, either teach 2 to 4 new exemplars or give additional training trials on already trained stimuli. If needed, select new exemplars for probes. Probe at least 10 untrained exemplars. Alternate probes and treatment until the probe criterion is met.

Scripts for Probe Trials		Note
Clinician	[*untrained stimulus: seat belt*] "What is this?"	No modeling or prompts
Child	"Seat belt."	A correct, generalized response
Clinician	Scores the response as correct.	No reinforcement
Clinician	[*untrained stimulus: asphalt*] "The street is made of _____?"	The second probe trial
Child	"Asphalt."	A correct, generalized response
Clinician	Scores the response as correct.	No reinforcement

Name:		Date:	Session #:
Age:		**Clinician:**	
Diagnosis: Articulation/Phonologic Disorder		**Word-final /lt/ probe**	
Untrained Stimuli		**Score: + correct; – incorrect or no responses**	
1. seat belt			
2. asphalt			
3. guilt			
4. bolt			
5. felt			
6. malt			
7. tilt			
8. fan belt			
9. result			
10. bank vault			
11. somersault			
12. insult			
Percent correct: (Criterion: 90%)			

If the child does not meet the probe criterion, give additional training on already trained exemplars or teach a few new exemplars. Subsequently, readminister the probe trials. When the child meets the 90% correct probe criterion for the exemplars, shift training to the sentence or conversational level or to another phoneme.

/lz/ in Word-Final Positions

Baserate Protocols

Use stimuli from the **Stimulus Book, *Volume 7***.

At the beginning of each trial, place a relevant stimulus (an object, a picture, or a printed word if the child can read) in front of the child. Point to the stimulus as you ask an evoking question. Do not respond in any way to the child's correct, incorrect, or lack of responses.

Scripts For Evoked Baserate Trial		Note
Clinician	[*stimulus: balls*] "What are these?"	Evoked trial
Child	"bɑəz."	Vowelization of /l/ in /lz/ cluster
Clinician	Pulls the stimulus toward her; records the response.	No corrective feedback
Clinician	[*stimulus: nails*] "What are these?"	The next evoked trial
Child	"neioz."	Vowelization of /l/ in /lz/ cluster
Clinician	Pulls the stimulus toward her; records the response.	No corrective feedback

Administer the modeled baserate trials only after completing the evoked trials on all 20 (or more) exemplars.

Scripts For Modeled Baserate Trial		Note
Clinician	[*stimulus: balls*] "What are these? Say, *balls.*"	Modeled trial
Child	"Balls."	Correct response
Clinician	Pulls the stimulus toward her; records the response.	No reinforcement
Clinician	[*stimulus: nails*] "What are these? Say, *nails.*"	The next modeled trial
Child	"neioz."	Vowelization of /l/ in /lz/ cluster
Clinician	Pulls the stimulus toward her; records the response.	No corrective feedback

Use the recording sheet with exemplars shown on the next page to establish the baserates; print it from the CD.

/lz/ in Word-Final Positions

Baserate Exemplars and Recording Sheet

Use stimuli from the **Stimulus Book,** *Volume 7.*

Print this page from the CD or photocopy this page for your clinical use.

Name/Age:	Date:
Goal: To establish the baserate production of /lz/ in word-final positions.	Clinician:

Scoring: Correct: ✓   Incorrect or no response: X

/lz/ in word-final positions	Evoked	Modeled
1. balls		
2. nails		
3. rolls		
4. holes		
5. dolls		
6. baseballs		
7. cymbals		
8. seashells		
9. noodles		
10. pretzels		
11. bells		
12. seals		
13. moles		
14. poles		
15. pails		
16. needles		
17. jewels		
18. footballs		
19. toenails		
20. petals		
Percent correct baserate		

Replace or add new exemplars as you see fit for a given child. After establishing the baserates, begin production teaching. Follow the protocols given on the next page.

/lz/ in Word-Final Positions

Treatment Protocols

Use stimuli from the **Stimulus Book,** *Volume 7.*

Teach 6 to 8 exemplars using the following script.

Place a relevant stimulus (an object, a picture, or a printed word if the child can read) in front of the child and point to the stimulus as you ask an evoking question.

Scripts For Modeled Discrete Trial Training		Note
Clinician	[*stimulus: balls*] "What are these? Say, *ba**lls**.*"	Modeling; the target vocally emphasized
Child	"baəz."	A wrong response
Clinician	"Oops. That's not right. You said *baəz*, but you should have said *ba**lls***. You left out the **l** sound before the **z** sound at the end."	Corrective feedback
Clinician	[*the same stimulus*] "What are these? Say, *ba**lls***. Remember to say the **l** sound before the **z** sound at the end of *ba**lls**.*"	The next trial
Child	"Balls."	A correct response
Clinician	"That was perfect! You said the **l** sound before the **z** sound at the end of the word!"	Verbal praise

Repeat the trials until the child gives 5 consecutively correct, imitated responses.

When the child imitates 5 correct responses in sequence, fade the modeling.

Scripts For Fading the Modeling		Note
Clinician	[*stimulus: balls*] "What are these? Don't forget the *l* sound before the *z* sound at the end."	Only a prompt
Child	"baəz."	A wrong response
Clinician	"Uh, oh, you forgot the *l*! It's *balls*, not *baəz*. Put the *l* before the *z* at the end."	Corrective feedback
Clinician	[*the same stimulus*] "What are these? The word ends with . . ." [*silently models the articulatory posture for the /lz/ cluster.*]	The next trial; a partial modeling
Child	"Balls."	A correct response
Clinician	"That was magnificent! You said *balls*, not *baəz*."	Verbal praise
Clinician	[*the same stimulus*] "What is this?"	Typical question; evoked trial
Child	"Balls."	A correct response
Clinician	"Alright! You said it perfectly! You are working very hard."	Verbal praise

If the wrong responses persist on 4 to 5 evoked trials, reinstate partial or full modeling for a few trials, again fade the modeling, and re-present the evoked trials.

When the child meets the tentative learning criterion of 10 consecutively correct, nonimitated responses for a given stimulus item, move on to the next stimulus item. With this procedure, teach 6 to 8 exemplars shown on the following recording sheet. Use different exemplars as you see fit for a given child.

/lz/ in Word-Final Positions

Treatment Exemplars and Recording Sheet

Use stimuli from the **Stimulus Book,** *Volume 7.*

Print this page from CD or photocopy this page for your clinical use.

Name/Age:	Date:
Goal: Production of /lz/ in word-final positions with 90% accuracy when asked an evoking question while showing a stimulus.	Clinician:

Scoring: Correct: ✓   Incorrect or no response: X

Target skills	Discrete Trials														
	1	2	3	4	5	6	7	8	9	10	11	12	13	14	15
1. balls															
2. nails															
3. rolls															
4. holes															
5. dolls															
6. baseballs															
7. cymbals															
8. seashells															

When the child has met the learning criterion of 10 consecutively correct evoked (nonimitated) responses for each of the 6 to 8 target exemplars, conduct a probe to see if the production has generalized to previously baserated but untrained exemplars.

If the probes do not meet the 90% correct criterion for untrained exemplars, teach additional exemplars and then probe again.

/lz/ in Word-Final Positions

Probe Protocols and Recording Sheet

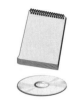

Use stimuli from the **Stimulus Book,** *Volume 7.*

Print this page from the CD or photocopy this page for your clinical use.

On the probes, present only the untrained exemplars (UT). When the child fails to meet the 90% correct probe criterion, either teach 2 to 4 new exemplars or give additional training trials on already trained stimuli. If needed, select new exemplars for probes. Probe at least 10 untrained exemplars. Alternate probes and treatment until the probe criterion is met.

Scripts for Probe Trials		Note
Clinician	[*untrained stimulus: noodles*] "What are these?"	No modeling or prompts
Child	"Noodles."	A correct, generalized response
Clinician	Scores the response as correct.	No reinforcement
Clinician	[*untrained stimulus: pretzels*] "What are these?"	The second probe trial
Child	"pretsoz."	A wrong probe response
Clinician	Scores the response as incorrect.	No corrective feedback

Name:	Date:	Session #:
Age:	**Clinician:**	
Diagnosis: Articulation/Phonologic Disorder	**Word-final /lz/ probe**	
Untrained Stimuli	**Score: + correct; – incorrect or no responses**	
1. noodles		
2. pretzels		
3. bells		
4. seals		
5. moles		
6. poles		
7. pails		
8. needles		
9. jewels		
10. footballs		
11. toenails		
12. petals		
Percent correct: (Criterion: 90%)		

If the child does not meet the probe criterion, give additional training on already trained exemplars or teach a few new exemplars. Subsequently, readminister the probe trials. When the child meets the 90% correct probe criterion for the exemplars, shift training to the sentence or conversational level or to another phoneme.

/rd/ in Word-Final Positions

Baserate Protocols

Use stimuli from the **Stimulus Book,** *Volume 7.*

At the beginning of each trial, place a relevant stimulus (an object, a picture, or a printed word if the child can read) in front of the child. Point to the stimulus as you ask an evoking question. Do not respond in any way to the child's correct, incorrect, or lack of responses.

Scripts For Evoked Baserate Trial		Note
Clinician	[*stimulus: card*] "What is this?"	Evoked trial
Child	"cɑəd."	Vowelization of /r/ in /rd/ cluster
Clinician	Pulls the stimulus toward her; records the response.	No corrective feedback
Clinician	[*stimulus: cord*] "What is this?"	The next evoked trial
Child	"coəd."	Vowelization of /r/ in /rd/ cluster
Clinician	Pulls the stimulus toward her; records the response.	No corrective feedback

Administer the modeled baserate trials only after completing the evoked trials on all 20 (or more) exemplars.

Scripts For Modeled Baserate Trial		Note
Clinician	[*stimulus: card*] "What is this? Say, *card.*"	Modeled trial
Child	"cɑəd."	Vowelization of /r/ in /rd/ cluster
Clinician	Pulls the stimulus toward her; records the response.	No corrective feedback
Clinician	[*stimulus: cord*] "What is this? Say, *cord.*"	The next modeled trial
Child	"coəd."	Vowelization of /r/ in /rd/ cluster
Clinician	Pulls the stimulus toward her; records the response.	No corrective feedback

Use the recording sheet with exemplars shown on the next page to establish the baserates; print it from the CD.

/rd/ in Word-Final Positions

Baserate Exemplars and Recording Sheet

Use stimuli from the **Stimulus Book,** *Volume 7.*

Print this page from the CD or photocopy this page for your clinical use.

Name/Age:	Date:
Goal: To establish the baserate production of /rd/ in word-final positions.	Clinician:

Scoring: Correct: ✓   Incorrect or no response: X

/rd/ in word-final positions	Evoked	Modeled
1. card		
2. cord		
3. yard		
4. hard		
5. gourd		
6. award		
7. front yard		
8. barnyard		
9. cardboard		
10. postcard		
11. scored		
12. lard		
13. stared		
14. guard		
15. board		
16. keyboard		
17. night guard		
18. bodyguard		
19. diving board		
20. backyard		
Percent correct baserate		

Replace or add new exemplars as you see fit for a given child. After establishing the baserates, begin production teaching. Follow the protocols given on the next page.

/rd/ in Word-Final Positions

Treatment Protocols

Use stimuli from the **Stimulus Book,** *Volume 7.*

Teach 6 to 8 exemplars using the following script.

Place a relevant stimulus (an object, a picture, or a printed word if the child can read) in front of the child and point to the stimulus as you ask an evoking question.

Scripts For Modeled Discrete Trial Training		Note
Clinician	[*stimulus: card*] "What is this? Say, *card*."	Modeling; the target vocally emphasized
Child	"caəd."	A wrong response
Clinician	"No. That's not correct. You said *caəd*, but it's a *card*. You need to say the **r** sound before the **d** sound at the end of the word."	Corrective feedback
Clinician	[*the same stimulus*] "What is this? Say, *card*. Don't forget the **r** sound before the **d** sound at the end."	The next trial
Child	"Card."	A correct response
Clinician	"Stupendous! You remembered to say the **r** sound before the **d** sound in the word *card*.	Verbal praise

Repeat the trials until the child gives 5 consecutively correct, imitated responses.

When the child imitates 5 correct responses in sequence, fade the modeling.

Scripts For Fading the Modeling		Note
Clinician	[*stimulus: card*] "What is this? Don't forget the r sound before the d sound at the end."	Only a prompt
Child	"caəd."	A wrong response
Clinician	"Gee, you forgot the r sound! It's a *card*, not caəd. Say the r before the d at the end."	Corrective feedback
Clinician	[*the same stimulus*] "What is this? It ends with . . . " [*silently models the articulatory posture for the /rd/ cluster.*]	The next trial; a partial modeling
Child	"Card."	A correct response
Clinician	"That's great! You said card, not caəd."	Verbal praise
Clinician	[*the same stimulus*] "What is this?"	Typical question; evoked trial
Child	"Card."	A correct response
Clinician	"I like it! You said it correctly! Keep up the good work!"	Verbal praise

If the wrong responses persist on 4 to 5 evoked trials, reinstate partial or full modeling for a few trials, again fade the modeling, and re-present the evoked trials.

When the child meets the tentative learning criterion of 10 consecutively correct, nonimitated responses for a given stimulus item, move on to the next stimulus item. With this procedure, teach 6 to 8 exemplars shown on the following recording sheet. Use different exemplars as you see fit for a given child.

/rd/ in Word-Final Positions

Treatment Exemplars and Recording Sheet

Use stimuli from the **Stimulus Book,** *Volume 7.*

Print this page from CD or photocopy this page for your clinical use.

Name/Age:	Date:
Goal: Production of /rd/ in word-final positions with 90% accuracy when asked an evoking question while showing a stimulus.	Clinician:

Scoring: Correct: ✓   Incorrect or no response: X

Target skills	Discrete Trials														
	1	2	3	4	5	6	7	8	9	10	11	12	13	14	15
1. card															
2. cord															
3. yard															
4. hard															
5. gourd															
6. award															
7. front yard															
8. barnyard															

When the child has met the learning criterion of 10 consecutively correct evoked (nonimitated) responses for each of the 6 to 8 target exemplars, conduct a probe to see if the production has generalized to previously baserated but untrained exemplars.

If the probes do not meet the 90% correct criterion for untrained exemplars, teach additional exemplars and then probe again.

/rd/ in Word-Final Positions

Probe Protocols and Recording Sheet

Use stimuli from the **Stimulus Book,** *Volume 7.*

Print this page from the CD or photocopy this page for your clinical use.

On the probes, present only the untrained exemplars (UT). When the child fails to meet the 90% correct probe criterion, either teach 2 to 4 new exemplars or give additional training trials on already trained stimuli. If needed, select new exemplars for probes. Probe at least 10 untrained exemplars. Alternate probes and treatment until the probe criterion is met.

Scripts for Probe Trials		Note
Clinician	[*untrained stimulus: cardboard*] "A box is made of _____?"	No modeling or prompts
Child	"Cardboard."	A correct, generalized response
Clinician	Scores the response as correct.	No reinforcement
Clinician	[*untrained stimulus: postcard*] "What is this?"	The second probe trial
Child	"A postcard."	A correct, generalized response
Clinician	Scores the response as correct.	No reinforcement

Name:	Date:	Session #:
Age:	**Clinician:**	
Diagnosis: Articulation/Phonologic Disorder	**Word-final /rd/ probe**	
Untrained Stimuli	**Score: + correct; – incorrect or no responses**	
1. cardboard		
2. postcard		
3. scored		
4. lard		
5. stared		
6. guard		
7. board		
8. key board		
9. night guard		
10. bodyguard		
11. diving board		
12. backyard		
Percent correct: (Criterion: 90%)		

If the child does not meet the probe criterion, give additional training on already trained exemplars or teach a few new exemplars. Subsequently, readminister the probe trials. When the child meets the 90% correct probe criterion for the exemplars, shift training to the sentence or conversational level or to another phoneme.

/rk/ in Word-Final Positions

Baserate Protocols

Use stimuli from the **Stimulus Book,** *Volume 7.*

At the beginning of each trial, place a relevant stimulus (an object, a picture, or a printed word if the child can read) in front of the child. Point to the stimulus as you ask an evoking question. Do not respond in any way to the child's correct, incorrect, or lack of responses.

Scripts For Evoked Baserate Trial		Note
Clinician	[*stimulus: fork*] "What is this?"	Evoked trial
Child	"foke."	Omission of /r/ in /rk/ cluster
Clinician	Pulls the stimulus toward her; records the response.	No corrective feedback
Clinician	[*stimulus: park*] "What is this?"	The next evoked trial
Child	"A pak."	Omission of /r/ in /rk/ cluster
Clinician	Pulls the stimulus toward her; records the response.	No corrective feedback

Administer the modeled baserate trials only after completing the evoked trials on all 20 (or more) exemplars.

Scripts For Modeled Baserate Trial		Note
Clinician	[*stimulus: fork*] "What is this? Say, *fork.*"	Modeled trial
Child	"Fork."	Correct response
Clinician	Pulls the stimulus toward her; records the response.	No reinforcement
Clinician	[*stimulus: park*] "What is this? Say, *park.*"	The next modeled trial
Child	"Park."	Correct response
Clinician	Pulls the stimulus toward her; records the response.	No reinforcement

Use the recording sheet with exemplars shown on the next page to establish the baserates; print it from the CD.

/rk/ in Word-Final Positions

Baserate Exemplars and Recording Sheet

Use stimuli from the **Stimulus Book,** *Volume 7.*

Print this page from the CD or photocopy this page for your clinical use.

Name/Age:	Date:
Goal: To establish the baserate production of /rk/ in word-final positions.	Clinician:

Scoring: Correct: ✓   Incorrect or no response: X

/rk/ in word-final positions	Evoked	Modeled
1. fork		
2. park		
3. bark		
4. cork		
5. ark		
6. bookmark		
7. birthmark		
8. skylark		
9. check mark		
10. pitchfork		
11. shark		
12. mark		
13. stork		
14. pork		
15. lark		
16. monarch		
17. postmark		
18. city park		
19. landmark		
20. quotation mark		
Percent correct baserate		

Replace or add new exemplars as you see fit for a given child. After establishing the baserates, begin production teaching. Follow the protocols given on the next page.

/rk/ in Word-Final Positions

Treatment Protocols

Use stimuli from the **Stimulus Book, Volume 7**.

Teach 6 to 8 exemplars using the following script.

Place a relevant stimulus (an object, a picture, or a printed word if the child can read) in front of the child and point to the stimulus as you ask an evoking question.

Scripts For Modeled Discrete Trial Training		Note
Clinician	[*stimulus: fork*] "What is this? Say, *fork*."	Modeling; the target vocally emphasized
Child	"foke."	A wrong response
Clinician	"I'm sorry. That's not right. You said *foke*, but it's a *fork*." You need to say the /r/ sound before the /k/ sound, *fork*.	Corrective feedback
Clinician	[*the same stimulus*] "What is this? Say, *fork*. Don't forget the *r* sound before the *k* at the end."	The next trial
Child	"Fork."	A correct response
Clinician	"Excellent! You didn't miss the *r*!"	Verbal praise

Repeat the trials until the child gives 5 consecutively correct, imitated responses.

When the child imitates 5 correct responses in sequence, fade the modeling.

Scripts For Fading the Modeling		Note
Clinician	[*stimulus: fork*] "What is this? Don't forget to say the *r* sound before the *k* sound at the end."	Only a prompt
Child	"foke."	A wrong response
Clinician	"Oh, oh, you forgot to say the *r* in the word! It's a *fork*, not *foke*. Remember to put the *r* before the *k* at the end."	Corrective feedback
Clinician	[*the same stimulus*] "What is this? It ends with . . . " [*silently models the articulatory posture for the target sound.*]	The next trial; a partial modeling
Child	"Fork."	A correct response
Clinician	"That's great! You said *fork*, not *foke*."	Verbal praise
Clinician	[*the same stimulus*] "What is this?"	Typical question; evoked trial
Child	"Fork."	A correct response
Clinician	"Excellent job! You said it correctly!" Keep up the good work.	Verbal praise

If the wrong responses persist on 4 to 5 evoked trials, reinstate partial or full modeling for a few trials, again fade the modeling, and re-present the evoked trials.

When the child meets the tentative learning criterion of 10 consecutively correct, nonimitated responses for a given stimulus item, move on to the next stimulus item. With this procedure, teach 6 to 8 exemplars shown on the following recording sheet. Use different exemplars as you see fit for a given child.

/rk/ in Word-Final Positions

Treatment Exemplars and Recording Sheet

Use stimuli from the **Stimulus Book,** *Volume 7.*

Print this page from CD or photocopy this page for your clinical use.

Name/Age:	Date:
Goal: Production of /rk/ in word-final positions with 90% accuracy when asked an evoking question while showing a stimulus.	Clinician:

Scoring: Correct: ✓   Incorrect or no response: X

Target skills	Discrete Trials														
	1	2	3	4	5	6	7	8	9	10	11	12	13	14	15
1. fork															
2. park															
3. bark															
4. cork															
5. ark															
6. bookmark															
7. birthmark															
8. skylark															

When the child has met the learning criterion of 10 consecutively correct evoked (nonimitated) responses for each of the 6 to 8 target exemplars, conduct a probe to see if the production has generalized to previously baserated but untrained exemplars.

If the probes do not meet the 90% correct criterion for untrained exemplars, teach additional exemplars and then probe again.

/rk/ in Word-Final Positions

Probe Protocols and Recording Sheet

Use stimuli from the **Stimulus Book,** *Volume 7.*

Print this page from the CD or photocopy this page for your clinical use.

On the probes, present only the untrained exemplars (UT). When the child fails to meet the 90% correct probe criterion, either teach 2 to 4 new exemplars or give additional training trials on already trained stimuli. If needed, select new exemplars for probes. Probe at least 10 untrained exemplars. Alternate probes and treatment until the probe criterion is met.

Scripts for Probe Trials		Note
Clinician	[*untrained stimulus: check mark*] "What is this?"	No modeling or prompts
Child	"A check mark."	A correct, generalized response
Clinician	Scores the response as correct.	No reinforcement
Clinician	[*untrained stimulus: pitchfork*] "What is this?"	The second probe trial
Child	"Pitchfork."	A correct, generalized response
Clinician	Scores the response as correct.	No reinforcement

Name:	Date:	Session #:
Age:	**Clinician:**	
Diagnosis: Articulation/Phonologic Disorder	**Word-final /rk/ probe**	
Untrained Stimuli	**Score: + correct; – incorrect or no responses**	
1. check mark		
2. pitchfork		
3. shark		
4. mark		
5. stork		
6. pork		
7. park		
8. monarch		
9. postmark		
10. city park		
11. landmark		
12. quotation mark		
Percent correct: (Criterion: 90%)		

If the child does not meet the probe criterion, give additional training on already trained exemplars or teach a few new exemplars. Subsequently, readminister the probe trials. When the child meets the 90% correct probe criterion for the exemplars, shift training to the sentence or conversational level or to another phoneme.

/rn/ in Word-Final Positions

Baserate Protocols

Use stimuli from the **Stimulus Book, Volume 7.**

At the beginning of each trial, place a relevant stimulus (an object, a picture, or a printed word if the child can read) in front of the child. Point to the stimulus as you ask an evoking question. Do not respond in any way to the child's correct, incorrect, or lack of responses.

Scripts For Evoked Baserate Trial		Note
Clinician	[*stimulus: barn*] "What is this?"	Evoked trial
Child	"A bɑn."	Vowelization of /r/ in /rn/ cluster
Clinician	Pulls the stimulus toward her; records the response.	No corrective feedback
Clinician	[*stimulus: corn*] "What is this?"	The next evoked trial
Child	"coən."	Vowelization of /r/ in /rn/ cluster
Clinician	Pulls the stimulus toward her; records the response.	No corrective feedback

Administer the modeled baserate trials only after completing the evoked trials on all 20 (or more) exemplars.

Scripts For Modeled Baserate Trial		Note
Clinician	[*stimulus: barn*] "What is this? Say, *barn*."	Modeled trial
Child	"bɑn."	Vowelization of /r/ in /rn/ cluster
Clinician	Pulls the stimulus toward her; records the response.	No corrective feedback
Clinician	[*stimulus: corn*] "What is this? Say, *corn*."	The next modeled trial
Child	"coən."	Vowelization of /r/ in /rn/ cluster
Clinician	Pulls the stimulus toward her; records the response.	No corrective feedback

Use the recording sheet with exemplars shown on the next page to establish the baserates; print it from the CD.

/rn/ in Word-Final Positions

Baserate Exemplars and Recording Sheet

Use stimuli from the **Stimulus Book,** *Volume 7.*

Print this page from the CD or photocopy this page for your clinical use.

Name/Age:	Date:
Goal: To establish the baserate production of /rn/ in word-final positions.	Clinician:

Scoring: Correct: ✓   Incorrect or no response: X

/rn/ in word-final positions	Evoked	Modeled
1. barn		
2. corn		
3. yarn		
4. farm		
5. horn		
6. acorn		
7. adorn		
8. newborn		
9. popcorn		
10. unicorn		
11. worn		
12. thorn		
13. born		
14. mourn		
15. torn		
16. long horn		
17. French horn		
18. fog horn		
19. airborne		
20. Capricorn		
Percent correct baserate		

Replace or add new exemplars as you see fit for a given child. After establishing the baserates, begin production teaching. Follow the protocols given on the next page.

/rn/ in Word-Final Positions

Treatment Protocols

Use stimuli from the **Stimulus Book,** *Volume 7.*

Teach 6 to 8 exemplars using the following script.

Place a relevant stimulus (an object, a picture, or a printed word if the child can read) in front of the child and point to the stimulus as you ask an evoking question.

Scripts For Modeled Discrete Trial Training		Note
Clinician	[*stimulus: barn*] "What is this? Say, *barn.*"	Modeling; the target vocally emphasized
Child	"ban."	A wrong response
Clinician	"No. That's not correct. You said *ban*, but you should have said *barn*. You left out the **r** sound before the **n** sound. You need to say the **r** and the **n** together at the end."	Corrective feedback
Clinician	[*the same stimulus*] "What is this? Say, *barn*. Don't forget the **r** sound before the **n** sound at the end."	The next trial
Child	"Barn."	A correct response
Clinician	"That was fantastic! You didn't miss the **r** at the end of the word!"	Verbal praise

Repeat the trials until the child gives 5 consecutively correct, imitated responses.

When the child imitates 5 correct responses in sequence, fade the modeling.

Scripts For Fading the Modeling		Note
Clinician	[*stimulus: barn*] "What is this? Don't forget the *r* sound before the *n* sound at the end of the word."	Only a prompt
Child	"ban."	A wrong response
Clinician	"Oops, you forgot the *r* sound in the word *barn!* You said *ban*, but it should be *barn*. Put the *r* sound before the *n* sound at the end."	Corrective feedback
Clinician	[*the same stimulus*] "What is this? It ends with . . . " [*silently models the articulatory posture for the target sound.*]	The next trial; a partial modeling
Child	"Barn."	A correct response
Clinician	"There you go! You said *barn*, not *ban*."	Verbal praise
Clinician	[*the same stimulus*] "What is this?"	Typical question; evoked trial
Child	"Barn."	A correct response
Clinician	"Beautifully done! You are working very hard!"	Verbal praise

If the wrong responses persist on 4 to 5 evoked trials, reinstate partial or full modeling for a few trials, again fade the modeling, and re-present the evoked trials.

When the child meets the tentative learning criterion of 10 consecutively correct, nonimitated responses for a given stimulus item, move on to the next stimulus item. With this procedure, teach 6 to 8 exemplars shown on the following recording sheet. Use different exemplars as you see fit for a given child.

/rn/ in Word-Final Positions

Treatment Exemplars and Recording Sheet

Use stimuli from the **Stimulus Book,** *Volume 7.*

Print this page from CD or photocopy this page for your clinical use.

Name/Age:	Date:
Goal: Production of /rn/ in word-final positions with 90% accuracy when asked an evoking question while showing a stimulus.	Clinician:

Scoring: Correct: ✓   Incorrect or no response: X

Target skills	Discrete Trials														
	1	2	3	4	5	6	7	8	9	10	11	12	13	14	15
1. barn															
2. corn															
3. yarn															
4. farm															
5. horn															
6. acorn															
7. adorn															
8. newborn															

When the child has met the learning criterion of 10 consecutively correct evoked (nonimitated) responses for each of the 6 to 8 target exemplars, conduct a probe to see if the production has generalized to previously baserated but untrained exemplars.

If the probes do not meet the 90% correct criterion for untrained exemplars, teach additional exemplars and then probe again.

/rn/ in Word-Final Positions

Probe Protocols and Recording Sheet

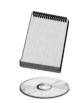

Use stimuli from the **Stimulus Book,** *Volume 7.*

Print this page from the CD or photocopy this page for your clinical use.

On the probes, present only the untrained exemplars (UT). When the child fails to meet the 90% correct probe criterion, either teach 2 to 4 new exemplars or give additional training trials on already trained stimuli. If needed, select new exemplars for probes. Probe at least 10 untrained exemplars. Alternate probes and treatment until the probe criterion is met.

Scripts for Probe Trials		Note
Clinician	[*untrained stimulus: popcorn*] "What is this?"	No modeling or prompts
Child	"popcoən."	A wrong probe response
Clinician	Scores the response as incorrect.	No corrective feedback
Clinician	[*untrained stimulus: unicorn*] "What is this?"	The second probe trial
Child	"A unicoən."	A wrong probe response
Clinician	Scores the response as incorrect.	No corrective feedback

Name:	Date:	Session #:
Age:	**Clinician:**	
Diagnosis: Articulation/Phonologic Disorder	**Word-final /rn/ probe**	
Untrained Stimuli	**Score: + correct; – incorrect or no responses**	
1. popcorn		
2. unicorn		
3. worn		
4. thorn		
5. born		
6. mourn		
7. torn		
8. long horn		
9. French horn		
10. fog horn		
11. airborne		
12. Capricorn		
Percent correct: (Criterion: 90%)		

If the child does not meet the probe criterion, give additional training on already trained exemplars or teach a few new exemplars. Subsequently, readminister the probe trials. When the child meets the 90% correct probe criterion for the exemplars, shift training to the sentence or conversational level or to another phoneme.

/rt/ in Word-Final Positions

Baserate Protocols

*Use stimuli from the **Stimulus Book, Volume 7**.*

At the beginning of each trial, place a relevant stimulus (an object, a picture, or a printed word if the child can read) in front of the child. Point to the stimulus as you ask an evoking question. Do not respond in any way to the child's correct, incorrect, or lack of responses.

Scripts For Evoked Baserate Trial		Note
Clinician	[*stimulus: heart*] "What is this?"	Evoked trial
Child	"hot."	Vowelization of /r/ in /rt/ cluster
Clinician	Pulls the stimulus toward her; records the response.	No corrective feedback
Clinician	[*stimulus: short*] "This girl is tall, but this girl is _____?"	The next evoked trial
Child	"shoǝt."	Vowelization of /r/ in /rt/ cluster
Clinician	Pulls the stimulus toward her; records the response.	No corrective feedback

Administer the modeled baserate trials only after completing the evoked trials on all 20 (or more) exemplars.

Scripts For Modeled Baserate Trial		Note
Clinician	[*stimulus: heart*] "What is this? Say, *heart*."	Modeled trial
Child	"Heart."	Correct response
Clinician	Pulls the stimulus toward her; records the response.	No reinforcement
Clinician	[*stimulus: short*] "This girl is short? Say, *short*."	The next modeled trial
Child	"shoǝt."	Vowelization of /r/ in /rt/ cluster
Clinician	Pulls the stimulus toward her; records the response.	No corrective feedback

Use the recording sheet with exemplars shown on the next page to establish the baserates; print it from the CD.

/rt/ in Word-Final Positions

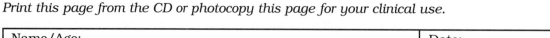

Baserate Exemplars and Recording Sheet

Use stimuli from the **Stimulus Book,** *Volume 7.*

Print this page from the CD or photocopy this page for your clinical use.

Name/Age:			Date:	
Goal: To establish the baserate production of /rt/ in word-final positions.			Clinician:	

Scoring: Correct: ✓   Incorrect or no response: X

/rt/ in word-final positions	Evoked	Modeled
1. heart		
2. short		
3. tart		
4. cart		
5. art		
6. distort		
7. passport		
8. tennis court		
9. air port		
10. pushcart		
11. dart		
12. part		
13. chart		
14. court		
15. fort		
16. seaport		
17. support		
18. resort		
19. oxcart		
20. report		
Percent correct baserate		

Replace or add new exemplars as you see fit for a given child. After establishing the baserates, begin production teaching. Follow the protocols given on the next page.

/rt/ in Word-Final Positions

Treatment Protocols

Use stimuli from the **Stimulus Book,** *Volume 7.*

Teach 6 to 8 exemplars using the following script.

Place a relevant stimulus (an object, a picture, or a printed word if the child can read) in front of the child and point to the stimulus as you ask an evoking question.

Scripts For Modeled Discrete Trial Training		Note
Clinician	[*stimulus: heart*] "What is this? Say, *heart*."	Modeling; the target vocally emphasized
Child	"hot."	A wrong response
Clinician	"No. That's not correct. You said *hot*, but it's a *heart*. You need to say the *r* sound before the *t* sound at the end of the word."	Corrective feedback
Clinician	[*the same stimulus*] "What is this? Say, *heart*. Don't forget the *r* before the *t* at the end, *heart*."	The next trial
Child	"Heart."	A correct response
Clinician	"Excellent! You didn't miss the *r* at the end of the word!"	Verbal praise

Repeat the trials until the child gives 5 consecutively correct, imitated responses.

When the child imitates 5 correct responses in sequence, fade the modeling.

Scripts For Fading the Modeling		Note
Clinician	[*stimulus: heart*] "What is this? Don't forget to say the *r* sound before the *t* sound at the end."	Only a prompt
Child	"hot."	A wrong response
Clinician	"I'm sorry, you forgot the *r* in the word! It's a *heart*, not *hot*. Put the *r* before the *t* at the end."	Corrective feedback
Clinician	[*the same stimulus*] "What is this? It ends with . . . " [*silently models the articulatory posture for the target sound.*]	The next trial; a partial modeling
Child	"Heart."	A correct response
Clinician	"That's great! You said *heart*, not *hot*.	Verbal praise
Clinician	[*the same stimulus*] "What is this?"	Typical question; evoked trial
Child	"Heart."	A correct response
Clinician	"I like it! You said it correctly!"	Verbal praise

If the wrong responses persist on 4 to 5 evoked trials, reinstate partial or full modeling for a few trials, again fade the modeling, and re-present the evoked trials.

When the child meets the tentative learning criterion of 10 consecutively correct, nonimitated responses for a given stimulus item, move on to the next stimulus item. With this procedure, teach 6 to 8 exemplars shown on the following recording sheet. Use different exemplars as you see fit for a given child.

/rt/ in Word-Final Positions

Treatment Exemplars and Recording Sheet

*Use stimuli from the **Stimulus Book, Volume 7**.*

Print this page from CD or photocopy this page for your clinical use.

Name/Age:	Date:
Goal: Production of /rt/ in word-final positions with 90% accuracy when asked an evoking question while showing a stimulus.	Clinician:

Scoring: Correct: ✓ Incorrect or no response: X

Target skills	Discrete Trials														
	1	2	3	4	5	6	7	8	9	10	11	12	13	14	15
1. heart															
2. short															
3. tart															
4. cart															
5. art															
6. airport															
7. passport															
8. tennis court															

When the child has met the learning criterion of 10 consecutively correct evoked (nonimitated) responses for each of the 6 to 8 target exemplars, conduct a probe to see if the production has generalized to previously baserated but untrained exemplars.

If the probes do not meet the 90% correct criterion for untrained exemplars, teach additional exemplars and then probe again.

/rt/ in Word-Final Positions

Probe Protocols and Recording Sheet

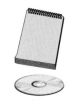

Use stimuli from the **Stimulus Book, Volume 7**.

Print this page from the CD or photocopy this page for your clinical use.

On the probes, present only the untrained exemplars (UT). When the child fails to meet the 90% correct probe criterion, either teach 2 to 4 new exemplars or give additional training trials on already trained stimuli. If needed, select new exemplars for probes. Probe at least 10 untrained exemplars. Alternate probes and treatment until the probe criterion is met.

Scripts for Probe Trials		Note
Clinician	[*untrained stimulus: airport*] "What is this?"	No modeling or prompts
Child	"No response."	Lack of generalization
Clinician	Scores it as *no response.*	No corrective feedback
Clinician	[*untrained stimulus: pushcart*] "What is this?"	The second probe trial
Child	"Pushcart."	A correct probe response
Clinician	Scores the response as correct.	No reinforcement

Name:	Date:	Session #:
Age:	**Clinician:**	
Diagnosis: Articulation/Phonologic Disorder	**Word-final /rt/ probe**	
Untrained Stimuli	**Score: + correct; – incorrect or no responses**	
1. airport		
2. pushcart		
3. dart		
4. part		
5. chart		
6. court		
7. fort		
8. seaport		
9. support		
10. resort		
11. oxcart		
12. report		
Percent correct: (Criterion: 90%)		

If the child does not meet the probe criterion, give additional training on already trained exemplars or teach a few new exemplars. Subsequently, readminister the probe trials. When the child meets the 90% correct probe criterion for the exemplars, shift training to the sentence or conversational level or to another phoneme.

/ks/ in Word-Final Positions

Baserate Protocols

Use stimuli from the **Stimulus Book,** *Volume 8.*

At the beginning of each trial, place a relevant stimulus (an object, a picture, or a printed word if the child can read) in front of the child. Point to the stimulus as you ask an evoking question. Do not respond in any way to the child's correct, incorrect, or lack of responses.

Scripts For Evoked Baserate Trial		Note
Clinician	[*stimulus: socks*] "What are these?"	Evoked trial
Child	"sots."	Substitution of /t/ for /k/ in /ks/ cluster
Clinician	Pulls the stimulus toward her; records the response.	No corrective feedback
Clinician	[*stimulus: bikes*] "What are these?"	The next evoked trial
Child	"bise."	Omission of /k/ in /ks/ cluster
Clinician	Pulls the stimulus toward her; records the response.	No corrective feedback

Administer the modeled baserate trials only after completing the evoked trials on all 20 (or more) exemplars.

Scripts For Modeled Baserate Trial		Note
Clinician	[*stimulus: socks*] "What are these? Say, *socks.*"	Modeled trial
Child	"Socks."	Correct response
Clinician	Pulls the stimulus toward her; records the response.	No reinforcement
Clinician	[*stimulus: bikes*] "What are these? Say, *bikes.*"	The next modeled trial
Child	"bise."	Omission of /k/ in /ks/ cluster
Clinician	Pulls the stimulus toward her; records the response.	No corrective feedback

Use the recording sheet with exemplars shown on the next page to establish the baserates; print it from the CD.

/ks/ in Word-Final Positions

Baserate Exemplars and Recording Sheet

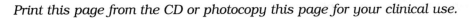

Use stimuli from the **Stimulus Book,** *Volume 8.*

Print this page from the CD or photocopy this page for your clinical use.

Name/Age:	Date:
Goal: To establish the baserate production of /ks/ in word-final positions.	Clinician:

Scoring: Correct: ✓   Incorrect or no response: X

/ks/ in word-final positions	Evoked	Modeled
1. socks		
2. bikes		
3. cheeks		
4. chicks		
5. fox		
6. icebox		
7. peacocks		
8. shamrocks		
9. artichokes		
10. toothpicks		
11. box		
12. ax		
13. sticks		
14. rocks		
15. blocks		
16. kayaks		
17. sandbox		
18. mailbox		
19. notebooks		
20. snowflakes		
Percent correct baserate		

Replace or add new exemplars as you see fit for a given child. After establishing the baserates, begin production teaching. Follow the protocols given on the next page.

/ks/ in Word-Final Positions

Treatment Protocols

*Use stimuli from the **Stimulus Book, Volume 8**.*

Teach 6 to 8 exemplars using the following script.

Place a relevant stimulus (an object, a picture, or a printed word if the child can read) in front of the child and point to the stimulus as you ask an evoking question.

Scripts For Modeled Discrete Trial Training		Note
Clinician	[*stimulus: socks*] "What are these? Say, so**cks**."	Modeling; the target vocally emphasized
Child	"sots."	A wrong response
Clinician	"No. That's not correct. You said *sots*, but it's so**cks**. You need to say the **k** sound, not the **t** sound, before the **s** at the end."	Corrective feedback
Clinician	[*the same stimulus*] "What are these? Say, so**cks**. Remember to say the **k** sound before the **s** at the end of the word so**cks**."	The next trial
Child	"Socks."	A correct response
Clinician	"Brilliant! You said the **k** sound before the **s** at the end. I knew you could do it!"	Verbal praise

Repeat the trials until the child gives 5 consecutively correct, imitated responses.

When the child imitates 5 correct responses in sequence, fade the modeling.

Scripts For Fading the Modeling		Note
Clinician	[*stimulus: socks*] "What are these? Don't forget to say the *k* sound before the *s* sound at the end."	Only a prompt
Child	"sots."	A wrong response
Clinician	"Bummer, you said the *t* sound before the *s* sound! They are *socks*, not *sots*. Say the *k* sound before the *s* at the end."	Corrective feedback
Clinician	[*the same stimulus*] "What are these? It ends with . . . " [*silently models the articulatory posture for the target sound.*]	The next trial; a partial modeling
Child	"Socks."	A correct response
Clinician	"That's terrific! You said socks, not sots."	Verbal praise
Clinician	[*the same stimulus*] "What are these?"	Typical question; evoked trial
Child	"Socks."	A correct response
Clinician	"Wow! You said it correctly!"	Verbal praise

If the wrong responses persist on 4 to 5 evoked trials, reinstate partial or full modeling for a few trials, again fade the modeling, and re-present the evoked trials.

When the child meets the tentative learning criterion of 10 consecutively correct, nonimitated responses for a given stimulus item, move on to the next stimulus item. With this procedure, teach 6 to 8 exemplars shown on the following recording sheet. Use different exemplars as you see fit for a given child.

/ks/ in Word-Final Positions

Treatment Exemplars and Recording Sheet

Use stimuli from the **Stimulus Book,** *Volume 8.*

Print this page from CD or photocopy this page for your clinical use.

Name/Age:	Date:
Goal: Production of /ks/ in word-final positions with 90% accuracy when asked an evoking question while showing a stimulus.	Clinician:

Scoring: Correct: ✓   Incorrect or no response: X

Target skills	Discrete Trials														
	1	2	3	4	5	6	7	8	9	10	11	12	13	14	15
1. socks															
2. bikes															
3. cheeks															
4. chick															
5. fox															
6. icebox															
7. peacocks															
8. shamrocks															

When the child has met the learning criterion of 10 consecutively correct evoked (nonimitated) responses for each of the 6 to 8 target exemplars, conduct a probe to see if the production has generalized to previously baserated but untrained exemplars.

If the probes do not meet the 90% correct criterion for untrained exemplars, teach additional exemplars and then probe again.

/ks/ in Word-Final Positions

Probe Protocols and Recording Sheet

Use stimuli from the **Stimulus Book,** *Volume 8.*

Print this page from the CD or photocopy this page for your clinical use.

On the probes, present only the untrained exemplars (UT). When the child fails to meet the 90% correct probe criterion, either teach 2 to 4 new exemplars or give additional training trials on already trained stimuli. If needed, select new exemplars for probes. Probe at least 10 untrained exemplars. Alternate probes and treatment until the probe criterion is met.

Scripts for Probe Trials		Note
Clinician	[*untrained stimulus: artichokes*] "What are these?"	No modeling or prompts
Child	"I think they're artichokes."	A correct, generalized response
Clinician	Scores the response as correct.	No reinforcement
Clinician	[*untrained stimulus: toothpicks*] "What are these?"	The second probe trial
Child	"toothpits."	A wrong probe response
Clinician	Scores the response as incorrect.	No corrective feedback

Name:	Date:	Session #:
Age:	**Clinician:**	
Diagnosis: Articulation/Phonologic Disorder	**Word-final /ks/ probe**	
Untrained Stimuli	**Score: + correct; – incorrect or no responses**	
1. artichokes		
2. toothpicks		
3. box		
4. ax		
5. stick		
6. rocks		
7. blocks		
8. kayaks		
9. sandbox		
10. mailbox		
11. notebooks		
12. snowflakes		
Percent correct: (Criterion: 90%)		

If the child does not meet the probe criterion, give additional training on already trained exemplars or teach a few new exemplars. Subsequently, readminister the probe trials. When the child meets the 90% correct probe criterion for the exemplars, shift training to the sentence or conversational level or to another phoneme.

/ns/ in Word-Final Positions

Baserate Protocols

Use stimuli from the **Stimulus Book,** *Volume 8.*

At the beginning of each trial, place a relevant stimulus (an object, a picture, or a printed word if the child can read) in front of the child. Point to the stimulus as you ask an evoking question. Do not respond in any way to the child's correct, incorrect, or lack of responses.

Scripts For Evoked Baserate Trial		Note
Clinician	[*stimulus: prince*] "A king's son is called a _____?"	Evoked trial
Child	"printh."	Lisping of /s/ in /ns/ cluster
Clinician	Pulls the stimulus toward her; records the response.	No corrective feedback
Clinician	[*stimulus: fence*] "What is this?"	The next evoked trial
Child	"fenth."	Lisping of /s/ in /ns/ cluster
Clinician	Pulls the stimulus toward her; records the response.	No corrective feedback

Administer the modeled baserate trials only after completing the evoked trials on all 20 (or more) exemplars.

Scripts For Modeled Baserate Trial		Note
Clinician	[*stimulus: prince*] "Who is this? Say, *prince.*"	Modeled trial
Child	"Prince."	Correct production
Clinician	Pulls the stimulus toward her; records the response.	No reinforcement
Clinician	[*stimulus: fence*] "What is this? Say, *fence.*"	The next modeled trial
Child	"Fence."	Correct production
Clinician	Pulls the stimulus toward her; records the response.	No reinforcement

Use the recording sheet with exemplars shown on the next page to establish the baserates; print it from the CD.

/ns/ in Word-Final Positions

Baserate Exemplars and Recording Sheet

Use stimuli from the **Stimulus Book,** *Volume 8.*

Print this page from the CD or photocopy this page for your clinical use.

Name/Age:	Date:
Goal: To establish the baserate production of /ns/ in word-final positions.	Clinician:

Scoring: Correct: ✓ Incorrect or no response: X

/ns/ in word-final positions	Evoked	Modeled
1. prince		
2. fence		
3. dance		
4. rinse		
5. bounce		
6. entrance		
7. silence		
8. audience		
9. ambulance		
10. patience		
11. prance		
12. science		
13. dense		
14. France		
15. glance		
16. balance		
17. incense		
18. appliance		
19. distance		
20. license		
Percent correct baserate		

Replace or add new exemplars as you see fit for a given child. After establishing the baserates, begin production teaching. Follow the protocols given on the next page.

/ns/ in Word-Final Positions

Treatment Protocols

Use stimuli from the **Stimulus Book,** *Volume 8.*

Teach 6 to 8 exemplars using the following script.

Place a relevant stimulus (an object, a picture, or a printed word if the child can read) in front of the child and point to the stimulus as you ask an evoking question.

Scripts For Modeled Discrete Trial Training		Note
Clinician	[*stimulus: prince*] "Who is this? Say, *pri**nce**.*"	Modeling; the target vocally emphasized
Child	"pri**nth**."	A wrong response
Clinician	"No. That's not correct. You said *pri**nth**,* but it's a *pri**nce**.* You need to say the **s** sound after the **n** sound."	Corrective feedback
Clinician	[*the same stimulus*] "What is this? Say, *pri**nce**.* Remember to say the **s** sound after the **n** sound at the end of the word."	The next trial
Child	"Prince."	A correct response
Clinician	"Super job! You said the **s** after the **n** at the end of the word!"	Verbal praise

Repeat the trials until the child gives 5 consecutively correct, imitated responses.

When the child imitates 5 correct responses in sequence, fade the modeling.

Scripts For Fading the Modeling		Note
Clinician	[*stimulus: prince*] "Who is this? Don't forget to say the s sound instead of the *th* sound after the *n*.	Only a prompt
Child	"pri**nth**."	A wrong response
Clinician	"Gee, you said the *th* instead of the *s*! It's a *prince*, not *printh*. Put the *s* sound after the *n* at the end."	Corrective feedback
Clinician	[*the same stimulus*] "Who is this? It ends with . . . " [*silently models the articulatory posture for the /ns/ cluster.*]	The next trial; a partial modeling
Child	"Prince."	A correct response
Clinician	"That's great! You said *prince*, not *printh*."	Verbal praise
Clinician	[*the same stimulus*] "Who is this?"	Typical question; evoked trial
Child	"Prince."	A correct response
Clinician	"Very good! You said it correctly! I knew you could do it."	Verbal praise

If the wrong responses persist on 4 to 5 evoked trials, reinstate partial or full modeling for a few trials, again fade the modeling, and re-present the evoked trials.

When the child meets the tentative learning criterion of 10 consecutively correct, nonimitated responses for a given stimulus item, move on to the next stimulus item. With this procedure, teach 6 to 8 exemplars shown on the following recording sheet. Use different exemplars as you see fit for a given child.

/ns/ in Word-Final Positions

Treatment Exemplars and Recording Sheet

Use stimuli from the **Stimulus Book,** *Volume 8.*

Print this page from CD or photocopy this page for your clinical use.

Name/Age:	Date:
Goal: Production of /ns/ in word-final positions with 90% accuracy when asked an evoking question while showing a stimulus.	Clinician:

Scoring: Correct: ✓   Incorrect or no response: X

Target skills	Discrete Trials														
	1	2	3	4	5	6	7	8	9	10	11	12	13	14	15
1. prince															
2. fence															
3. dance															
4. rinse															
5. bounce															
6. entrance															
7. silence															
8. audience															

When the child has met the learning criterion of 10 consecutively correct evoked (nonimitated) responses for each of the 6 to 8 target exemplars, conduct a probe to see if the production has generalized to previously baserated but untrained exemplars.

If the probes do not meet the 90% correct criterion for untrained exemplars, teach additional exemplars and then probe again.

/ns/ in Word-Final Positions

Probe Protocols and Recording Sheet

Use stimuli from the **Stimulus Book, *Volume 8*.**

Print this page from the CD or photocopy this page for your clinical use.

On the probes, present only the untrained exemplars (UT). When the child fails to meet the 90% correct probe criterion, either teach 2 to 4 new exemplars or give additional training trials on already trained stimuli. If needed, select new exemplars for probes. Probe at least 10 untrained exemplars. Alternate probes and treatment until the probe criterion is met.

Scripts for Probe Trials		Note
Clinician	[*untrained stimulus: ambulance*] "What is this?"	No modeling or prompts
Child	"Ambulance."	A correct, generalized response
Clinician	Scores the response as correct.	No reinforcement
Clinician	[*untrained stimulus: patience*] "When the food is not ready, you should show some _____?"	The second probe trial
Child	"patienth."	A wrong probe response
Clinician	Scores the response as incorrect.	No corrective feedback

Name:	Date:	Session #:
Age:	**Clinician:**	
Diagnosis: Articulation/Phonologic Disorder	**Word-final /ns/ probe**	
Untrained Stimuli	**Score: + correct; – incorrect or no responses**	
1. ambulance		
2. patience		
3. prance		
4. science		
5. dense		
6. France		
7. glance		
8. balance		
9. incense		
10. appliance		
11. distance		
12. license		
Percent correct: (Criterion: 90%)		

If the child does not meet the probe criterion, give additional training on already trained exemplars or teach a few new exemplars. Subsequently, readminister the probe trials. When the child meets the 90% correct probe criterion for the exemplars, shift training to the sentence or conversational level or to another phoneme.

/ps/ in Word-Final Positions
Baserate Protocols

Use stimuli from the **Stimulus Book, Volume 8**.

At the beginning of each trial, place a relevant stimulus (an object, a picture, or a printed word if the child can read) in front of the child. Point to the stimulus as you ask an evoking question. Do not respond in any way to the child's correct, incorrect, or lack of responses.

Scripts For Evoked Baserate Trial		Note
Clinician	[*stimulus: lips*] "What are these?"	Evoked trial
Child	"lip."	Omission of /s/ in /ps/ cluster
Clinician	Pulls the stimulus toward her; records the response.	No corrective feedback
Clinician	[*stimulus: ships*] "What are these?"	The next evoked trial
Child	"ship."	Omission of /s/ in /ps/ cluster
Clinician	Pulls the stimulus toward her; records the response.	No corrective feedback

Administer the modeled baserate trials only after completing the evoked trials on all 20 (or more) exemplars.

Scripts For Modeled Baserate Trial		Note
Clinician	[*stimulus: lips*] "What are these? Say, *lips.*"	Modeled trial
Child	"Lips."	Correct response
Clinician	Pulls the stimulus toward her; records the response.	No reinforcement
Clinician	[*stimulus: ships*] "What are these? Say, *ships.*"	The next modeled trial
Child	"Ships."	Correct response
Clinician	Pulls the stimulus toward her; records the response.	No reinforcement

Use the recording sheet with exemplars shown on the next page to establish the baserates; print it from the CD.

/ps/ in Word-Final Positions

Baserate Exemplars and Recording Sheet

Use stimuli from the **Stimulus Book,** *Volume 8.*

Print this page from the CD or photocopy this page for your clinical use.

Name/Age:	Date:
Goal: To establish the baserate production of /ps/ in word-final positions.	Clinician:

Scoring: Correct: ✓   Incorrect or no response: X

/ps/ in word-final positions	Evoked	Modeled
1. lips		
2. ships		
3. cups		
4. caps		
5. maps		
6. biceps		
7. collapse		
8. tulips		
9. raindrops		
10. cantaloupes		
11. pups		
12. scoops		
13. mops		
14. chips		
15. jumps		
16. antelopes		
17. push-ups		
18. turnips		
19. sit-ups		
20. forceps		
Percent correct baserate		

Replace or add new exemplars as you see fit for a given child. After establishing the baserates, begin production teaching. Follow the protocols given on the next page.

/ps/ in Word-Final Positions

Treatment Protocols

Use stimuli from the **Stimulus Book,** *Volume 8.*

Teach 6 to 8 exemplars using the following script.

Place a relevant stimulus (an object, a picture, or a printed word if the child can read) in front of the child and point to the stimulus as you ask an evoking question.

Scripts For Modeled Discrete Trial Training		Note
Clinician	[*stimulus: lip*] "What are these? Say, *li**ps**.*"	Modeling; the target vocally emphasized
Child	"lip."	A wrong response
Clinician	"No. That's not correct. You said *lip*, but it's *li**ps**. You need to say the **s** sound after the **p** at the end."	Corrective feedback
Clinician	[*the same stimulus*] "What are these? Say, *li**ps**. Don't forget the **s** at the end."	The next trial
Child	"Lips."	A correct response
Clinician	"I knew you could do it! You didn't miss the **s** at the end of the word!"	Verbal praise

Repeat the trials until the child gives 5 consecutively correct, imitated responses.

When the child imitates 5 correct responses in sequence, fade the modeling.

Scripts For Fading the Modeling		Note
Clinician	[*stimulus: lips*] "What are these? Don't forget to say the *s* after the *p* at the end."	Only a prompt
Child	"lip."	A wrong response
Clinician	"Oops, you forgot to say the *s* after the *p*! It's *lips*, not *lip*. Put the s at the end."	Corrective feedback
Clinician	[*the same stimulus*] "What are these? It ends with . . . " [*silently models the articulatory posture for the /ps/ cluster.*]	The next trial; a partial modeling
Child	"Lips."	A correct response
Clinician	"Bravo! You said *lips*, not *lip*."	Verbal praise
Clinician	[*the same stimulus*] "What are these?"	Typical question; evoked trial
Child	"Lips."	A correct response
Clinician	"Fantastic work! You said it correctly!"	Verbal praise

If the wrong responses persist on 4 to 5 evoked trials, reinstate partial or full modeling for a few trials, again fade the modeling, and re-present the evoked trials.

When the child meets the tentative learning criterion of 10 consecutively correct, nonimitated responses for a given stimulus item, move on to the next stimulus item. With this procedure, teach 6 to 8 exemplars shown on the following recording sheet. Use different exemplars as you see fit for a given child.

/ps/ in Word-Final Positions

Treatment Exemplars and Recording Sheet

Use stimuli from the **Stimulus Book,** *Volume 8.*

Print this page from CD or photocopy this page for your clinical use.

Name/Age:	Date:
Goal: Production of /ps/ in word-final positions with 90% accuracy when asked an evoking question while showing a stimulus.	Clinician:

Scoring: Correct: ✓   Incorrect or no response: X

Target skills	Discrete Trials														
	1	2	3	4	5	6	7	8	9	10	11	12	13	14	15
1. lips															
2. ships															
3. cups															
4. caps															
5. maps															
6. biceps															
7. collapse															
8. tulips															

When the child has met the learning criterion of 10 consecutively correct evoked (nonimitated) responses for each of the 6 to 8 target exemplars, conduct a probe to see if the production has generalized to previously baserated but untrained exemplars.

If the probes do not meet the 90% correct criterion for untrained exemplars, teach additional exemplars and then probe again.

<h1 style="text-align:center">/ps/ in Word-Final Positions</h1>

Probe Protocols and Recording Sheet

Use stimuli from the **Stimulus Book, Volume 8.**

Print this page from the CD or photocopy this page for your clinical use.

On the probes, present only the untrained exemplars (UT). When the child fails to meet the 90% correct probe criterion, either teach 2 to 4 new exemplars or give additional training trials on already trained stimuli. If needed, select new exemplars for probes. Probe at least 10 untrained exemplars. Alternate probes and treatment until the probe criterion is met.

Scripts for Probe Trials		Note
Clinician	[*untrained stimulus: raindrops*] "What are these?"	No modeling or prompts
Child	"raindrop."	A wrong probe response
Clinician	Scores the response as incorrect.	No corrective feedback
Clinician	[*untrained stimulus: cantaloupes*] "What are these?"	The second probe trial
Child	"cantaloupe."	A wrong probe response
Clinician	Scores the response as incorrect.	No corrective feedback

Name:	Date:	Session #:
Age:	**Clinician:**	
Diagnosis: Articulation/Phonologic Disorder	**Word-final /ps/ probe**	
Untrained Stimuli	**Score: + correct; – incorrect or no responses**	
1. raindrops		
2. cantaloupes		
3. pups		
4. scoops		
5. mops		
6. ships		
7. jumps		
8. antelopes		
9. push-ups		
10. turnips		
11. sit-ups		
12. forceps		
Percent correct: (Criterion: 90%)		

If the child does not meet the probe criterion, give additional training on already trained exemplars or teach a few new exemplars. Subsequently, readminister the probe trials. When the child meets the 90% correct probe criterion for the exemplars, shift training to the sentence or conversational level or to another phoneme.

/st/ in Word-Final Positions

Baserate Protocols

Use stimuli from the **Stimulus Book,** *Volume 8.*

At the beginning of each trial, place a relevant stimulus (an object, a picture, or a printed word if the child can read) in front of the child. Point to the stimulus as you ask an evoking question. Do not respond in any way to the child's correct, incorrect, or lack of responses.

Scripts For Evoked Baserate Trial		Note
Clinician	[*stimulus: nest*] "What is this?"	Evoked trial
Child	"nes."	Omission of /t/ in /st/ cluster
Clinician	Pulls the stimulus toward her; records the response.	No corrective feedback
Clinician	[*stimulus: wrist*] "What is this?"	The next evoked trial
Child	"wris."	Omission of /t/ in /st/ cluster
Clinician	Pulls the stimulus toward her; records the response.	No corrective feedback

Administer the modeled baserate trials only after completing the evoked trials on all 20 (or more) exemplars.

Scripts For Modeled Baserate Trial		Note
Clinician	[*stimulus: nest*] "What is this? Say, *nest*."	Modeled trial
Child	"nes."	Omission of /t/ in /st/ cluster
Clinician	Pulls the stimulus toward her; records the response.	No corrective feedback
Clinician	[*stimulus: wrist*] "What is this? Say, *wrist*."	The next modeled trial
Child	"Wrist."	Correct production
Clinician	Pulls the stimulus toward her; records the response.	No reinforcement

Use the recording sheet with exemplars shown on the next page to establish the baserates; print it from the CD.

/st/ in Word-Final Positions

Baserate Exemplars and Recording Sheet

Use stimuli from the **Stimulus Book,** *Volume 8.*

Print this page from the CD or photocopy this page for your clinical use.

Name/Age:	Date:
Goal: To establish the baserate production of /st/ in word-final positions.	Clinician:

Scoring: Correct: ✓   Incorrect or no response: X

/st/ in word-final positions	Evoked	Modeled
1. nest		
2. wrist		
3. ghost		
4. chest		
5. beast		
6. biggest		
7. forest		
8. smallest		
9. dentist		
10. breakfast		
11. toast		
12. vest		
13. fast		
14. waist		
15. west		
16. oldest		
17. artist		
18. locust		
19. longest		
20. gatepost		
Percent correct baserate		

Replace or add new exemplars as you see fit for a given child. After establishing the baserates, begin production teaching. Follow the protocols given on the next page.

/st/ in Word-Final Positions

Treatment Protocols

Use stimuli from the **Stimulus Book, Volume 8.**

Teach 6 to 8 exemplars using the following script.

Place a relevant stimulus in front of the child (an object, a picture, or a printed word if the child can read) and ask a question as you point to the stimulus.

Scripts For Modeled Discrete Trial Training		Note
Clinician	[*stimulus: nest*] "What is this? Say, *ne**st**.*"	Modeling; the target vocally emphasized
Child	"nes."	A wrong response
Clinician	"No. That's not correct. You said *nes*, but it's a *ne**st**.* You need to say the *t* sound after the *s* at the end, *ne**st**.*"	Corrective feedback
Clinician	[*the same stimulus*] "What is this? Say, *ne**st**.* Don't forget the *t* sound after the *s* sound at the end."	The next trial
Child	"Nest."	A correct response
Clinician	"Fabulous! You didn't miss the *t* this time!"	Verbal praise

Repeat the trials until the child gives 5 consecutively correct, imitated responses.

When the child imitates 5 correct responses in sequence, fade the modeling.

Scripts For Fading the Modeling		Note
Clinician	[*stimulus: nest*] "What is this? Don't forget the *t* after the *s* at the end."	Only a prompt
Child	"nes."	A wrong response
Clinician	"Uh, oh, you forgot the *t* after the *s*! It's a *nest*, not *nes*. Put the *t* at the end."	Corrective feedback
Clinician	[*the same stimulus*] "What is this? It ends with . . . " [*silently models the articulatory posture for the /st/ cluster.*]	The next trial; a partial modeling
Child	"Nest."	A correct response
Clinician	"You've got it! You said *nest*, not *nes*."	Verbal praise
Clinician	[*the same stimulus*] "What is this?"	Typical question; evoked trial
Child	"Nest."	A correct response
Clinician	"Way to go! You said it correctly!"	Verbal praise

If the wrong responses persist on 4 to 5 evoked trials, reinstate partial or full modeling for a few trials, again fade the modeling, and re-present the evoked trials.

When the child meets the tentative learning criterion of 10 consecutively correct, nonimitated responses for a given stimulus item, move on to the next stimulus item. With this procedure, teach 6 to 8 exemplars shown on the following recording sheet. Use different exemplars as you see fit for a given child.

/st/ in Word-Final Positions

Treatment Exemplars and Recording Sheet

Use stimuli from the **Stimulus Book,** *Volume 8.*

Print this page from CD or photocopy this page for your clinical use.

Name/Age:	Date:
Goal: Production of /st/ in word-final positions with 90% accuracy when asked an evoking question while showing a stimulus.	Clinician:

Scoring: Correct: ✓ Incorrect or no response: X

Target skills	Discrete Trials														
	1	2	3	4	5	6	7	8	9	10	11	12	13	14	15
1. nest															
2. wrist															
3. ghost															
4. chest															
5. beast															
6. biggest															
7. forest															
8. smallest															

When the child has met the learning criterion of 10 consecutively correct evoked (nonimitated) responses for each of the 6 to 8 target exemplars, conduct a probe to see if the production has generalized to previously baserated but untrained exemplars.

If the probes do not meet the 90% correct criterion for untrained exemplars, teach additional exemplars and then probe again.

/st/ in Word-Final Positions

Probe Protocols and Recording Sheet

Use stimuli from the **Stimulus Book,** *Volume 8.*

Print this page from the CD or photocopy this page for your clinical use.

On the probes, present only the untrained exemplars (UT). When the child fails to meet the 90% correct probe criterion, either teach 2 to 4 new exemplars or give additional training trials on already trained stimuli. If needed, select new exemplars for probes. Probe at least 10 untrained exemplars. Alternate probes and treatment until the probe criterion is met.

Scripts for Probe Trials		Note
Clinician	[*untrained stimulus: dentist*] "What is this?"	No modeling or prompts
Child	"A dentist."	A correct, generalized response
Clinician	Scores the response as correct.	No reinforcement
Clinician	[*untrained stimulus: breakfast*] "In the morning we eat _____?"	The second probe trial
Child	"breakfas."	A wrong probe response
Clinician	Scores the response as incorrect.	No corrective feedback

Name:	Date:	Session #:
Age:	**Clinician:**	
Diagnosis: Articulation/Phonologic Disorder	**Word-final /st/ probe**	
Untrained Stimuli	**Score: + correct; – incorrect or no responses**	
1. dentist		
2. breakfast		
3. toast		
4. vest		
5. fast		
6. waist		
7. west		
8. oldest		
9. artist		
10. locust		
11. longest		
12. gatepost		
Percent correct: (Criterion: 90%)		

If the child does not meet the probe criterion, give additional training on already trained exemplars or teach a few new exemplars. Subsequently, readminister the probe trials. When the child meets the 90% correct probe criterion for the exemplars, shift training to the sentence or conversational level or to another phoneme.

/ts/ in Word-Final Positions

Baserate Protocols

*Use stimuli from the **Stimulus Book, Volume 8**.*

At the beginning of each trial, place a relevant stimulus (an object, a picture, or a printed word if the child can read) in front of the child. Point to the stimulus as you ask an evoking question. Do not respond in any way to the child's correct, incorrect, or lack of responses.

Scripts For Evoked Baserate Trial		Note
Clinician	[*stimulus: goats*] "What are these?"	Evoked trial
Child	"goaks."	Substitution of /k/ for /t/ in /ks/ cluster
Clinician	Pulls the stimulus toward her; records the response.	No corrective feedback
Clinician	[*stimulus: bats*] "What are these?"	The next evoked trial
Child	"backs."	Substitution of /k/ for /t/ in /ks/ cluster
Clinician	Pulls the stimulus toward her; records the response.	No corrective feedback

Administer the modeled baserate trials only after completing the evoked trials on all 20 (or more) exemplars.

Scripts For Modeled Baserate Trial		Note
Clinician	[*stimulus: goats*] "What are these? Say, *goats*."	Modeled trial
Child	"goaks."	Substitution of /k/ for /s/ in /ks/ cluster
Clinician	Pulls the stimulus toward her; records the response.	No corrective feedback
Clinician	[*stimulus: bats*] "What are these? Say, *bats*."	The next modeled trial
Child	"backs."	Substitution of /k/ for /s/ in /ks/ cluster
Clinician	Pulls the stimulus toward her; records the response.	No corrective feedback

Use the recording sheet with exemplars shown on the next page to establish the baserates; print it from the CD.

/ts/ in Word-Final Positions

Baserate Exemplars and Recording Sheet

Use stimuli from the **Stimulus Book,** *Volume 8.*

Print this page from the CD or photocopy this page for your clinical use.

Name/Age:	Date:
Goal: To establish the baserate production of /ts/ in word-final positions.	Clinician:

Scoring: Correct: ✓   Incorrect or no response: X

/ts/ in word-final positions	Evoked	Modeled
1. goats		
2. bats		
3. plates		
4. boots		
5. pants		
6. biscuits		
7. carrots		
8. ice skates		
9. peanuts		
10. doughnuts		
11. pots		
12. boats		
13. seats		
14. spots		
15. roots		
16. violets		
17. pockets		
18. pirates		
19. planets		
20. tickets		
Percent correct baserate		

Replace or add new exemplars as you see fit for a given child. After establishing the baserates, begin production teaching. Follow the protocols given on the next page.

/ts/ in Word-Final Positions

Treatment Protocols

Use stimuli from the **Stimulus Book,** *Volume 8.*

Teach 6 to 8 exemplars using the following script.

Place a relevant stimulus in front of the child (an object, a picture, or a printed word if the child can read) and ask a question as you point to the stimulus.

Scripts For Modeled Discrete Trial Training		Note
Clinician	[*stimulus: goats*] "What are these? Say, *goats.*"	Modeling; the target vocally emphasized
Child	"goaks."	A wrong response
Clinician	"No. That's not right. You said *goaks*, but it's *goats*." You need to say the *t* sound, not the *k*, before the *s* sound at the end."	Corrective feedback
Clinician	[*the same stimulus*] "What are these? Say, *goats*. Don't forget to say the *t* sound before the *s* at the end, *goats*."	The next trial
Child	"Goats."	A correct response
Clinician	"Fabulous! You didn't miss the *t* this time!"	Verbal praise

Repeat the trials until the child gives 5 consecutively correct, imitated responses.

When the child imitates 5 correct responses in sequence, fade the modeling.

Scripts For Fading the Modeling		Note
Clinician	[*stimulus: goats*] "What are these? Don't forget to say the *t* sound before the *s* sound at the end."	Only a prompt
Child	"goaks."	A wrong response
Clinician	"Uh, oh, you said the *k* sound before the *s* sound! It's *goats*, not *goaks*. Put the *t* sound before the *s* sound at the end."	Corrective feedback
Clinician	[*the same stimulus*] "What are these? The word ends with . . . " [*silently models the articulatory posture for the /ts/cluster.*]	The next trial; a partial modeling
Child	"Goats."	A correct response
Clinician	"That's great! You said *goats*, not *goaks*."	Verbal praise
Clinician	[*the same stimulus*] "What are these?"	Typical question; evoked trial
Child	"Goats."	A correct response
Clinician	"Outstanding job! You said it correctly!"	Verbal praise

If the wrong responses persist on 4 to 5 evoked trials, reinstate partial or full modeling for a few trials, again fade the modeling, and re-present the evoked trials.

When the child meets the tentative learning criterion of 10 consecutively correct, nonimitated responses for a given stimulus item, move on to the next stimulus item. With this procedure, teach 6 to 8 exemplars shown on the following recording sheet. Use different exemplars as you see fit for a given child.

/ts/ in Word-Final Positions

Treatment Exemplars and Recording Sheet

*Use stimuli from the **Stimulus Book, Volume 8**.*

Print this page from CD or photocopy this page for your clinical use.

Name/Age:	Date:
Goal: Production of /ts/ in word-final positions with 90% accuracy when asked an evoking question while showing a stimulus.	Clinician:

Scoring: Correct: ✓   Incorrect or no response: X

Target skills	Discrete Trials														
	1	2	3	4	5	6	7	8	9	10	11	12	13	14	15
1. goats															
2. bats															
3. plates															
4. boots															
5. pants															
6. biscuits															
7. carrots															
8. ice skates															

When the child has met the learning criterion of 10 consecutively correct evoked (nonimitated) responses for each of the 6 to 8 target exemplars, conduct a probe to see if the production has generalized to previously baserated but untrained exemplars.

If the probes do not meet the 90% correct criterion for untrained exemplars, teach additional exemplars and then probe again.

/ts/ in Word-Final Positions

Probe Protocols and Recording Sheet

Use stimuli from the **Stimulus Book,** *Volume 8.*

Print this page from the CD or photocopy this page for your clinical use.

On the probes, present only the untrained exemplars (UT). When the child fails to meet the 90% correct probe criterion, either teach 2 to 4 new exemplars or give additional training trials on already trained stimuli. If needed, select new exemplars for probes. Probe at least 10 untrained exemplars. Alternate probes and treatment until the probe criterion is met.

Scripts for Probe Trials		Note
Clinician	[*untrained stimulus: peanuts*] "What are these?"	No modeling or prompts
Child	"Peanuts."	A correct, generalized response
Clinician	Scores the response as correct.	No reinforcement
Clinician	[*untrained stimulus: doughnuts*] "What are these?"	The second probe trial
Child	"Doughnuts."	A correct, generalized response
Clinician	Scores the response as correct.	No reinforcement

Name:	Date:	Session #:
Age:	Clinician:	
Diagnosis: Articulation/Phonologic Disorder	Word-final /ts/ probe	
Untrained Stimuli	**Score: + correct; – incorrect or no responses**	
1. peanuts		
2. doughnuts		
3. pots		
4. boats		
5. seats		
6. spots		
7. roots		
8. violets		
9. pockets		
10. pirates		
11. planets		
12. tickets		
Percent correct: (Criterion: 90%)		

If the child does not meet the probe criterion, give additional training on already trained exemplars or teach a few new exemplars. Subsequently, readminister the probe trials. When the child meets the 90% correct probe criterion for the exemplars, shift training to the sentence or conversational level or to another phoneme.

/bz/ in Word-Final Positions

Baserate Protocols

Use stimuli from the **Stimulus Book,** *Volume 8.*

At the beginning of each trial, place a relevant stimulus (an object, a picture, or a printed word if the child can read) in front of the child. Point to the stimulus as you ask an evoking question. Do not respond in any way to the child's correct, incorrect, or lack of responses.

Scripts For Evoked Baserate Trial		Note
Clinician	[*stimulus: bibs*] "What are these?"	Evoked trial
Child	"bib."	Omission of /z/ in /bz/ cluster
Clinician	Pulls the stimulus toward her; records the response.	No corrective feedback
Clinician	[*stimulus: cubs*] "What are these?"	The next evoked trial
Child	"cub."	Omission of /z/ in /bz/ cluster
Clinician	Pulls the stimulus toward her; records the response.	No corrective feedback

Administer the modeled baserate trials only after completing the evoked trials on all 20 (or more) exemplars.

Scripts For Modeled Baserate Trial		Note
Clinician	[*stimulus: bibs*] "What are these? Say, *bibs*."	Modeled trial
Child	"bib."	Omission of /z/ in /bz/ cluster
Clinician	Pulls the stimulus toward her; records the response.	No corrective feedback
Clinician	[*stimulus: cubs*] "What are these? Say, *cubs*."	The next modeled trial
Child	"cub."	Omission of /z/ in /bz/ cluster
Clinician	Pulls the stimulus toward her; records the response.	No corrective feedback

Use the recording sheet with exemplars shown on the next page to establish the baserates; print it from the CD.

/bz/ in Word-Final Positions

Baserate Exemplars and Recording Sheet

Use stimuli from the **Stimulus Book,** *Volume 8.*

Print this page from the CD or photocopy this page for your clinical use.

Name/Age:	Date:
Goal: To establish the baserate production of /bz/ in word-final positions.	Clinician:

Scoring: Correct: ✓   Incorrect or no response: X

/bz/ in word-final positions	Evoked	Modeled
1. bibs		
2. cubs		
3. knobs		
4. crabs		
5. ribs		
6. earlobes		
7. cobwebs		
8. golf clubs		
9. bathrobes		
10. bathtubs		
11. cubes		
12. webs		
13. robes		
14. tubs		
15. tubes		
16. doorknobs		
17. ice cubes		
18. bear cubs		
19. spareribs		
20. sand crabs		
Percent correct baserate		

Replace or add new exemplars as you see fit for a given child. After establishing the baserates, begin production teaching. Follow the protocols given on the next page.

/bz/ in Word-Final Positions

Treatment Protocols

Use stimuli from the **Stimulus Book,** *Volume 8.*

Teach 6 to 8 exemplars using the following script.

Place a relevant stimulus (an object, a picture, or a printed word if the child can read) in front of the child and point to the stimulus as you ask an evoking question.

Scripts For Modeled Discrete Trial Training		Note
Clinician	[*stimulus: bibs*] "What are these? Say, *bi**bs**.*"	Modeling; the target vocally emphasized
Child	"bib."	A wrong response
Clinician	"I'm sorry. That's not right. You said *bib*, but it's *bi**bs**. You need to say the **/z/** sound after the **b** sound at the end."	Corrective feedback
Clinician	[*the same stimulus*] "What are these? Say, *bi**bs**. Don't forget the **/z/** sound after the **b** at the end."	The next trial
Child	"Bibs."	A correct response
Clinician	"Excellent! You didn't miss the **/z/** at the end of the word!"	Verbal praise

Repeat the trials until the child gives 5 consecutively correct, imitated responses.

When the child imitates 5 correct responses in sequence, fade the modeling.

Scripts For Fading the Modeling		Note
Clinician	[*stimulus: bibs*] "What are these? Don't forget to say the /z/ sound after the *b* at the end."	Only a prompt
Child	"bib."	A wrong response
Clinician	"Oops, you forgot the /z/! It's *bibs*, not *bib*. Put the /z/ at the end."	Corrective feedback
Clinician	[*the same stimulus*] "What are these? The word ends with . . . " [*silently models the articulatory posture for the /bz/ cluster.*]	The next trial; a partial modeling
Child	"Bibs."	A correct response
Clinician	"Very good! You said *bibs*, not *bib*."	Verbal praise
Clinician	[*the same stimulus*] "What are these?"	Typical question; evoked trial
Child	"Bibs."	A correct response
Clinician	"Thumbs up! You said it perfectly!"	Verbal praise

If the wrong responses persist on 4 to 5 evoked trials, reinstate partial or full modeling for a few trials, again fade the modeling, and re-present the evoked trials.

When the child meets the tentative learning criterion of 10 consecutively correct, nonimitated responses for a given stimulus item, move on to the next stimulus item. With this procedure, teach 6 to 8 exemplars shown on the following recording sheet. Use different exemplars as you see fit for a given child.

/bz/ in Word-Final Positions

Treatment Exemplars and Recording Sheet

*Use stimuli from the **Stimulus Book, Volume 8**.*

Print this page from CD or photocopy this page for your clinical use.

Name/Age:	Date:
Goal: Production of /bz/ in word-final positions with 90% accuracy when asked an evoking question while showing a stimulus.	Clinician:

Scoring: Correct: ✓   Incorrect or no response: X

Target skills	Discrete Trials														
	1	2	3	4	5	6	7	8	9	10	11	12	13	14	15
1. bibs															
2. cubs															
3. knobs															
4. crabs															
5. ribs															
6. earlobes															
7. cobwebs															
8. golf clubs															

When the child has met the learning criterion of 10 consecutively correct evoked (nonimitated) responses for each of the 6 to 8 target exemplars, conduct a probe to see if the production has generalized to previously baserated but untrained exemplars.

If the probes do not meet the 90% correct criterion for untrained exemplars, teach additional exemplars and then probe again.

/bz/ in Word-Final Positions

Probe Protocols and Recording Sheet

Use stimuli from the **Stimulus Book,** *Volume 8.*

Print this page from the CD or photocopy this page for your clinical use.

On the probes, present only the untrained exemplars (UT). When the child fails to meet the 90% correct probe criterion, either teach 2 to 4 new exemplars or give additional training trials on already trained stimuli. If needed, select new exemplars for probes. Probe at least 10 untrained exemplars. Alternate probes and treatment until the probe criterion is met.

Scripts for Probe Trials		Note
Clinician	[*untrained stimulus: bathrobes*] "What are these?"	No modeling or prompts
Child	"bathrobes."	A correct, generalized response
Clinician	Scores the response as correct.	No reinforcement
Clinician	[*untrained stimulus: bathtubs*] "What are these?"	The second probe trial
Child	"bathtubs."	A correct, generalized response
Clinician	Scores the response as correct.	No reinforcement

Name:	Date:	Session #:
Age:	**Clinician:**	
Diagnosis: Articulation/Phonologic Disorder	**Word-final /bz/ probe**	
Untrained Stimuli	**Score: + correct; – incorrect or no responses**	
1. bathrobes		
2. bathtubs		
3. cubes		
4. webs		
5. robes		
6. tubs		
7. tubes		
8. doorknobs		
9. ice cubes		
10. bear cubs		
11. spear ribs		
12. sand crabs		
Percent correct: (Criterion: 90%)		

If the child does not meet the probe criterion, give additional training on already trained exemplars or teach a few new exemplars. Subsequently, readminister the probe trials. When the child meets the 90% correct probe criterion for the exemplars, shift training to the sentence or conversational level or to another phoneme.

/dz/ in Word-Final Positions

Baserate Protocols

Use stimuli from the **Stimulus Book, Volume 8**.

At the beginning of each trial, place a relevant stimulus (an object, a picture, or a printed word if the child can read) in front of the child. Point to the stimulus as you ask an evoking question. Do not respond in any way to the child's correct, incorrect, or lack of responses.

Scripts For Evoked Baserate Trial		Note
Clinician	[*stimulus: kids*] "What are these?"	Evoked trial
Child	"kith."	Substitution of /θ/ for /dz/ cluster
Clinician	Pulls the stimulus toward her; records the response.	No corrective feedback
Clinician	[*stimulus: toads*] "What are these?"	The next evoked trial
Child	"tothe."	Substitution of /θ/ for /dz/ cluster
Clinician	Pulls the stimulus toward her; records the response.	No corrective feedback

Administer the modeled baserate trials only after completing the evoked trials on all 20 (or more) exemplars.

Scripts For Modeled Baserate Trial		Note
Clinician	[*stimulus: kids*] "What are these? Say, *kids*."	Modeled trial
Child	"kiz."	Omission of /d/ in /dz/ cluster
Clinician	Pulls the stimulus toward her; records the response.	No corrective feedback
Clinician	[*stimulus: toads*] "What is this? Say, *toads*."	The next modeled trial
Child	"toes."	Omission of /d/ in /dz/ cluster
Clinician	Pulls the stimulus toward her; records the response.	No corrective feedback

Use the recording sheet with exemplars shown on the next page to establish the baserates; print it from the CD.

/dz/ in Word-Final Positions

Baserate Exemplars and Recording Sheet

Use stimuli from the **Stimulus Book,** *Volume 8.*

Print this page from the CD or photocopy this page for your clinical use.

Name/Age:	Date:
Goal: To establish the baserate production of /dz/ in word-final positions.	Clinician:

Scoring: Correct: ✓   Incorrect or no response: X

/dz/ in word-final positions	Evoked	Modeled
1. kids		
2. toads		
3. slides		
4. lids		
5. seeds		
6. rides		
7. weeds		
8. grades		
9. woods		
10. beads		
11. adds		
12. sheds		
13. shades		
14. suds		
15. loads		
16. crowds		
17. heads		
18. lads		
19. feeds		
20. reads		
Percent correct baserate		

Replace or add new exemplars as you see fit for a given child. After establishing the baserates, begin production teaching. Follow the protocols given on the next page.

/dz/ in Word-Final Positions

Treatment Protocols

Use stimuli from the **Stimulus Book, Volume 8.**

Teach 6 to 8 exemplars using the following script.

Place a relevant stimulus (an object, a picture, or a printed word if the child can read) in front of the child and point to the stimulus as you ask an evoking question.

Scripts For Modeled Discrete Trial Training		Note
Clinician	[*stimulus: kids*] "What are these? Say, *ki**ds**.*"	Modeling; the target vocally emphasized
Child	"kiz."	A wrong response
Clinician	"No. That's not correct. You said *kiz*, but it's *ki**ds**. You need to say the **d** sound before the /z/ at the end, *ki**ds**.*"	Corrective feedback
Clinician	[*the same stimulus*] "What are these? Say, *ki**ds**. Don't forget to say the **d** sound before the /z/ at the end."	The next trial
Child	"Kids."	A correct response
Clinician	"You've got it! You didn't forget the **d** sound this time."	Verbal praise

Repeat the trials until the child gives 5 consecutively correct, imitated responses.

When the child imitates 5 correct responses in sequence, fade the modeling.

Scripts For Fading the Modeling		Note
Clinician	[*stimulus: kids*] "What are these? Don't forget the *d* before the /z/ at the end."	Only a prompt
Child	"kiz."	A wrong response
Clinician	"Bummer, you forgot the *d* sound before the /z/! It's *kids*, not *kiz*. Say the *d* before the /z/ at the end."	Corrective feedback
Clinician	[*the same stimulus*] "What are these? The word ends with . . . " [*silently models the articulatory posture for the /dz/ cluster.*]	The next trial; a partial modeling
Child	"Kids."	A correct response
Clinician	"That's great! You said *kids*, not *kiz*."	Verbal praise
Clinician	[*the same stimulus*] "What are these?"	Typical question; evoked trial
Child	"Kids."	A correct response
Clinician	"Spectacular! You said it perfectly! I knew you could do it."	Verbal praise

If the wrong responses persist on 4 to 5 evoked trials, reinstate partial or full modeling for a few trials, again fade the modeling, and re-present the evoked trials.

When the child meets the tentative learning criterion of 10 consecutively correct, nonimitated responses for a given stimulus item, move on to the next stimulus item. With this procedure, teach 6 to 8 exemplars shown on the following recording sheet. Use different exemplars as you see fit for a given child.

/dz/ in Word-Final Positions

Treatment Exemplars and Recording Sheet

Use stimuli from the **Stimulus Book,** *Volume 8.*

Print this page from CD or photocopy this page for your clinical use.

Name/Age:	Date:
Goal: Production of /dz/ in word-final positions with 90% accuracy when asked an evoking question while showing a stimulus.	Clinician:

Scoring: Correct: ✓   Incorrect or no response: X

Target skills	Discrete Trials														
	1	2	3	4	5	6	7	8	9	10	11	12	13	14	15
1. kids															
2. toads															
3. slides															
4. lids															
5. seeds															
6. rides															
7. weeds															
8. grades															

When the child has met the learning criterion of 10 consecutively correct evoked (nonimitated) responses for each of the 6 to 8 target exemplars, conduct a probe to see if the production has generalized to previously baserated but untrained exemplars.

If the probes do not meet the 90% correct criterion for untrained exemplars, teach additional exemplars and then probe again.

/dz/ in Word-Final Positions

Probe Protocols and Recording Sheet

Use stimuli from the **Stimulus Book, Volume 8.**

Print this page from the CD or photocopy this page for your clinical use.

On the probes, present only the untrained exemplars (UT). When the child fails to meet the 90% correct probe criterion, either teach 2 to 4 new exemplars or give additional training trials on already trained stimuli. If needed, select new exemplars for probes. Probe at least 10 untrained exemplars. Alternate probes and treatment until the probe criterion is met.

Scripts for Probe Trials		Note
Clinician	[*untrained stimulus: woods*] "Bears that don't live in the zoo live in the _____?"	No modeling or prompts
Child	"Woods."	A correct, generalized response
Clinician	Scores the response as correct.	No reinforcement
Clinician	[*untrained stimulus: beads*] "What are these?"	The second probe trial
Child	"Beads."	A correct, generalized response
Clinician	Scores the response as correct.	No reinforcement

Name:	Date:	Session #:
Age:	**Clinician:**	
Diagnosis: Articulation/Phonologic Disorder	**Word-final /dz/ probe**	
Untrained Stimuli	**Score: + correct; – incorrect or no responses**	
1. woods		
2. beads		
3. adds		
4. sheds		
5. shades		
6. suds		
7. loads		
8. crowds		
9. heads		
10. lads		
11. feeds		
12. reads		
Percent correct: (Criterion: 90%)		

If the child does not meet the probe criterion, give additional training on already trained exemplars or teach a few new exemplars. Subsequently, readminister the probe trials. When the child meets the 90% correct probe criterion for the exemplars, shift training to the sentence or conversational level or to another phoneme.

/gz/ in Word-Final Positions

Baserate Protocols

*Use stimuli from the **Stimulus Book, Volume 8**.*

At the beginning of each trial, place a relevant stimulus (an object, a picture, or a printed word if the child can read) in front of the child. Point to the stimulus as you ask an evoking question. Do not respond in any way to the child's correct, incorrect, or lack of responses.

Scripts For Evoked Baserate Trial		Note
Clinician	[*stimulus: pigs*] "What are these?"	Evoked trial
Child	"pids."	Substitution of /d/ for /g/ in /gz/ cluster
Clinician	Pulls the stimulus toward her; records the response.	No corrective feedback
Clinician	[*stimulus: dogs*] "What are these?"	The next evoked trial
Child	"dods."	Substitution of /d/ for /g/ in /gz/ cluster
Clinician	Pulls the stimulus toward her; records the response.	No corrective feedback

Administer the modeled baserate trials only after completing the evoked trials on all 20 (or more) exemplars.

Scripts For Modeled Baserate Trial		Note
Clinician	[*stimulus: pigs*] "What are these? Say, *pigs*."	Modeled trial
Child	"pids."	Substitution of /d/ for /g/ in /gz/ cluster
Cliician	Pulls the stimulus toward her; records the response.	No corrective feedback
Clinician	[*stimulus: dogs*] "What are these? Say, *dogs*."	The next modeled trial
Child	"Dogs."	Correct response
Clinician	Pulls the stimulus toward her; records the response.	No reinforcement

Use the recording sheet with exemplars shown on the next page to establish the baserates; print it from the CD.

/gz/ in Word-Final Positions

Baserate Exemplars and Recording Sheet

Use stimuli from the **Stimulus Book,** *Volume 8.*

Print this page from the CD or photocopy this page for your clinical use.

Name/Age:	Date:
Goal: To establish the baserate production of /gz/ in word-final positions.	Clinician:

Scoring: Correct: ✓   Incorrect or no response: X

/gz/ in word-final positions	Evoked	Modeled
1. pigs		
2. dogs		
3. legs		
4. jogs		
5. hugs		
6. bags		
7. bugs		
8. digs		
9. wigs		
10. eggs		
11. wags		
12. tugs		
13. mugs		
14. pegs		
15. rags		
16. lugs		
17. sags		
18. begs		
19. rugs		
20. jugs		
Percent correct baserate		

Replace or add new exemplars as you see fit for a given child. After establishing the baserates, begin production teaching. Follow the protocols given on the next page.

/gz/ in Word-Final Positions

Treatment Protocols

Use stimuli from the **Stimulus Book,** *Volume 8.*

Teach 6 to 8 exemplars using the following script.

Place a relevant stimulus in front of the child (an object, a picture, or a printed word if the child can read) and ask a question as you point to the stimulus.

Scripts For Modeled Discrete Trial Training		Note
Clinician	[*stimulus: pigs*] "What are these? Say, *pigs.*"	Modeling; the target vocally emphasized
Child	"pids."	A wrong response
Clinician	"No. That's not correct. You said *pids*, but it's *pigs*. You need to say the ***g*** sound, not the *d* sound before the /z/."	Corrective feedback
Clinician	[*the same stimulus*] "What are these? Say, *pigs*. Don't forget to say the ***g*** sound before the /z/ at the end of the word."	The next trial
Child	"Pigs."	A correct response
Clinician	"I knew you could do it! You said the ***g*** sound before the /z/.	Verbal praise

Repeat the trials until the child gives 5 consecutively correct, imitated responses.

When the child imitates 5 correct responses in sequence, fade the modeling.

Scripts For Fading the Modeling		Note
Clinician	[*stimulus: pigs*] "What are these? Don't forget the *g* sound before the *s* at the end."	Only a prompt
Child	"pids."	A wrong response
Clinician	"Gee, you said the *d* instead of the *g* sound! It's *pigs*, not *pids*. Remember to say the *g* sound before the /z/ at the end."	Corrective feedback
Clinician	[*the same stimulus*] "What are these? The word ends with . . . " [*silently models the articulatory posture for the /gz/ cluster.*]	The next trial; a partial modeling
Child	"Pigs."	A correct response
Clinician	"That's great! You said *pigs*, not *pids*."	Verbal praise
Clinician	[*the same stimulus*] "What are these?"	Typical question; evoked trial
Child	"Pigs."	A correct response
Clinician	"Stupendous! You said it correctly!"	Verbal praise

If the wrong responses persist on 4 to 5 evoked trials, reinstate partial or full modeling for a few trials, again fade the modeling, and re-present the evoked trials.

When the child meets the tentative learning criterion of 10 consecutively correct, nonimitated responses for a given stimulus item, move on to the next stimulus item. With this procedure, teach 6 to 8 exemplars shown on the following recording sheet. Use different exemplars as you see fit for a given child.

/gz/ in Word-Final Positions

Treatment Exemplars and Recording Sheet

Use stimuli from the **Stimulus Book,** *Volume 8.*

Print this page from CD or photocopy this page for your clinical use.

Name/Age:	Date:
Goal: Production of /gz/ in word-final positions with 90% accuracy when asked an evoking question while showing a stimulus.	Clinician:

Scoring: Correct: ✓   Incorrect or no response: X

Target skills	Discrete Trials														
	1	2	3	4	5	6	7	8	9	10	11	12	13	14	15
1. pigs															
2. dogs															
3. legs															
4. jogs															
5. hugs															
6. bags															
7. bugs															
8. digs															

When the child has met the learning criterion of 10 consecutively correct evoked (nonimitated) responses for each of the 6 to 8 target exemplars, conduct a probe to see if the production has generalized to previously baserated but untrained exemplars.

If the probes do not meet the 90% correct criterion for untrained exemplars, teach additional exemplars and then probe again.

/gz/ in Word-Final Positions

Probe Protocols and Recording Sheet

Use stimuli from the **Stimulus Book,** *Volume 8.*

Print this page from the CD or photocopy this page for your clinical use.

On the probes, present only the untrained exemplars (UT). When the child fails to meet the 90% correct probe criterion, either teach 2 to 4 new exemplars or give additional training trials on already trained stimuli. If needed, select new exemplars for probes. Probe at least 10 untrained exemplars. Alternate probes and treatment until the probe criterion is met.

Scripts for Probe Trials		Note
Clinician	[*untrained stimulus: wigs*] "What are these?"	No modeling or prompts
Child	"wids."	A wrong probe response
Clinician	Scores the response as incorrect.	No corrective feedback
Clinician	[*untrained stimulus: eggs*] "What are these?"	The second probe trial
Child	"eds."	A wrong probe response
Clinician	Scores the response as incorrect.	No corrective feedback

Name:	Date:	Session #:
Age:	**Clinician:**	
Diagnosis: Articulation/Phonologic Disorder	**Word-final /gz/ probe**	
Untrained Stimuli	**Score: + correct; – incorrect or no responses**	
1. wigs		
2. eggs		
3. wags		
4. tugs		
5. mugs		
6. pegs		
7. rags		
8. lugs		
9. sags		
10. begs		
11. rugs		
12. jugs		
Percent correct: (Criterion: 90%)		

If the child does not meet the probe criterion, give additional training on already trained exemplars or teach a few new exemplars. Subsequently, readminister the probe trials. When the child meets the 90% correct probe criterion for the exemplars, shift training to the sentence or conversational level or to another phoneme.

/mz/ in Word-Final Positions

Baserate Protocols

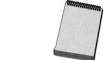

Use stimuli from the **Stimulus Book,** *Volume 8.*

At the beginning of each trial, place a relevant stimulus (an object, a picture, or a printed word if the child can read) in front of the child. Point to the stimulus as you ask an evoking question. Do not respond in any way to the child's correct, incorrect, or lack of responses.

Scripts For Evoked Baserate Trial		Note
Clinician	[*stimulus: thumbs*] "What are these?"	Evoked trial
Child	"thumb."	Omission of /z/ in /mz/ cluster
Clinician	Pulls the stimulus toward her; records the response.	No corrective feedback
Clinician	[*stimulus: clams*] "What are these?"	The next evoked trial
Child	"I don't know."	Does not know word
Clinician	Pulls the stimulus toward her; records the response. Notes that child does not know word.	No corrective feedback

Administer the modeled baserate trials only after completing the evoked trials on all 20 (or more) exemplars.

Scripts For Modeled Baserate Trial		Note
Clinician	[*stimulus: thumbs*] "What are these? Say, *thumbs.*"	Modeled trial
Child	"Thumbs."	Correct response
Clinician	Pulls the stimulus toward her; records the response.	No reinforcement
Clinician	[*stimulus: clams*] "What are these? Say, *clams.*"	The next modeled trial
Child	"Clams."	Correct response
Clinician	Pulls the stimulus toward her; records the response.	No reinforcement

Use the recording sheet with exemplars shown on the next page to establish the baserates; print it from the CD.

/mz / in Word-Final Positions

Baserate Exemplars and Recording Sheet

Use stimuli from the **Stimulus Book,** *Volume 8.*

Print this page from the CD or photocopy this page for your clinical use.

Name/Age:	Date:
Goal: To establish the baserate production of /mz/ in word-final positions.	Clinician:

Scoring: Correct: ✓   Incorrect or no response: X

/mz/ in word-final positions	Evoked	Modeled
1. thumbs		
2. clams		
3. climbs		
4. dimes		
5. charms		
6. wind chimes		
7. bedrooms		
8. daydreams		
9. lambs		
10. games		
11. gums		
12. limes		
13. fumes		
14. palms		
15. chimes		
16. rooms		
17. beams		
18. teams		
19. rims		
20. exams		
Percent correct baserate		

Replace or add new exemplars as you see fit for a given child. After establishing the baserates, begin production teaching. Follow the protocols given on the next page.

/mz/ in Word-Final Positions

Treatment Protocols

*Use stimuli from the **Stimulus Book, Volume 8**.*

Teach 6 to 8 exemplars using the following script.

Place a relevant stimulus (an object, a picture, or a printed word if the child can read) in front of the child and point to the stimulus as you ask an evoking question.

Scripts For Modeled Discrete Trial Training		Note
Clinician	[*stimulus: thumbs*] "What are these? Say, *thu**mbs**.*"	Modeling; the target vocally emphasized
Child	"thumb."	A wrong response
Clinician	"No. That's not correct. You said *thumb*, but it's *thu**mbs***. There are two thumbs so you need to say the **/z/** sound after the **m** at the end."	Corrective feedback
Clinician	[*the same stimulus*] "What are these? Say, *thu**mbs**.*" Don't forget the **/z/** after the **m** at the end."	The next trial
Child	"Thumbs."	A correct response
Clinician	"Excellent! You remembered to say the **/z/** after the **m** this time. You said *thu**mbs**.*"	Verbal praise

Repeat the trials until the child gives 5 consecutively correct, imitated responses.

When the child imitates 5 correct responses in sequence, fade the modeling.

Scripts For Fading the Modeling		Note
Clinician	[*stimulus: thumbs*] "What are these? Don't forget the /z/ after the m at the end."	Only a prompt
Child	"thumb."	A wrong response
Clinician	"Oh, oh, you forgot the /z/! It's two *thumbs*, not one *thumb*. Put the /z/ after the m at the end."	Corrective feedback
Clinician	[*the same stimulus*] "What are these? The word ends with . . ." [*silently models the articulatory posture for the /mz/ cluster.*]	The next trial; a partial modeling
Child	"Thumbs."	A correct response
Clinician	"That's great! You said *thumbs*, not *thumb*."	Verbal praise
Clinician	[*the same stimulus*] "What are these?"	Typical question; evoked trial
Child	"Thumbs."	A correct response
Clinician	"Out of sight! You said it correctly!"	Verbal praise

If the wrong responses persist on 4 to 5 evoked trials, reinstate partial or full modeling for a few trials, again fade the modeling, and re-present the evoked trials.

When the child meets the tentative learning criterion of 10 consecutively correct, nonimitated responses for a given stimulus item, move on to the next stimulus item. With this procedure, teach 6 to 8 exemplars shown on the following recording sheet. Use different exemplars as you see fit for a given child.

/mz/ in Word-Final Positions

Treatment Exemplars and Recording Sheet

Use stimuli from the **Stimulus Book, *Volume 8***.

Print this page from CD or photocopy this page for your clinical use.

Name/Age:	Date:
Goal: Production of /mz/ in word-final positions with 90% accuracy when asked an evoking question while showing a stimulus.	Clinician:

Scoring: Correct: ✓ Incorrect or no response: X

Target skills	Discrete Trials														
	1	2	3	4	5	6	7	8	9	10	11	12	13	14	15
1. thumbs															
2. clams															
3. climbs															
4. dimes															
5. charms															
6. wind chimes															
7. bedrooms															
8. daydreams															

When the child has met the learning criterion of 10 consecutively correct evoked (nonimitated) responses for each of the 6 to 8 target exemplars, conduct a probe to see if the production has generalized to previously baserated but untrained exemplars.

If the probes do not meet the 90% correct criterion for untrained exemplars, teach additional exemplars and then probe again.

/mz/ in Word-Final Positions

Probe Protocols and Recording Sheet

Use stimuli from the **Stimulus Book, Volume 8.**

Print this page from the CD or photocopy this page for your clinical use.

On the probes, present only the untrained exemplars (UT). When the child fails to meet the 90% correct probe criterion, either teach 2 to 4 new exemplars or give additional training trials on already trained stimuli. If needed, select new exemplars for probes. Probe at least 10 untrained exemplars. Alternate probes and treatment until the probe criterion is met.

Scripts for Probe Trials		Note
Clinician	[*untrained stimulus: lambs*] "Baby sheep are called _____?"	No modeling or prompts
Child	"lamb."	A wrong probe response
Clinician	Scores the response as incorrect.	No corrective feedback
Clinician	[*untrained stimulus: games*] "Kids like to play fun _____?"	The second probe trial
Child	"game."	A wrong probe response
Clinician	Scores the response as incorrect.	No corrective feedback

Name:	Date:	Session #:
Age:	**Clinician:**	
Diagnosis: Articulation/Phonologic Disorder	**Word-final /mz/ probe**	
Untrained Stimuli	**Score: + correct; – incorrect or no responses**	
1. lambs		
2. games		
3. gums		
4. limbs		
5. fumes		
6. palms		
7. chimes		
8. rooms		
9. beams		
10. teams		
11. rims		
12. exams		
Percent correct: (Criterion: 90%)		

If the child does not meet the probe criterion, give additional training on already trained exemplars or teach a few new exemplars. Subsequently, readminister the probe trials. When the child meets the 90% correct probe criterion for the exemplars, shift training to the sentence or conversational level or to another phoneme.

/nz/ in Word-Final Positions

Baserate Protocols

Use stimuli from the **Stimulus Book,** *Volume 8.*

At the beginning of each trial, place a relevant stimulus (an object, a picture, or a printed word if the child can read) in front of the child. Point to the stimulus as you ask an evoking question. Do not respond in any way to the child's correct, incorrect, or lack of responses.

Scripts For Evoked Baserate Trial		Note
Clinician	[*stimulus: bones*] "What are these?"	Evoked trial
Child	"bodes."	Substitution of /d/ for /n/ in /nz/ cluster
Clinician	Pulls the stimulus toward her; records the response.	No corrective feedback
Clinician	[*stimulus: cones*] "What are these?"	The next evoked trial
Child	"codes."	Substitution of /d/ for /n/ in /nz/ cluster
Clinician	Pulls the stimulus toward her; records the response.	No corrective feedback

Administer the modeled baserate trials only after completing the evoked trials on all 20 (or more) exemplars.

Scripts For Modeled Baserate Trial		Note
Clinician	[*stimulus: bones*] "What are these? Say, *bones.*"	Modeled trial
Child	"Bones."	Correct response
Clinician	Pulls the stimulus toward her; records the response.	No reinforcement
Clinician	[*stimulus: cones*] "What are these? Say, *cones.*"	The next modeled trial
Child	"codes."	Substitution of /d/ for /n/ in /nz/ cluster
Clinician	Pulls the stimulus toward her; records the response.	No corrective feedback

Use the recording sheet with exemplars shown on the next page to establish the baserates; print it from the CD.

/nz/ in Word-Final Positions

Baserate Exemplars and Recording Sheet

Use stimuli from the **Stimulus Book,** *Volume 8.*

Print this page from the CD or photocopy this page for your clinical use.

Name/Age:	Date:
Goal: To establish the baserate production of /nz/ in word-final positions.	Clinician:

Scoring: Correct: ✓   Incorrect or no response: X

/nz/ in word-final positions	Evoked	Modeled
1. bones		
2. cones		
3. buns		
4. cans		
5. crowns		
6. balloons		
7. buttons		
8. ribbons		
9. wagons		
10. napkins		
11. coins		
12. chains		
13. pens		
14. planes		
15. trains		
16. pigeons		
17. mountains		
18. chickens		
19. muffins		
20. blue jeans		
Percent correct baserate		

Replace or add new exemplars as you see fit for a given child. After establishing the baserates, begin production teaching. Follow the protocols given on the next page.

/nz/ in Word-Final Positions

Treatment Protocols

Use stimuli from the **Stimulus Book,** *Volume 8.*

Teach 6 to 8 exemplars using the following script.

Place a relevant stimulus (an object, a picture, or a printed word if the child can read) in front of the child and point to the stimulus as you ask an evoking question.

Scripts For Modeled Discrete Trial Training		Note
Clinician	[*stimulus: bones*] "What are these? Say, ***bones***."	Modeling; the target vocally emphasized
Child	"bodes."	A wrong response
Clinician	"No. That's not correct. You said *bodes*, but it's *bones*."	Corrective feedback
Clinician	[*the same stimulus*] "What are these? Say ***bones***. You need to say the ***n*** sound instead of the *d* before the /z/ at the end, ***bones***."	The next trial
Child	"Bones."	A correct response
Clinician	"Excellent! You said the ***n*** sound before the /z/ at the end."	Verbal praise

Repeat the trials until the child gives 5 consecutively correct, imitated responses.

When the child imitates 5 correct responses in sequence, fade the modeling.

Scripts For Fading the Modeling		Note
Clinician	[*stimulus: bones*] "What are these? Remember to say the *n* sound before the /z/ sound at the end of the word."	Only a prompt
Child	"bodes."	A wrong response
Clinician	"Gee, you said the *d* instead of the *n*! It's *bones*, not *bodes*. Remember to say the *n* sound."	Corrective feedback
Clinician	[*the same stimulus*] "What are these? The word ends with . . . " [*silently models the articulatory posture for the /nz/ cluster.*]	The next trial; a partial modeling
Child	"Bones."	A correct response
Clinician	"That's fantastic! You said *bones*, not *bodes*."	Verbal praise
Clinician	[*the same stimulus*] "What are these?"	Typical question; evoked trial
Child	"Bones."	A correct response
Clinician	"Great job! You said it correctly! You are working very hard."	Verbal praise

If the wrong responses persist on 4 to 5 evoked trials, reinstate partial or full modeling for a few trials, again fade the modeling, and re-present the evoked trials.

When the child meets the tentative learning criterion of 10 consecutively correct, nonimitated responses for a given stimulus item, move on to the next stimulus item. With this procedure, teach 6 to 8 exemplars shown on the following recording sheet. Use different exemplars as you see fit for a given child.

/nz/ in Word-Final Positions

Treatment Exemplars and Recording Sheet

Use stimuli from the **Stimulus Book,** *Volume 8.*

Print this page from CD or photocopy this page for your clinical use.

Name/Age:	Date:
Goal: Production of /nz/ in word-final positions with 90% accuracy when asked an evoking question while showing a stimulus.	Clinician:

Scoring: Correct: ✓ Incorrect or no response: X

Target skills	Discrete Trials														
	1	2	3	4	5	6	7	8	9	10	11	12	13	14	15
1. bones															
2. cones															
3. buns															
4. cans															
5. crowns															
6. balloons															
7. buttons															
8. ribbons															

When the child has met the learning criterion of 10 consecutively correct evoked (nonimitated) responses for each of the 6 to 8 target exemplars, conduct a probe to see if the production has generalized to previously baserated but untrained exemplars.

If the probes do not meet the 90% correct criterion for untrained exemplars, teach additional exemplars and then probe again.

/nz/ in Word-Final Positions

Probe Protocols and Recording Sheet

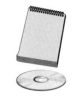

Use stimuli from the **Stimulus Book, Volume 8.**

Print this page from the CD or photocopy this page for your clinical use.

On the probes, present only the untrained exemplars (UT). When the child fails to meet the 90% correct probe criterion, either teach 2 to 4 new exemplars or give additional training trials on already trained stimuli. If needed, select new exemplars for probes. Probe at least 10 untrained exemplars. Alternate probes and treatment until the probe criterion is met.

Scripts for Probe Trials		Note
Clinician	[*untrained stimulus: wagons*] "What are these?"	No modeling or prompts
Child	"Wagons."	A correct, generalized response
Clinician	Scores the response as correct.	No reinforcement
Clinician	[*untrained stimulus: napkins*] "What are these?"	The second probe trial
Child	"Napkins."	A correct, generalized response
Clinician	Scores the response as correct.	No reinforcement

Name:	Date:	Session #:
Age:	**Clinician:**	
Diagnosis: Articulation/Phonologic Disorder	**Word-final /nz/ probe**	
Untrained Stimuli	**Score: + correct; – incorrect or no responses**	
1. wagons		
2. napkins		
3. coins		
4. chains		
5. pens		
6. planes		
7. trains		
8. pigeons		
9. mountains		
10. chickens		
11. muffins		
12. blue jeans		
Percent correct: (Criterion: 90%)		

If the child does not meet the probe criterion, give additional training on already trained exemplars or teach a few new exemplars. Subsequently, readminister the probe trials. When the child meets the 90% correct probe criterion for the exemplars, shift training to the sentence or conversational level or to another phoneme.

Glossary

acoustic phonetics: Branch of phonetics dedicated to the study of the science of sound. See *acoustics.*

acoustics: A branch of phonetics, which pertains to the study of the science of sound. It includes the study of the origin, transmission, modification, and effects of sound vibrations.

adaptation: In articulation, the process by which sounds are affected by or take on the properties of other surrounding sounds. The perceptual property of the sound may be unaffected.

addition: A form of articulation error; a superfluous sound that does not belong in a word (e.g., "biga" for *big*).

advanced word forms: Words used by a young child that have an advanced pronunciation in comparison to the rest of the child's phonologic system. The use of such forms may disappear as the child's phonologic system matures. Synonym: *progressive idioms.*

affricates: A group of consonants with the characteristics of stops and fricatives.

age of customary production: The age at which approximately 50% of children produce a particular singleton sound.

age of mastery: The age at which approximately 90% of children produce a particular singleton sound.

allographs: Different letters (alphabetic symbols) and letter combinations that can be used to represent the same sound (phoneme) in a specific language.

allophones: Variations of a phoneme.

allophonic variations: Articulatory or perceptual variations of the same phoneme, often caused by the sound's phonetic environment, that do not change the meaning of a word.

alternating motion rates: Alternating repetitive movements of the tongue. Part of diadochokinetic testing by successive repetition of the same syllable sequence (e.g., /pʌ pʌ pʌ pʌ/, /tʌ tʌ tʌ tʌ/, and /kʌ kʌ kʌ kʌ/).

alveolar process: The outer edges of the maxillary bone (upper jaw) that house the molar, bicuspid, and cuspid teeth.

alveolar ridge: A ridge on the maxilla that overlies the roots of the teeth, most often located behind the upper anterior teeth. In most people it serves as the point of articulation for English sounds /s/, /z/, /t/, /d/, /n/, /l/.

alveolar sounds: Consonant sounds /s/, /z/, /t/, /d/, /n/, /l/ made by placing the tongue against the alveolar ridge.

ankyloglossia: Limited movement of the tongue tip due to an abnormally short lingual frenulum; also known as tongue-tie.

antecedent event: A stimulus presented before a target response is produced or attempted.

anterior feature: Distinctive feature characteristic of sounds made in the front region of the mouth, generally at the alveolar ridge or forward. See *distinctive features.*

anticipatory substitution: Sound substitution created by the coarticulatory effects of a sound that follows the target sound.

applied phonetics: A branch of phonetics dedicated to the practical application of the knowledge gained from experimental, articulatory, acoustic, and perceptual phonetics.

approximants: Sounds produced by an "approximating" contact between the two articulators that form them; includes liquids and glides.

apraxia: A disorder of sequenced movements of body parts in the absence of muscle weakness, incoordination, or paralysis; an acquired motor programming disorder. See also *oral apraxia, limb apraxia,* and *apraxia of speech.*

apraxia of speech: A sensorimotor disorder of speech, characterized by impaired ability to position the speech muscles and sequence the muscle movements (respiratory, laryngeal, and oral) necessary for volitional production of sounds and words.

arresting sound: A consonant sound that closes a syllable.

articulation: In speech, movement of the speech mechanism to produce the sound of speech. One of the four basic processes involved in speech production.

articulation disorders: Problems in producing speech sounds.

articulator-bound features: Sound features produced by the action of a single articulator.

articulator-free features: Sound features produced by the actions of multiple articulators.

articulators: Organs of the speech production mechanism; help produce meaningful sound by interrupting the flow of exhaled air or by narrowing the space for its passage. The articulators include the lips, tongue, velum, jaw, hard palate, alveolar ridge, and teeth.

articulatory phonetics: A branch of phonetics that focuses on how a speaker of a language makes speech sounds.

assessment: In articulation, the process that is followed and the procedures that are used to identify the presence or absence of an articulation or phonologic disorder.

assimilation: The effect one speech sound has on another when produced in close sequence, such that the sounds become more like each other. The effect can be so extensive that it can be perceptually identified. See also *progressive assimilation* and *regressive assimilation.*

ataxic dysarthria: A motor speech disorder associated with ataxia. See also *dysarthria.*

audible nasal emission: Noise that can be heard of the air escaping through the nose.

auditory bombardment: Procedure by which a child is provided with amplified auditory stimulation for a particular sound that is being taught.

back feature: A distinctive feature that characterizes sounds made in the back part of the oral cavity; the body of the tongue is retracted from the neutral position /ə/ during the production of sounds containing the back distinctive feature.

baselines: Measures of a client's target behaviors or treatment objectives before those behaviors are taught; they help the clinician establish client improvement, clinical effectiveness, and professional accountability.

baserating: The process followed by a clinician to obtain baseline measures of a client's target behaviors before those behaviors are taught. See also *baselines.*

behavioral approach. A treament method that explicitly uses the principles and procedures operant conditioning and learning.

behavioral principles: Concepts and procedures of operant conditioning and learning; frequently used in the treatment of communication disorders.

bilabial: Involving both lips; bilabial sounds are produced primarily by the two lips.

bilingual: Of two languages; often refers to a person who speaks two languages.

binary classification system: A (+) and (–) value system that identifies whether a specific feature is present or absent in a sound. See also *distinctive features.*

blends: Two or more juxtaposed consonants with no vowel separation (e.g., /tr/, /pl/, /str/). See also *cluster.*

broad phonetic transcription: Orthographic (written) representation of phonemes or spoken speech with special phonetic symbols enclosed between virgules (slash marks); may be interpretable only by someone familiar with the phonetic symbols (e.g., /bot/ for *boat*; /ʃɪp/ for *ship*).

carryover: The regular use of newly learned speech or language skills in everyday situations.

cavity: A hollow space within the body; a structure within the body containing other structures, as in the oral cavity, which contains the tongue, hard palate, soft palate, and so forth.

centering diphthongs: Diphthongs in which one of the stressed vowels combines with schwar /ɚ/. Synonym: *rhotic diphthongs.*

Class I malocclusion: Misalignment of some individual teeth while the two arches are normally aligned.

Class II malocclusion: The upper jaw is protruded and the lower jaw is retracted or receded.

Class III malocclusion: upper jaw is receded and the lower jaw is protruded.

cleft palate: Failure of the premaxilla to fuse with the maxillary bone and/or failure of the palatine process to fuse at the midline.

closed syllable: Vowel followed by a singleton consonant or consonant cluster.

closed-syllable word: A word that ends in a singleton consonant or consonant cluster (e.g., *pot, stop, must, last*).

cluster: Two or more juxtaposed consonant sounds with no vowel separation. See also *blends.*

cluster reduction: Omission of one or more consonants of a cluster (e.g., "top" for *stop*).

cluster simplification: Omission or substitution of one or more sound segments in a consonant cluster. Can be considered a phonologic process if it occurs frequently in a child's phonologic system.

coarticulation: Articulatory movements for one phone that are carried over into the production of previous or subsequent phones; influence of one phone on another in perception or production.

coda: Consonant segment or consonant cluster that follows the nucleus (vowel or diphthong) of a syllable.

cognates: Consonants produced in the same place and manner, except that one is voiceless and the other is voiced; in phonetic transcription they are typically written in pairs, with the voiceless sound given first (e.g., /p-b/, /wh-w/, /f-v/, /t-d/, /s-z/, /k-g/) /s-z/.

compensatory articulation: Correct or markedly improved production of sounds through unusual methods of articulation by a child with defective speech structures.

complementary distribution: Sounds that cannot be interchanged in a certain position; allophones that together cover all possible positional occurrences but do not appear in the same linguistic environment.

concurrent treatment: Simultaneously training a target sound at different levels of response complexity.

consonant: A conventional speech sound made by certain movements of the articulatory muscles that alter, interrupt, or obstruct the expired airstream; defined according to manner of production, place of articulation, and voicing dimensions.

consonantal feature: A distinctive feature applied to sounds that have a marked constriction along the midline region of the vocal tract. Includes all consonant sounds except /h/, /w/, and /j/.

consonant deletion: A phonologic process that describes the omission of initial or final consonants of words; a phonologic problem. See also *final-consonant deletion* and *initial-consonant deletion*.

consonant harmony: An assimilation phonologic process that affects manner of production or place of articulation; includes labial assimilation, velar assimilation, nasal assimilation, and alveolar assimilation.

consonant sequence reduction: The omission of one or more sound segments from two or more adjoining consonants.

contextual testing: A special assessment procedure that helps identify a facilitative phonetic context for correct production of a particular phoneme.

contextual training: A method of teaching speech sounds using contexts in which a target sound is correctly produced.

contiguous assimilation: A type of assimilation in which the affected sound and the sound that caused the change are adjacent to each other, with no interfering sound between them.

continuant: Distinctive feature applied to sounds made with an incomplete point of constriction; flow of air is not entirely stopped. Continuant sounds are /w/, /f/, /v/, /t/, /d/, /s/, /z/, /l/, /s/, /z/, /j/, /r/.

contrast therapy approach: A cognitive-linguistic approach to the treatment of articulation and phonologic disorders; incorporates structured activities to increase awareness of the semantic distinction between the error production and the target.

coronal feature: A distinctive feature used in reference to sounds made with the tongue blade raised above the neutral position required for the production of /ə/. Includes consonants /t/, /d/, /s/, /z/, /n/, /l/, /r/.

corrective feedback: A treatment procedure by which a client is provided with specific verbal, visual, or written feedback about the acceptability of a response immediately after the response is made; helps reduce incorrect responses; includes such verbal statements as "No, that's not correct!"

criterion of performance: The level of accuracy (e.g., 80% correct) in the production of a target behavior taught in treatment.

denasalization: Substitution of an oral sound for a nasal sound (e.g., "tep" for *ten*); a problem of articulation.

developmental apraxia of speech (DAS): A childhood motor speech disorder affecting the motor programming of the articulators; it primarily affects articulation and prosody. Also termed *developmental verbal dyspraxia*.

diacritical markers: Special symbols used in narrow phonetic transcription to depict the articulatory or perceptual features of a phone.

diadochokinetic syllable rates: The speed at which a speaker can repeat selected syllables (e.g., pʌ-tə-kə).

diadochokinetic testing: A special procedure used to evaluate the client's ability to rapidly alternate and sequence repetitive articulatory movements; helps assess the functional and structural integrity of the lips, jaw, and tongue through rapid repetitions of syllables.

dialect: Variation of speech within a specific language. Every dialect may have its own unique phonologic, semantic, morphologic, syntactic, and pragmatic characteristics.

direct replication: A type of treatment research in which the same researcher repeats his or her own earlier study with little or no modification in the treatment procedure to see if the results are reliable; most of the behavioral treatment techniques described in the protocols have been directly replicated and shown to produce reliable results.

diphthong: A combination of two pure vowels. See also *monophthong.*

discrete trials: A highly researched behavioral treatment procedure in which the client is given repeated and temporally separated opportunities to produce a response; often a discrete trial includes instructions, exhibition of pictures or other stimuli, questions, modeling, and prompts that the clinician delivers and then waits for a few seconds for the child to respond; each of the child's attempts is scored as correct or wrong; trials are repeated until the child meets a learning criterion; known to be efficient and effective in establishing various skills, including language skills in children (and adults); helps measure skills reliably.

discriminative stimuli: Persons, objects, and physical settings that are associated with a reinforced response; the response is more likely to occur in the presence of such stimuli.

distinctive feature approach: An articulation-phonologic treatment approach based on the distinctive features or phonemic contrasts of sounds; the goal of treatment is to establish missing distinctive features that create contrasts between words.

distinctive features: Unique characteristics that distinguish one phoneme from another.

distortions: Imprecise productions of speech sounds.

doubling: A phonologic process characterized by reduplication or doubling of a syllable; often alters a single-syllable word form into a multisyllable production (e.g., [dada] for *dog* and [baba] for *ball*).

dysarthria: A group of motor speech disorders due to paralysis, weakness, or incoordination of speech muscles caused by central or peripheral nerve damage. There are seven types of dysarthria: flaccid, ataxic, spastic, hypokinetic, hyperkinetic, unilateral upper motor neuron, and mixed.

elicited responses: Reflexive responses triggered by stimuli; for example, the dilation of the pupil in response to light. See also *evoked responses.*

evidence-based practice: The use of treatment methods that are supported by controlled and replicated research evidence; may include such other considerations as the clinician's best judgment, cost, and social acceptability of the procedures offered.

evoked responses: Responses that are not imitated, not reflexive, but learned; they are produced in relation to various discriminative stimuli; a response to such typical questions as "What is this?" are called *evoked.*

evoked trial: A structured opportunity for the production of the target behavior; may be baserate or treatment trials; the clinician asks a typical question, but does not model the response; more naturalistic than the imitative trials; when a client gives 10 consecutively correct, evoked responses, the clinicians may consider a particular exemplar trained and move on to the next examplar.

exemplar: A response that illustrates the target behavior.

experimental phonetics: A branch of phonetics dedicated to the development of scientific methods for the study of speech sounds.

extinction: Terminating the reinforcer for a response while no other attempt is made to stop it; the same as ignoring it; the clinician may use extinction in place of corrective feedback, although the latter may be more effective.

facilitative phonetic context: A surrounding sound or group of sounds that has a positive influence on the production of a misarticulated sound.

final-consonant deletion: A phonologic process affecting the production of final consonants. Patterned deletion of consonant sounds in the final position of words.

final conversational probe: An assessment of generalized production of phonemes taught in treatment sessions; a speech sample recorded while providing no reinforcement for correct productions or corrective feedback for incorrect productions helps establish generalized production of target phonemes.

fixed-ratio reinforcement (FR): Used in the treatment of articulation disorders, the fixed ratio requires the production of a certain number of correct responses before receiving reinforcement; a FR of 5 means that every fifth response is reinforced.

flaccid dysarthria: A type of dysarthria associated with disorders of the lower motor neuron. Speech is characterized by marked hypernasality and nasal emission; breathiness may be present during phonation; audible inspiration may be perceived; consonant production is imprecise.

flaccid paralysis: Muscles that are too soft and flabby, caused by a lesion in the lower motoneurons.

follow-up assessment: Any assessment of a client's articulation skills following initial dismissal from treatment; necessary to assess response maintenance; when the follow-up assessment shows a decline in target skills, booster therapy may be arranged.

frenulum: A small cord of tissue that extends from the floor of the mouth to the midline inferior surface of the tongue blade; if too short, it may restrict the elevation and extension of the tongue, which may or may not affect articulation.

frequency of occurrence: In articulation and phonology, the number of times a particular phonologic process occurs.

fricatives: A category of speech sounds that are produced by severely constricting the oral cavity and forcing the air through the point of constriction.

fronting: Substituting sounds produced in the front of the mouth for sounds produced in the back of the mouth; classified as a phonologic process that occurs in both normally developing children and children with phonologic disorders.

frozen word forms: Words that children continue to mispronounce despite the development of a more advanced phonologic system; such words are likely related to names of familiar people or pets and are used often. Synonym: *regressive idioms.*

functional articulation disorders: Disorders that do not have a demonstrable organic or neurologic cause.

generalization: The production of untrained (new) behaviors following training of similar behaviors, or the production of trained behaviors when shown new stimuli not used in training; assessed through the probe procedure.

glides: Speech sounds that are produced by gradually changing the shape of the articulators.

glottal sounds: Sounds that are produced by keeping the vocal folds open and letting the air pass through; because this results in friction noise, glottals are also fricatives.

glottis: An opening that results when the vocal folds are abducted.

hard palate: The roof of the mouth and the floor of the nasal cavity. The point of constriction for several sounds including /ʃ/, /ʒ/, /dʒ/, /tʃ/.

high feature: Distinctive feature term referring to sounds made with the tongue elevated above the neutral position required for /ə/. The high-consonant sounds are /ʃ/, /ʒ/, /j/, /tʃ/, /dʒ/, /k/, /g/, /ŋ/.

homonymy: The loss of linguistic contrast between two or more words due to the presence of phonologic processes. A child who substitutes a single phoneme for multiple phonemes is likely to exhibit this serious problem. For example, a child who substitutes /t/ for /s/, /k/, /ch/, and /tr/ will will say *tip* for *sip, Kip, chip,* and *trip.*

idiopathic: Of unknown cause or origin.

idiosyncratic processes: Phonologic processes that are unique to an individual child and are not common in the normal course of development.

imitation: In articulation therapy, the client's response to the clinician's model of the target production; used to baserate target sound productions; often the initial mode of response in treatment sessions.

inappropriate communicative behaviors: A client's typical behaviors in place of appropriate speech–language behaviors; in articulation therapy, a client's sound substitutions, omissions, or distortions; in phonologic therapy, a child's absence of distinctive features or use of phonologic processes.

independent analysis: In articulation-phonologic assessment, a description of the client's speech production errors without reference to the adult model; most clinically useful with very young children or children with significantly decreased speech intelligibility.

Individualized Education Program: Federally and state-mandated program for children with disabilities and special needs who qualify for special education services in the public school system.

Individualized Family Service Plan. An individualized education plan for a child with an emphasis on family needs, services, and family members participation.

Individuals with Disabilities Education Act: Federal legislation that demands the provision of special education services to children with disabilities and special needs in the public schools; includes children with speech and language disorders.

informative feedback: Increasing behaviors by providing feedback on the progress a child is making in learning a skill; an excellent form of verbal social reinforcement; the clinician might say, "Last time, you said 5 out of 10 words correctly; but today, you said 9 out of 10 words correctly!"

initial-consonant deletion: A phonologic process affecting the production of initial consonants; patterned deletion of consonant sounds in the initial position of words.

instructions: In speech–language treatment, verbal stimuli that help facilitate a client's actions (i.e., production of a target sound).

intelligibility: How understandable a person's speech is to family members, strangers, and other listeners.

interdental sound: Sound made by lightly placing the tip of the tongue between the upper and lower central incisors; English interdental sounds include voiced /ð/ and voiceless /θ/.

intermittent schedule of reinforcement: Various ways of reinforcing only some of the correct responses while others go unreinforced; effective in strengthening newly learned skills; clinician typically reinforces all responses to begin with and thins out reinforcement by offering it to only some.

International Phonetic Alphabet (IPA): A set of phonetic symbols, each of which stands for only one speech sound.

interrupted feature: Distinctive feature term applied to sounds produced by complete blockage of the airstream at their point of constriction; such sounds are the stops /t/, /d/, /k/, /g/, /p/, /b/ and the affricates /tʃ/, /dʒ/.

intervocalic: In articulation, singleton consonants or consonant blends that occur between vowels or diphthongs.

kinesthetic cues: on the position of the articulators or their correct pattern of movements to teach the correct production of a speech sound.

key words: A word or words in which a typically misarticulated sound is made correctly; can be used in therapy to stabilize the production of the sound across words.

labiodental sounds: Sounds that are produced by the lips and teeth.

language: A system of symbols and codes in communication; a form of social behavior shaped and maintained by a verbal community.

laterals: Sounds that are produced by letting air escape through the sides of the tongue; English /l/ is a lateral.

lax vowels: Vowel sounds that are made without added muscle tension and have a short duration. The vowels typically described as lax include /ɪ/, /ɛ/, /æ/, /ʊ/, /ɑ/, /ɚ/, /ə/, /ʌ/.

levels of treatment: Treatment at varied complexity of response topography: words, phrases, sentences, or conversational speech.

lingua-alveolar sounds: Sounds produced by raising the tip of the tongue to make contact with the alveolar ridge, which is immediately behind the front teeth.

linguadental sounds: Sounds produced by the tongue as it makes contact with the upper teeth.

linguapalatal sounds: Sounds produced by the tongue as it comes in contact with the hard palate, which is located just behind the alveolar ridge.

linguavelar sounds: Sounds produced by the back of the tongue as it rises to make contact with the velum (soft palate).

linguistic-based approaches: In articulation-phonologic therapy, treatment programs or approaches with the underlying philosophy that children's production errors result from phonologic processes or rules of the adult system that have not yet been learned or fully acquired, or have been suppressed.

liquids: Speech sounds produced with the least restriction of the oral cavity; also called semivowels. English /r/ and /l/ are liquids.

long-term goals: Broadly defined speech and language behaviors that a client needs to learn to improve his or her overall communication competence.

low feature: Distinctive feature term used to describe sounds made with the tongue lowered for the neutral position of /ə/. In American English, only the consonant /h/ has the low feature.

maintenance: The continued production of clinically established skills over time and across situations; to have the child maintain correct production of target phonemes, the clinician needs to train the family members, teachers, and others to evoke, prompt, and reinforce them in natural settings.

maintenance strategies: Techniques that help extend treatment to natural settings; parent training and self-control strategies in monitoring correct productions of phoneme are the most effective.

malocclusions: Deviations in the shape and dimensions of the upper and lower jaw bones, the positioning of individual teeth, and the relation between the two jaws.

mandible: The lower jaw, which forms the floor of the mouth and houses the lower set of teeth.

manner of production: The degree of and type of constriction of the vocal tract while producing certain speech sounds.

manual guidance: Any procedure in which the clinician uses his or her hands and fingers to physically guide and shape a correct response from a client.

marginal babbling: Infant vocal productions characterized by CV and VC syllable sequences that begin at about 4 months of age.

maximal contrast method (maximal opposition): A method of selecting word pairs for phonologic treatment that contain multiple feature contrasts or maximal opposition between contrasted phonemes.

metathesis: A phonologic process characterized by the reversal of two sounds in a word that may or may not be adjacent to each other (e.g., [pots] for *post*).

metathetic error: The reversal of two sounds within a word that may or may not be adjacent to each other.

minimal pairs: Morphemes that are similar except for one sound (e.g., *mit/sit, hot/pot, bake/bait*); a method of selecting word pairs for treatment.

modeled trial: A baserate or treatment trial in which the clinician models the correct production of a target phoneme in words or phrases and the client is instructed to imitate the modeled production; most treatment begins with a modeled trial; modeling is faded as the child's imitation becomes relatively stable.

modeling: A treatment procedure used to facilitate a target production; the clinician models the target behavior and the client is instructed to imitate the clinician; used on both baserate and treatment trials; treatment begins with modeling; faded in gradual steps.

monophthong: Term used in reference to pure vowels.

morphophonemics: Sound alterations that result from joining one morpheme with another; morphophonemic rules specify how sounds are produced in combination in morphemes.

moto-kinesthetic cues: Cues provided by the clinician to teach the placement of sounds. The clinician touches and manipulates the client's articulators to facilitate correct production of the target sound. Moto-kinesthetic cues are often accompanied by auditory and visual cues.

moto-kinesthetic method: A procedure of teaching the correct production of speech sounds; the clinician manually moves the articulators to provide motor and kinesthetic feedback to the client.

motor-based approaches: In articulation therapy, treatment programs or approaches that focus on teaching the motor behaviors associated with the production of speech sounds; often considered "traditional" articulation treatment approaches.

motor speech disorders: Also known as neurogenic speech disorders; result from central or peripheral nervous system damage. Apraxia of speech and dysarthria are motor speech disorders.

multiple contrast method (the multiple opposition): A method of selecting target sounds for treatment that is similar to the minimal pair approach but differs from it by creating minimal pairs for all or most of the errors simultaneously.

multiple-phoneme approach: A highly structured motor-based articulation approach developed to meet the needs of children with multiple articulation errors; key features of the multiple phoneme approach are the simultaneous teaching of multiple phonemes, a systematic application of behavioral principles, and an analysis of sound production in conversational speech.

myofunctional therapy: Treatment aimed at correcting a tongue thrust or myofunctional imbalance.

narrow phonetic transcription: A detailed form of recording a speech sound or utterance using the symbols of the International Phonetic Alphabet and special diacritic markers; transcription enclosed in brackets to highlight the allophonic features or variations of a phoneme (e.g., [kʰ]out] for *coat* would indicate an aspirated production of the /k/ sound).

nasal emission: Excessive airflow through the nose that can often be measured and perceived; heard most frequently during the production of voiceless plosives and fricatives; typically indicative of an incomplete seal between the oral and the nasal cavities; often associated with cleft palate speech and some types of dysarthria.

nasal feature: A distinctive feature applied to sounds resonated in the nasal cavity. The nasal sounds include /m/, /n/, and /ŋ/.

nasals: Speech sounds with nasal resonance added to them; produced while keeping the velopharyngeal port open.

noncontiguous assimilation: A type of assimilation in which the assimilated sound and the sound causing the assimilation are separated by an intervening sound.

nonphonemic diphthong: Diphthongs that do not contrast meaning in words when they are interchanged with their pure-vowel counterpart; the only two American English nonphonemic diphthongs are /ei/ and /ou/.

nonverbal corrective feedback: A treatment procedure by which corrective feedback is provided through nonverbal means such as facial expressions, gestures, and other signals to decrease incorrect productions of a phoneme.

nonverbal prompts: Various signals or gestures the clinician gives to evoke the correct production of a target behavior; the clinician, for example, may silently demonstrate the articulatory postures involved in the production of various target sounds (e.g., the lip closure for the production of such bilabial sounds as /p/ or /b/); an effective means of fading verbal modeling.

normative data: research data that show the various ages at which children master specific skills; ages at which children master the phonemes of their language.

obstruents: Distinctive feature term used for consonants that are made with complete closure or narrow constriction of the oral cavity so that the airstream is stopped or friction noise is produced; obstruents include stops, fricatives, and affricates.

occlusion: The manner in which the upper and lower dental arches meet each other.

omission: An absence of a required sound in a word position; a type of articulation error.

onset: One of the components of the syllable; the consonant or consonant cluster that initiates the syllable.

open syllable: A syllable that ends in a vowel or a diphthong.

open-syllable word: A word that ends with an open syllable. See also *open syllable*.

operational definition: A definition that describes that which is being defined in observable and measurable terms; most treatment targets are defined operationally (e.g., *the production of the plural morpheme in words at 90% accuracy*).

oral apraxia: An inability to move the muscles of oral structures for nonspeech purposes in the absence of muscle weakness, incoordination, or paralysis. See also *apraxia of speech* and *limb apraxia.*

organic: Relating to an organ or structure of the body.

organic articulation disorder: An inability to produce correctly all or some of the standard sounds of a language as a result of anatomic, physiologic, or neurologic causes.

orofacial examination: A procedure conducted to rule out gross organic problems of the face and mouth that may be associated with disorders of communication.

paired-stimuli approach: A motor-based articulation treatment approach that depends on the identification of a key word to teach correct production of a target sound in other contexts.

partial assimilation: In articulation, a physiologic occurrence in which a sound takes on some of the characteristics of a neighboring sound.

partial model: A modeled stimulus that provides only a portion of the correct response; just enough for the child to imitate the response; a method to fade the influence of the full model; useful in promoting more spontaneous or naturalistic response.

pattern analysis: In articulation-phonologic assessment, the clinician's attempt to identify any patterned or systematic modifications in the client's speech production errors.

percentage of occurrence: When conducting a phonologic process analysis, the actual percentage with which the child uses a particular phonologic process; calculated by determining the number of times the child uses a particular phonologic process and dividing that number by the total number of opportunities for occurrence of the process.

pharyngeal fricatives: Consonant sounds produced by lingual-pharyngeal contact and an unusual tongue configuration; often an associated compensatory error in children with cleft palate.

phonate: To produce sound.

phone: In the study of speech production, a single speech sound represented by a single symbol in a phonetic system.

phoneme: A group or family of very closely related speech sounds that vary slightly in their production but are sufficiently similar acoustically that the listener perceives them as the same sound. For example, whether *t* in cat is aspirated or unaspirated, the listener perceives the sound as /t/.

phoneme isolation: A phonologic awareness skill in identifying whehter a specfic sound occurs in the beginning, end, or middle of a word.

phoneme manipulation: A phonologic awareness skill in deleting, adding, or substituting a sound in a word to create other words.

phonemic awareness: A person's underlying knowledge that words are created by sounds and sound combinations. Synonym: *phonologic awareness.*

phonemic diphthong: A diphthong that cannot be reduced to its pure-vowel components without affecting the meaning of the words in which they occur.

phonemic inventory: In a phonologic analysis, an inventory of sounds that a child uses contrastively to signal a difference in the meanings of words.

phonemic transcription: Recording of a speech sound or speech unit into phonemic symbols, which are enclosed between virgules (slash marks); such recording indicates the phoneme to which the sound belongs. Synonym: *broad transcription.*

phonemics: Study of the sound system and sound differences in a language.

phonetic inventory: A person's repertoire of speech sounds; sounds that a person can produce with appropriate articulation although not always contrastively.

phonetic placement method: A procedure of teaching a target sound by describing and demonstrating in front of a mirror how that sound is produced correctly.

phonetic transcription: See *narrow phonetic transcription.*

phonetics: Study of speech sounds, their production and acoustic properties, and the written symbols used to represent their production.

phonologic awareness: See *phonemic awareness.*

phonologic disorders: Errors of many phonemes that form patterns or clusters.

phonologic process analysis: In articulation-phonologic assessment, the classification of sound errors according to operating phonologic processes and their frequecuncies.

phonologic processes: Many ways or patterns of simplifying difficult sound productions by omissions or substitutions.

phonology: The study of speech sounds, sound patterns, and the rules used to create words with those sounds.

phonotactics: Rules for how sounds can be combined to form syllables and how those sounds can be distributed; some rules vary across languages.

physical prompts: In articulation therapy, visual signs or gestures that help a client visualize correct production of the target sound.

physical stimulus generalization: In articulation-phonologic therapy, a client's production of the target sounds in untrained words.

place of articulation: One of three factors used to classify consonants; refers to the place of articulatory contact or constriction.

plosive sound: A stop consonant produced when the impounded air pressure behind the point of constriction is released through the oral cavity; not all stop consonants are plosive in nature.

positive reinforcement: A method of increasing a response by presenting something desirable immediately after that response is made; a frequently used positive reinforcer is verbal praise.

postvocalic: A consonant or consonant blend produced after a vowel or a diphthong; postvocalic sounds terminate the syllable.

pressure consonants: Consonant sounds produced with a buildup of intraoral pressure, which include fricatives, stops, and affricates.

primary reinforcement: A method of increasing target skills by providing such consequences as food and drink; may be useful in treating articulation disorders in young children or those with developmental disability; always paired with social reinforcement (e.g., verbal praise) so that the primary reinforcment may be eventually faded out.

probe: An assessment of generalized productions of clinically established speech sound productions; a final test of success of treatment; only untrained stimuli are presented during probes; no reinforcement or corrective feedback is offered on probe trials or assessment; the protocols include probes for most target phonemes or phoneme clusters.

probe criterion: Generally, 90% correct responses given to untrained stimuli; correct production of trained phonemes in untrained words, phrases, sentences, and conversational speech; an indication of successful treatment.

probe procedure: A clinical procedure used to assess the generalized production of the trained target behavior to untrained sounds, words, sentences, audiences, settings, and so forth.

prognosis: A statement about the future course of a disorder when certain therapeutic steps are taken or when nothing is done.

programmed learning: A method of mastering various skills by the systematic use of operant conditioning principles.

progressive assimilation: A type of assimilation in which a sound takes on the articulatory or acoustic qualities of a preceding sound.

prompts: A hint; may be verbal (e.g., vocal emphasis on the target sound as illustrated in the protocols) or nonverbal (e.g., a silent articulatory gesture); another special stimulus that is added or layered over other evoking or modeling stimuli; less than a full model; useful in fading modeling; known to be effective in teaching skills.

protocols: Detailed and scripted plans for treatment; specification of the roles of the clinician and the client in baserate, treatment, and probe trials or sessions; scripts the clinician can follow in treating a disorder.

punisher: In behavior modification terms, any stimulus that decreases a behavior when it is presented upon the behavior's occurrence.

punishment: A procedure designed to decrease the frequency of selected behaviors by arranging an immediate consequence for those behaviors.

pure vowels: Vowel sounds that maintain a relatively unchanged quality across the syllables in which they are produced.

range of motion: The limitations within which a motion or movement may occur.

raspberries: In speech and language development, bilabial fricative sounds produced by young infants in the vocal play stage.

regressive assimilation: A type of assimilation in which a sound takes on some or all of the articulatory or acoustic features of a following sound.

regressive substitution: Sound substitution in which a phoneme is affected by a sound that occurs earlier in the word; a speech characteristic of verbal apraxia.

reinforcers: Events that follow a response and thereby make that response more likely in the future; consequences provided contingent upon a correct response that consists of verbal praise, objects, or opportunities for certain favorite activities; to be delivered immediately after a response is made; should increase the correct response rate to be called a reinforcer; the most powerful treatment technique.

relational analysis: A comparison of a child's productions to the adult target forms within a specific linguistic community to identify errors of articulation and the operation of phonologic processes.

releasing sound: A consonant sound that begins the syllable.

replicated: Treatment research that is repeated by either the same researcher (direct replication) or other researchers (systematic replication); helps demonstrate that the results of the original treatment research were reliable.

response cost: An effective method to decrease incorrect responses; presenting a token for correct production of phonemes and taking one away for each incorect production; tokens the client retains are exchanged for a gift at the end of the session.

rhotic: Distinctive feature term used for the /r/ consonant and its various allophonic variations.

rhotic diphthongs: See *centering diphthongs.*

rhyme: A collective term for the nucleus and coda components of a syllable.

rhyming: A phonologic awareness skill in identifying words that sound alike or rhyme.

round feature: Distinctive feature term applied to sounds made with the lips rounded or protruded; includes the consonants /r/ and /w/ and the vowels /u/, /ʊ/, /o/, /ɔ/, and /ɝ/.

schwa: Name for the neutral vowel /ə/.

schwar: Name for the vowel /ɚ/.

screening: A brief procedure that helps determine whether a person should be assessed at length or not.

secondary reinforcement: The use of social consequences to increase skills; verbal praise, included in almost all protocols, is a form of secondary reinforcement; based on past learning (unlike primary reinforcement).

semivowel: A consonant sound made by maintaining the vocal tract briefly in the vowel-like position needed for the following vowel in a syllable; term used for /w/, /j/, and sometimes /l/ and /r/.

sensorimotor approach: Motor-based articulation approach based on the assumption that the syllable is the basic unit of training and that phonetic contexts can be used to facilitate correct production of the target sound. Synonym: *McDonald's sensorimotor approach.*

sensory-perceptual training: A step typically included in the traditional articulation therapy approach; the goal is to increase the client's awareness of his own sound errors by incorporating ear-training activities such as sound identification and discrimination.

sequential motion rates: Rapid movements from one articulatory posture to another by repetition of different syllable chains. Part of diadochokinetic testing by repetitive movement of the syllable sequence /pʌ-tə-kə/.

setting generalization: Production of clinically established responses in such nonclinical settings as home, school, and social situations; a goal of all treatment.

shaping: See *successive approximation.*

short-term objectives: In articulation-phonologic therapy, the sounds, phonologic rules, and other behaviors selected for training that support the long-term goals or final target behaviors.

sibilants: Distinctive feature term applied to high-frequency consonant sounds that have a more strident quality and longer duration than most other consonants; most phoneticians classify /s/, /z/, /ʃ/, /ʒ/, /tʃ/, /dʒ/ in this category.

silent nasal emission: Inaudible leakage of air through the nose during the production of non-nasal speech sounds.

sonorant: A consonant sound produced with a relatively unobstructed flow of air at the point of constriction: /m/, /n/, /ŋ/, /l/, /r/, /j/, and /w/.

sound approximation: Production of a misarticulated sound that approaches the target or standard production of that phoneme.

sound segmentation: A phonologic awareness skill to break down a word into its individual sound components.

speech: Production of phonemes; articulated sounds and syllables. See also *language*.

speech-language pathologist: A specialist in the study, assessment, and treatment of speech-language (communication) disorders.

speech-language pathology: The study of human communication and its disorders and the assessment and treatment of those disorders.

speech perception: The identification of speech sounds from acoustic cues.

stimulability: The extent to which a misarticulated sound can be produced correctly by imitation or other cues.

stimulus generalization: The production of already learned responses in relation to novel but similar stimuli; correct production of clinically established phonemes in relation to untrained pictures or physical stimuli; assessed through probes.

stopping: Phonologic process term used to describe patterned substitutions of stop consonants for fricatives and affricates.

stops: Speech sounds produced by completely stopping the airflow; also known as stop-plosives.

stress: A suprasegmental device that gives prominence to certain syllables within a sequence of syllables.

stridents: Consonant sounds that are made by forcing the airstream through a small opening, which results in intense noise: /f/, /v/, /s/, /z/, /ʃ/, /ʒ/, /tʃ/, /dʒ/.

substitution: The production of a wrong sound in place of a right one.

successive approximation: A treatment technique for establishing a target behavior not in the client's repertoire; the client's target responses are progressively shaped to match the final target behavior; helps teach more complex skills by by building upon a series of simpler skills; teaching the child to first prduce the phoneme in syllables and then in words is an example of successive approximation. Synonym: *shaping*.

syllabic speech sound: A vowel sound that creates the syllable; sometimes refers to consonants that take on a syllable-forming status (e.g., /l/ in the second syllable of the word *handle*).

syllable: The combination of a consonant and a vowel.

syllable word shapes: Organization of consonants and vowels in a syllable (e.g., CVC = consonant, vowel, consonant; CCVC = consonant, consonant, vowel, consonant).

systematic replication: Treatment research in which previous studies are repeated in different settings, by different researchers, using different clients to show that the technique will yield similar results under varied conditions and with different clinicians; techniques that are systematically replicated may be recommended for general practice; most techniques included in the protocols have been systematically replicated.

target behavior: A behavior that a client is taught and expected to learn; correct production of phonemes in words, phrases, and syllables.

tense feature: Distinctive feature term applied to sounds that are made with a relatively greater degree of tension or contraction at the root of the tongue, including the consonants /p/, /t/, /k/, /tʃ/, /dʒ/, /ʃ/, /f/, /s/, /l/, /θ/ and vowels /i/, /e/, /o/, /u/, /ʌ/, /ɝ/.

textual cues or prompts: Printed words, phrases, or sentences (with or without pictures) used to evoke target phonemes during treatment; helpful in integrating articulation treatment with literacy skill training.

time-out: A procedure used to decrease the frequency of an error response; every time an error response is made, the clinician avoids eye contact and imposes a brief period (usually 5 seconds) of silence; an effective procedure.

tongue thrust: A pattern of deviant or reverse swallow in which the tongue pushes against the teeth.

total assimilation: In articulation, a physiologic occurrence in which a sound takes on all the characteristics of a neighboring sound, thus becoming identical to a neighboring sound (e.g., the *k* of *cat* totally assimilating to the *t* that follows to produce "tat").

traditional treatment approach: A highly strucured classic approach to the treatment of articulation disorders that progresses from sensory perceptual training to production training and then from the sound in isolation to the maintenance of learned behaviors in nonclinical settings across time.

training broad approach: An articulation-phonologic treatment approach in which several target sounds are taught at the same time.

transfer: The extension of newly learned behaviors from one setting (usually the clinical setting) to various other settings.

treatment objectives: The skills selected for training.

treatment procedures: Special techniques a clinician uses to effect changes in client behaviors.

unrounded vowels: Vowels made without lip rounding: /i/, /ɪ/, /ɛ/, /e/, /ɑ/, /æ/, /ɚ/, /ə/, /ʌ/.

untrained stimuli (probe stimuli): Novel stimuli, not used in treatment sessions, but can evoke the same target phoneme; help assess generalized productions; protocols give probe stimuli for all target phonemes.

velar fronting: Phonologic process characterized by the substitution of alveolar consonants for velar sounds; typical substitutions include d/g, t/k, and n/ŋ; however, others may be observed.

velopharyngeal closure: The physiologic act of closing the nasal cavity from the oral cavity so that air is directed through the mouth rather than the nose; closure is achieved by intricate upward, backward, and lateral movements of the velum and various pharyngeal muscles.

velopharyngeal port: The structure that connects the oral and nasal passages; it may be closed or opened by various muscle actions.

velum: The soft palate; formed by muscles that help raise or lower it.

verbal apraxia: Difficulty in initiating and executing the movement patterns necessary to produce speech when there is no paralyis, weakness, or incoordination of speech muscles; thought to be due to the brain's disturbed motor planning.

verbal corrective feedback: Verbal information provided to a client when a target or other behavior is inadequate, inappropriate, or unacceptable.

verbal prompt: A verbal "hint" or "cue" used to draw a target response from a client; it may include the use of vocal emphasis and the provision of verbal information (e.g., "When you make your *s*, remember that your tongue stays inside your mouth").

virgules: Slash marks used to enclose phonemic symbols.

vocal emphasis: A treatment technique by which a clinician increases his or her vocal intensity to highlight a target behavior; in articulation therapy, a clinician would say the target sound more loudly or prolong production of the target sound.

vocalic: Distinctive feature term used for sounds made without marked constriction of the vocal tract; includes all vowels and the consonants /l/ and /r/.

vocalis muscles: The vibrating parts of the vocal folds; also known as the thyroarytenoid muscles.

voiced sounds: Sounds made with vocal fold vibration.

voiceless sounds: Sounds made without vocal fold vibration.

volitional speech: Speech productions made under voluntary control.

vowel: A speech sound produced with an unrestricted passage of the airstream through the oral cavity; a syllable-forming sound.

vowel quadrilateral: A schematic representation of the tongue positions for the four extreme points of vowel production /i/, /u/, /æ/, and /ɑ/.

References

Bailey, J. S., Timbers, G. D., Phillips, E. L., & Wolf, M. M. (1971). Modification of articulation errors of predelinquents by their peers. *Journal of Applied Behavior Analysis, 4,* 266–281.

Baker, R. D., & Ryan, B. P. (1971). *Programmed conditioning for articulation.* Monterey, CA: Monterey Learning Systems.

Bennett, C. W. (1974). Articulation training in two hearing impaired girls. *Journal of Applied Behavior Analysis, 7,* 439–445.

Bernthal, N. W., & Bankson, J. E. (2004). *Articulation and phonological disorders* (5th ed.). Boston: Allyn & Bacon.

Costello, J. M., & Onstine, J. M. (1976). The modification of multiple articulation errors based on distinctive feature theory. *Journal of Speech and Hearing Disorders, 46,* 199–215.

Creaghead, N. A., Newman, P. W., & Secord, W. A. (Eds.). (1989). *Assessment and remediation of articulatory and phonological disorders* (2nd ed). Columbus, OH: Merrill Publishing Company.

Elbert, M., Dinnsen, D. A., Swartzlander, P., & Chin, S. B. (1990). Generalization to conversational speech. *Journal of Speech and Hearing Disorders, 55,* 694–699.

Elbert, M., & McReynolds, L. V. (1975). Transfer of /r/ across contexts. *Journal of Speech and Hearing Disorders, 40,* 380–387.

Fitch, J. L. (1973). Voice and articulation. In B. B. Lahey (Ed.), *The modification of language behavior* (pp. 130–177). Springfield, IL: Charles C. Thomas.

Gierut, J. (1989). Maximal opposition approach to phonological treatment. *Journal of Speech and Hearing Disorders, 54,* 9–19.

Gierut, J. (1990). A functional analysis of phonological contrast treatments. In L. B. Olswang, C. K. Thompson, S. F. Warren, & N. J. Minghetti (Eds.), *Treatment efficacy research in communication disorders* (p. 252). Washington, DC: American Speech–Language–Hearing Foundation.

Gierut, J. A. (1998). Treatment efficacy: Functional phonological disorders in children. *Journal of Speech, Language, and Hearing Research, 41,* S85–S100.

Gierut, J., A., Morrisette, M. L., Hughes, M. T., Rowland, S. (1996). Phonological treatment efficacy and developmental norms. *Language, Speech, and Hearing Services in Schools, 27,* 215–230.

Koegel, R. L., Koegel, L. K., & Ingham, J. C. (1986). Programming rapid generalization of correct articulation through self–monitoring procedures. *Journal of Speech and Hearing Disorders, 51,* 24–32.

Koegel, R. L., Koegel, L. K., Voy, K. V., & Ingham, J. C. (1988). Within–clinic versus outside-of-clinic self-monitoring of articulation to promote generalization. *Journal of Speech and Hearing Disorders, 53,* 392–399.

McCabe, R. B., & Bradley, D. P. (1975). Systemic multiple phonemic approach to articulation therapy. *Acta Symbolica, 6,* 2–18.

McReynolds, L. V., & Elbert, M. F. (1981). Generalization of correct articulation in clusters. *Applied Psycholinguistics, 2,* 119–132.

Mowrer, D. E. (1989). *The behavioral approach to treatment.* In N. A. Creaghead, P. W. Newman, & W. A. Secord (Eds.), *Assessment and remediation of articulatory and phonological disorders* (2nd ed.). Columbus, OH: Merrill Publishing Company.

Peña–Brooks, A., & Hegde, M. N. (2007). *Assessment and treatment of articulation and phonological disorders in children* (2nd ed.). Austin, TX: Pro-Ed.

Skelton, S. L. (2004). Concurrent task sequencing in single-phoneme phonologic treatment and generalization. *Journal of Communication Disorders, 37,* 131-155.

Sommers, R. K., Logsdon, B. S., & Wright, J. M. (1992). A review and critical analysis of treatment research related to articulation and phonological disorders. *Journal of Communication Disorders, 25,* 3–22.

Williams, A. L. (2000). Multiple oppositions: Theoretical foundations for an alternative contrastive intervention approach. *American Journal of Speech–Language Pathology, 9,* 282–288.

Williams, A. L. (2003). *Speech disorders resource guide for preschool children.* Clifton Park, NY: Thomson Delmar Learning.

Williams, G. C., & McReynolds, L. V. (1975). The relationship between discrimination and articulation training in children with misarticulation. *Journal of Speech and Hearing Research, 18,* 401–412.

Wright, P. W. D., Esq. (2004). The individuals with disabilities education improvement act of 2004. Retrieved March 15, 2006, from http://www.wrightslaw.com.

Appendix A

Cumulative Progress Recording Sheet

On the next page, a cumulative progress recording sheet is provided. The clinician may individualize it and print it from the CD to chart a child's progress over several sessions.

Cumulative Progress Recording Sheet
Correct Response Rates in Treatment Sessions

Name:	DOB:
Clinician:	Diagnosis:
Objective/IEP statement:	

Dates of Treatment Sessions	**Percent Correct**	**Comments**	**Objective Met**	
			Yes ☐	No ☐
			Yes ☐	No ☐
			Yes ☐	No ☐
			Yes ☐	No ☐
			Yes ☐	No ☐
			Yes ☐	No ☐
			Yes ☐	No ☐
			Yes ☐	No ☐
			Yes ☐	No ☐
			Yes ☐	No ☐
			Yes ☐	No ☐
			Yes ☐	No ☐
			Yes ☐	No ☐
			Yes ☐	No ☐
			Yes ☐	No ☐
			Yes ☐	No ☐
			Yes ☐	No ☐
			Yes ☐	No ☐
			Yes ☐	No ☐
			Yes ☐	No ☐

Appendix B

Sample Cumulative Progress Recording Sheet

On the next page, an example is provided of how a cumulative progress recording sheet may be filled.

Example Cumulative Progress Recording Sheet
Correct Response Rates in Treatment Sessions

Name: *Raman Smith Garcia*	DOB: *01/01/07*
Clinician: *Rachel Gutierrez Bhatt*	Diagnosis: *Mild Articulation Disorder*
Objective/IEP statement: *Correct evoked productions of /s/ in word-initial positions at 90% accuracy in three consecutive clinic sessions.*	

Treatment Session Dates	Percent Correct	Comments	Objective Met	
01/22/07	30	1st 20 min group session	Yes ☐	No ☒
01/24/07	35	20 min group session	Yes ☐	No ☒
01/26/07	45	10 min individual session	Yes ☐	No ☒
01/29/07	53	20 min individual session	Yes ☐	No ☒
01/31/07	62	20 min individual session	Yes ☐	No ☒
02/02/07	65	15 min individual session/did not feel good	Yes ☐	No ☒
02/05/07	70	20 min group session	Yes ☐	No ☒
02/07/07	65	20 min group session/distracted & uncooperative	Yes ☐	No ☒
02/09/07	75	20 min group session	Yes ☐	No ☒
02/12/07	85	20 min group session	Yes ☐	No ☒
02/14/07	90	20 min group session	Yes ☒	No ☐
02/16/07	92	20 min group session	Yes ☒	No ☐
02/19/07	95	20 min group session	Yes ☒	No ☐
02/21/07		Treatment shifted to phrase level	Yes ☐	No ☐
			Yes ☐	No ☐
			Yes ☐	No ☐
			Yes ☐	No ☐
			Yes ☐	No ☐
			Yes ☐	No ☐
			Yes ☐	No ☐

Appendix C

Baserate Recording Sheet

On the next page, a template of a baserate recording sheet is provided. The clinician who wishes to baserate targets for which the exemplars are not provided in the protocols may use this template. The clinician may type in the exemplars, personalize the information on the sheet, and print it from the CD.

Baserate Recording Sheet

Name:	Date:	File #:
DOB/Age:	Clinician:	
Disorder:	Target Behavior:	
Goal:		

Target Responses	Trials	
	Evoked	Modeled
1.		
2.		
3.		
4.		
5.		
6.		
7.		
8.		
9.		
10.		
11.		
12.		
13.		
14.		
15.		
16.		
17.		
18.		
19.		
20.		
Percent correct baserate		

Note: + = Correct response; – = Incorrect response; 0 = no response.

Appendix D

Treatment Recording Sheet

On the next page, a template of a treatment recording sheet is provided. The clinician who wishes to teach targets for which the exemplars are not provided in the protocols may use this template. The clinician may type in the exemplars, personalize the information on the sheet, and print it from the CD.

Treatment Recording Sheet

Name:	Date:	File #: 4
DOB/Age:	Clinician:	
Disorder:	Target Behavior:	
Goal:		

Scoring: Correct: ✓   Incorrect or no response: X

Target skills	Discrete Trials														
	1	2	3	4	5	6	7	8	9	10	11	12	13	14	15
1.															
2.															
3.															
4.															
5.															
6.															
7.															
8.															
9.															
10.															

Appendix E

Probe Recording Sheet

On the next page, a template of a probe recording sheet is provided. The clinician who needs to probe for targets for which the exemplars are not provided in the protocols may use this template. The clinician may type in the exemplars, personalize the information on the sheet, and print it from the CD.

Probe Recording Sheet

Name:	Date: File #:
Age:	Clinician:
Disorder:	Target Behavior:

Name:	Date:	Session #:
Age:	Clinician:	
Disorder: Language	Target:	(Probe)

Untrained Stimuli (UT)	**Score: + correct; – incorrect or no responses**	
1.	(UT)	
2.	(UT)	
3.	(UT)	
4.	(UT)	
5.	(UT)	
6.	(UT)	
7.	(UT)	
8.	(UT)	
9.	(UT)	
10.	(UT)	
Percent correct probe (Criterion: 90%)		

Sound Category Index

CLUSTERS—FINAL

L-type

R-type

S-type

Z-type